UPDATES IN LIVER CANCER

Edited by **Hesham Mohamed Abdeldayem**

Updates in Liver Cancer
http://dx.doi.org/10.5772/62680
Edited by Hesham Mohamed Abdeldayem

Contributors
Shing Chung Hooi, Guo-Dong Lu, Tomohiro Kanayama, Ayumi Niwa, Kei Noguchi, Kazuhisa Ishida, Masayuki Niwa, Akira Hara, Hiroyuki Tomita, Asma Gomaa, Alzhraa Alkhatib, Shimaa Alkilany, Osama Lotfy El Abd, Imam Waked, Hesham Abdeldayem, Sebahat Basyigit, Abdullah Ozgur Yeniova, Ayse Kefeli, Irinel Popescu, Sorin Tiberiu Alexandrescu, Bolin Niu, Hie-Won Hann, Mandivavarira Maundura, Jonathan Koea, Ahmed Elsarawy, Chao-Long Chen, Chih-Che Lin, Rahul Anil Sheth, Nicolas Cardenas, Joshua Kuban, Giovanni Brandi

Published by InTech
Janeza Trdine 9, 51000 Rijeka, Croatia

Publishing Process Manager Romina Skomersic
Technical Editor SPi Global
Cover InTech Design team

First published April, 2017
Printed in Croatia
Legal deposit, Croatia: National and University Library in Zagreb

Additional hard copies can be obtained from orders@intechopen.com

Updates in Liver Cancer , Edited by Hesham Mohamed Abdeldayem
p. cm.
Print ISBN 978-953-51-3063-5
Online ISBN 978-953-51-3064-2

For EU product safety concerns:
IN TECH d.o.o., Prolaz Marije Krucifikse Kozulić 3, 51000 Rijeka, Croatia,
info@intechopen.com or visit our website at intechopen.com.

Meet the editor

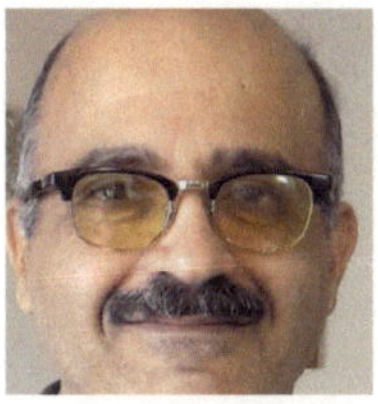

Professor Abdeldayem graduated from Kasr Al-Ainy School of Medicine in 1987. He got his training at Cairo University Hospitals, Menoufia University, University of Pittsburgh Medical Center, and King Abdulaziz Medical City. He joined the National Liver Institute in 1993. He has several publications in the fields of hepato-pancreato-biliary surgery and organ transplantation. He is a member of InTech's Editorial Advisory Board and an associate editor of *Frontiers in Surgery*. He currently holds the positions of professor of Surgery and vice dean for Postgraduate Studies and Research, at the National Liver Institute, Menoufia University, Egypt.

Contents

Preface

The incidence of liver cancer is increasing worldwide and still carries a guarded prognosis. Liver cancers result in considerable amount of financial and social burden. On the other hand, researches and clinical studies related to liver cancers continue to advance at a rapid pace.

The chapters in this book provide state-of-the-art reviews on the current knowledge and advances in research and management of liver cancers. It includes the most recent advances in that field, particularly, hepatocarcinogenesis and the potential role of intestinal microbiota, nonalcoholic steatohepatitis, cancer stem cells, aldehyde dehydrogenase-1, and hepatitis B virus. This book also discusses the methods of diagnosis of HCC, the minimally invasive therapies for liver cancers, living donor liver transplantation for HCC, surgical management of liver metastases from colorectal cancers, and assessment and optimization for the future liver remnant.

This book is written by recognized medical experts and researchers from North America, Europe, Asia, Oceania, and Africa. I wish to thank all the distinguished authors for their cooperation and desire to share their precious experience with the medical community. On their behalf, I wish to express hope that this publication will facilitate access to the latest scientific achievements in the field of gallbladder diseases all across the world.

I am particularly thankful to Ana Pantar, Romina Skomersic, and their colleagues at InTech, the publisher of one of the largest multidisciplinary open access collections of books covering the fields of science, for their expertise and support in bringing this edition to completion.

I would like to acknowledge the help of Professor Imam Waked and his colleagues at the Department of Liver Oncology, National Liver Institute, Menoufia University, Egypt, a dedicated center of excellence and a leading medical institution at the Middle East involved in the management of liver diseases and advanced training and research in hepatobiliary sciences.

Hesham Mohamed Abdeldayem
National Liver Institute
Menoufia University
Egypt

Chapter 1

Introductory Chapter: Updates on the Management of Hepatocellular Carcinoma

Asmaa Gomaa, Alzhraa Alkhatib, Shimaa Alkilany, Osama Lotfy El Abd, Hesham Abdeldayem and Imam Waked

Additional information is available at the end of the chapter

http://dx.doi.org/10.5772/67557

1. Introduction

Due to many factors, such as the frequent coexistence of chronic liver disease, the wide heterogeneity in HCC presentation, increased available therapeutic options with diverse responses to these therapies in addition to the variable biologic behavior of the tumor, it is crucial to manage HCC patients by multidisciplinary team [1–3].

2. Early stage HCC

Only 15–30% of patients present in early stage HCC and can receive curative treatments [4]. This is mainly due to liver cirrhosis associated with hepatocarcinoma, and the late presentation reported in most patients.

2.1. Resection

Surgical resection is the best treatment option for solitary tumors in patients without cirrhosis with postresection 5-year survival rates of 41–74% [5, 6]. A cirrhotic liver loses its regenerative potential and has less functional reserve [7, 8]. The best outcome after resection is achieved in cirrhotic patients with well-compensated Child-Pugh class-A cirrhosis, normal bilirubin, and no portal hypertension [20]. Poor prognosis is influenced by pathological findings, such as vascular invasion, presence of satellites, and poor differentiation. Anatomic resection margins of 2 cm are recommended as it provides better survival outcome than narrow resection margins <1 cm, provided that appropriate remnant liver volume is maintained [9]. The minimal critical remnant liver volume for resection is approximately 25% (15–40%) for noncirrhotic and 50% (25–90%) for cirrhotic livers. Preoperative portal vein embolization (PVE) is recommended when the estimated remnant liver volume unmet the minimal requirement.

Portal hypertension, hepatic venous pressure gradient (HVPG) ≥ 10 mmHg, was found to be the best predictor of postoperative liver decompensation and poor long-term outcomes in compensated cirrhotic patients undergoing hepatic resection [10]. Postresection tumor recurrences often have multifocal presentations and repeat resections are rarely ideal, instead, salvage liver transplantation, or other loco-regional therapies, with or without oral multi-kinase inhibitors are more suitable. Molecular biomarkers and gene signatures [11] can be used for better selection of patients for hepatic resection with low risk for late recurrence.

2.2. Liver transplantation (LTx)

LTx is a potentially curative treatment and the best treatment option for patients with decompensated cirrhosis, and it allows the removal of the primary tumor and treats hepatic insufficiency by removing cirrhotic tissue simultaneously [12]. In an attempt to identify the most appropriate transplant patients, the Milan criteria have emerged as main inclusion criteria for LTx. LTx is recommended for the patients with single lesion not larger than 5 cm, or up to three lesions with each less than or equal 3 cm. Restriction to Milan criteria is compatible with early BCLC stage and results in a 5-year overall survival rate of 75% with a risk of recurrence less than 15% in specialized liver transplantation centers. The perioperative mortality and 1-year mortality are expected to be approximately 3 and ≤10%, respectively [5]. Milan criteria was found to be an independent prognostic factor for outcome after liver transplantation with 5-year survival rate similar to non-HCC patients (65–78%) [13].

MELD score, initially proposed for prediction of early mortality in patients with cirrhosis, is the standard method to prioritize assignment of cirrhotic patients to the LTx waiting list. However, the MELD score is not able to predict the drop-out rate and mortality in the patient with HCC; therefore, a "MELD exception" has been developed to assign extra points to the HCC patients on the basis of the tumor burden leading to increased percentage of LTx (30–40%) performed for HCC [14, 15]. Several priority scores have been assigned to these patients. Early proposals assigned 24 and 29 points to single <2 cm and single 2–5 cm or three nodules each <3 cm, respectively. In the current era, no extra points and 22 points are assigned to those patients, respectively. Several studies have investigated the effect of expanding the Milan criteria, the University of California San Francisco (UCSF) proposed criteria for LTx for HCC (one tumor ≤6.5 cm or up to three nodules with the largest ≤4.5 cm, and the total tumor diameter ≤8 cm). These criteria have been prospectively and retrospectively validate with an overall survival comparable to those within Milan criteria [16]. Modest expansion of Milan criteria to "up-to-seven" criteria was proposed. This pathology-based proposal (HCCs having the number 7 as the sum of the size of the largest tumor and the number of tumors in patients without microvascular invasion) [17] has been externally validated in an independent series [18] but requires prospective validation studies using pretransplant radiolog.

2.3. Local ablative therapy

Tumor ablation techniques induce their therapeutic effect by destroying tumor cells, either directly by exposing tumor cells to chemical substances (ethanol or acetic acid) or physically by modifying the temperature (heating or cooling).

2.4. Percutaneous ethanol injection (PEI)

PEI has been considered the most appropriate technique utilized for many years owing to its impacts on the natural history of HCC as shown in several studies. The major limitation of PEI is the high incidence of local recurrence (33–43%). PEI is indicated for the treatment of nodular-type HCC up to 5 cm and achieves complete necrosis in 50–90% of tumors 2–5 cm.

2.5. Radiofrequency ablation (RFA)

In the last decade, RFA appears to be superior to all other local ablative therapies and is now the first-line technique for ablation [19]. RFA is considered the standard of care for patients with very early and early stage tumors not suitable for or refusing surgery. Patients with Child-Pugh class A and tumor size of less than or equal 3 cm in diameter undergoing percutaneous ablation had the best prognosis [20]. RFA depends on energy production, via utilization of elevated frequency alternated currents, through an electrode inserted directly into the tumor that induces coagulative necrosis of the tumor with safety margins of the apparently healthy tissue around the lesion. RFA is less invasive, less expensive with lower complication rates and shorter hospital stay than surgical resection (**Figure 1**). However, RFA is size-dependent. RFA can produce a necrotic area of about 4 cm so it should be considered the first option for the treatment of small HCC measuring up to 3 cm. With development of technology, the use of

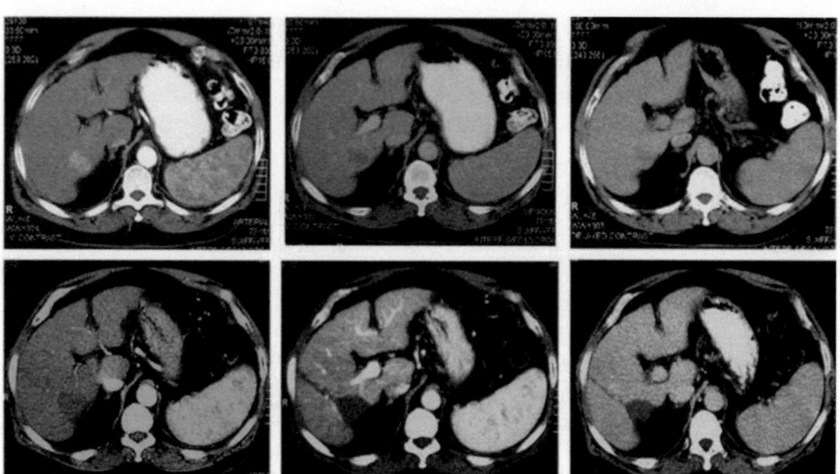

Figure 1. Above, left to right: Triphasic CT scan revealed enhancing right lobe focal lesion (segment VII) showing washout in the portovenous phase and in the delayed phase. Below, left to right: Post-RFA triphasic CT scan obtained 1 month later revealed complete necrosis with no residual enhancing tumor.

expandable tipped or cool-tip electrodes will achieve ablation of areas 5 cm or more in diameter effectively. Bipolar RF electrodes can create a larger (up to 8.4 cm) ablation in a short time [21].

2.6. Microwave ablation

Microwave ablation (MWA) is an emerging form of thermal ablation, alternative to RFA, evaluated for the treatment of HCC using electromagnetic waves with frequencies greater than 900 kHz [22]. MWA utilizes active ablation heating, enables continuous and uniform ablation, permitting generation of higher temperatures and larger ablation zones, thus leading to higher rates of tumor necrosis. Another advantage of MWA over RFA is that treatment outcome overcomes the "heat-sink" effect of vessels proximal to the tumor which can lead to incomplete ablation.

3. Intermediate stage HCC

3.1. Transarterial therapies

Transarterial therapies include TACE, transarterial embolization (TAE), transarterial bland embolization, transarterial chemotherapy, and transarterial radioembolization [23, 24]. TACE is currently considered the standard of care for patients with large multifocal lesions with compensated liver function, without evidence of vascular invasion or extra hepatic spread; however, TACE is recommended in Japan for HCC patients with vascular invasion if radiological portal invasion (Vp) is Vp1 or Vp2; distal to, or in the second-order branches of, the portal vein [25]. Success of TACE is controlled by the maximum and sustained retention of the chemical agent used (**Figure 2**). Lipiodol has been widely used in TACE protocols due to the great hunger of HCC to lipiodol. However, there is no data validated the effect of lipiodol in achieving slow release of the chemotherapeutic agents leading to sustained concentration of chemotherapeutic agents in tumor. Moreover, this can be achieved by the use of embolic microspheres which have the ability to sequester chemotherapeutic agents and release them in a controlled manner over a 1-week period and a subsequent increase of the local concentration of the drug with minimal systemic toxicity. Occurrence of complications after TACE may be related to more extensive disease; requiring nonselective embolization, and poor liver reserve. Selection of patients is mandatory to prevent post-TACE-induced liver failure. For example, patients with total bilirubin >3 mg/dL were excluded from TACE in several studies. MELD score can be used to select best candidates for TACE [26].

3.2. TACE with drug-eluting beads

Special particles of various sizes (from 100 to 1000 μm) can be used with the characteristic not only of embolizing the tumor but also of releasing substances overtime (up to 30 days) that determine antiblastic necrosis. Embolic microspheres have the ability to actively sequester chemotherapeutic agents as doxorubicin hydrochloride from solution and release them in a controlled fashion over a 1-week period. The use of embolic microspheres has been shown to substantially diminish the amount of the chemotherapeutic agent that reaches the systemic circulation, increase the local concentration of the drug, and the antitumor efficacy with negligible systemic toxicity. Tolerance to conventional TACE has improved by the use of drug-eluting beads that obstruct arterial vessels and slowly release chemotherapy [27].

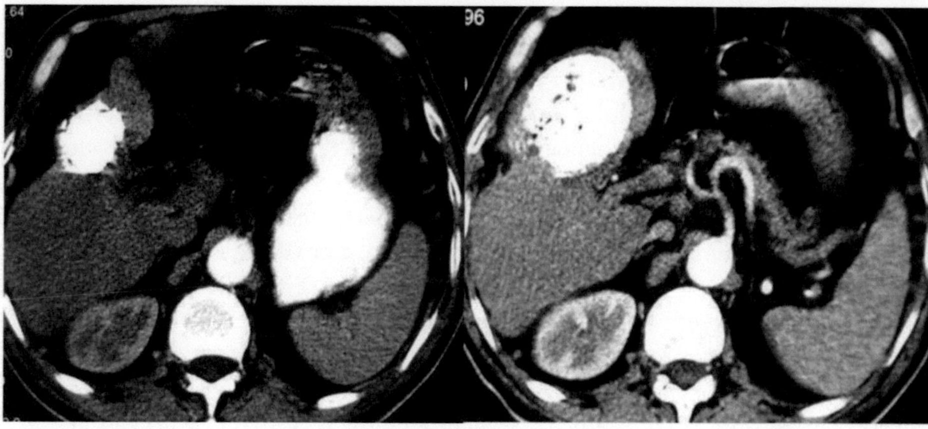

Figure 2. Left: Triphasic CT scan revealed enhancing right lobe focal lesion in the arterial phase. Right: Post TACE triphasic CT scan obtained 1 month showed complete cure.

3.3. Radioembolization

Selective internal radiation therapy (SIRT) has been emerged as a therapeutic option for intermediate-stage HCC. SIRT aims to selectively target radiation to liver tumors while limiting the dose to normal liver parenchyma, thus preventing ischemia to the liver tissue, SIRT exerts its effect through deposition of yttrium-90 ((90)Y) microspheres into the hepatic artery that feed the tumor in a 3:1 to 20:1 ratio compared with a normal liver, so that tumor nodules are treated irrespective of their number, size, or location [28].

4. Advanced stage HCC

4.1. Systemic therapy

Systemic therapy with hormonal agents such as octreotide and tamoxifen or with biological agents as interferon therapy [29], and thalidomide showed poor results.

Systemic chemotherapy showed contradictory results. HCC is one of the most chemo-resistant tumors; in addition, chemotherapy is poorly tolerated by patients with liver cirrhosis because of major side effects. Hence, no systemic chemotherapy was recommended for patients with advanced tumors. Cytotoxic agents such as 5-fluorouracil, cisplatin, doxorubicin, gemcitabine, capecitabin, and epirubicin or combined regimens showed a low response rate (<10%) with only marginal improvements in overall survival [30]. Cisplatin, interferon, doxorubicin, and fluorouracil (PIAF) used in combination showed promising activity in a phase II study but not in phase III. Moreover, patients treated with the PIAF regimen experienced significantly higher rate of myelotoxicity compared with doxorubicin.

4.2. Molecular targeted therapy

Hepatocarcinogenesis is associated with epigenetic and genetic alterations that eventually lead to an alteration in the molecular pathways resulting in uncontrolled growth of the hepatocytes [31].

4.2.1. Sorafenib

Multiple cellular kinases are involved in the development and progression of the HCC through induction of angiogenesis and cellular proliferation. Overexpression of surface tyrosine kinases or mutational activation of *Ras* oncogene leads to Ras/MAPK pathway activation, an important step in HCC proliferation and angiogenesis. Sorafenib is an orally administered multikinase inhibitor drug, inhibits vascular endothelial growth factor receptor (VEGFR)- (VEGFR-) 1, VEGFR-2, VEGFR-3, platelet-derived growth factor receptor (PDGFR), Ras/MAPK pathway, involving Raf-1 (C-Raf) and B-Raf (wild and mutant types), FMS-like tyrosine kinase-3 (Flt), and c-kit with antiproliferative and antiangiogenic activity [32, 33]. The European guidelines recommended sorafenib for unresectable, advanced, Child–Pugh class A or B HCC with PS 0–2 and vascular invasion or distant metastasis [5]. According to the Japanese guidelines, sorafenib is recommended for unresectable, advanced, Child–Pugh class A HCC with vascular invasion or distant metastasis, as well as for patients intolerant to TACE or in whom the procedure of TACE is technically difficult [34]. Sorafenib was generally well tolerated with mild toxicity, predominantly including diarrhea, fatigue, weight loss, rash, or superficial skin desquamation and hand-foot skin reaction, hair loss, anorexia, nausea, and abdominal pain.

4.2.2. Molecular targeted agents other than sorafenib

Since the survival benefit achieved with sorafenib (compared to placebo) was minimal, search for alternative therapies was mandatory. Other targeted agents in phase III trials revealed nonsuperior results of antiangiogenic tyrosine kinase inhibitors (TKI) sunitinib, linifanib, brivanib, or the combination of sorafenib with erlotinib [35] for sorafenib-naive advanced HCC patients compared to sorafenib and none have exceeded the benefits of sorafenib, in addition, brivanib [36], ramucirumab [37], and everolimus [38] have been tested as second line, in patients who were refractory or intolerant to first-line treatment with sorafenib, with no significant improvement in overall survival, although TTP was significantly longer in the brivanib arm than with placebo. A decision-making process is required to tailor first-line medical treatment with sorafenib in the advanced stage. This should include nutritional, functional, and comorbidity status of the patient.

Author details

Asmaa Gomaa[1,2], Alzhraa Alkhatib[1], Shimaa Alkilany[1], Osama Lotfy El Abd[3], Hesham Abdeldayem[4,*] and Imam Waked[1,2]

*Address all correspondence to: habdeldayem64@hotmail.com

1 Department of Oncology, National Liver Institute, Menoufia University, Egypt

2 Department of Hepatology, National Liver Institute, Menoufia University, Egypt

3 Department of Radiology, National Liver Institute, Menoufia University, Egypt

4 Department of Surgery, National Liver Institute, Menoufia University, Egypt

References

[1] Bruix, J., G.J. Gores, and V. Mazzaferro, *Hepatocellular carcinoma: clinical frontiers and perspectives*. Gut, 2014. **63**(5): pp. 844–55.

[2] Guy, J., et al., *Multidisciplinary management of hepatocellular carcinoma*. Clin Gastroenterol Hepatol, 2012. **10**(4): pp. 354–62.

[3] Kaseb, A.O., Y.M. Abaza, and R.E. Roses, *Multidisciplinary management of hepatocellular carcinoma*. Recent Results Cancer Res, 2013. **190**: pp. 247–59.

[4] Finn, R.S., *Development of molecularly targeted therapies in hepatocellular carcinoma: where do we go now?* Clin Cancer Res, 2010. **16**(2): pp. 390–7.

[5] Arii, S., et al., *Results of surgical and nonsurgical treatment for small-sized hepatocellular carcinomas: a retrospective and nationwide survey in Japan. The Liver Cancer Study Group of Japan*. Hepatology, 2000. **32**(6): pp. 1224–9.

[6] Grazi, G.L., et al., *Improved results of liver resection for hepatocellular carcinoma on cirrhosis give the procedure added value*. Ann Surg, 2001. **234**(1): pp. 71–8.

[7] Beard, R.E., et al., *A comparison of surgical outcomes for noncirrhotic and cirrhotic hepatocellular carcinoma patients in a Western institution*. Surgery, 2013. **154**(3): pp. 545–55.

[8] Bhoori, S., et al., *First-line treatment for hepatocellular carcinoma: resection or transplantation?* Transplant Proc, 2007. **39**(7): pp. 2271–3.

[9] Forner, A., et al., *Diagnosis of hepatic nodules 20 mm or smaller in cirrhosis: Prospective validation of the noninvasive diagnostic criteria for hepatocellular carcinoma*. Hepatology, 2008. **47**(1): pp. 97–104.

[10] Shi, M., et al., *Partial hepatectomy with wide versus narrow resection margin for solitary hepatocellular carcinoma: a prospective randomized trial*. Ann Surg, 2007. **245**(1): pp. 36–43.

[11] Bruix, J. and M. Sherman, *Management of hepatocellular carcinoma: an update*. Hepatology, 2011. **53**(3): pp. 1020–2.

[12] Nault, J.C., et al., *A hepatocellular carcinoma 5-gene score associated with survival of patients after liver resection*. Gastroenterology, 2013. **145**(1): pp. 176–87.

[13] Mazzaferro, V., et al., *Liver transplantation for hepatocellular carcinoma*. Ann Surg Oncol, 2008. **15**(4): pp. 1001–7.

[14] Raia, S., J.R. Nery, and S. Mies, *Liver transplantation from live donors*. Lancet, 1989. **2**(8661): p. 497.

[15] Mazzaferro, V., et al., *Milan criteria in liver transplantation for hepatocellular carcinoma: an evidence-based analysis of 15 years of experience*. Liver Transpl, 2011. **17**(2): p. 22365.

[16] Taniguchi, M., *Liver transplantation in the MELD era--analysis of the OPTN/UNOS registry*. Clin Transpl, 2012: p. 41–65.

[17] Raza, A. and G.K. Sood, *Hepatocellular carcinoma review: current treatment, and evidence-based medicine*. World J Gastroenterol, 2014. **20**(15): pp. 4115–27.

[18] Yao, F.Y., et al., *Excellent outcome following down-staging of hepatocellular carcinoma prior to liver transplantation: an intention-to-treat analysis*. Hepatology, 2008. **48**(3): pp. 819–27.

[19] Ravaioli, M., et al., *Liver transplantation for hepatocellular carcinoma: results of down-staging in patients initially outside the Milan selection criteria*. Am J Transplant, 2008. **8**(12): pp. 2547–57.

[20] Yao, F.Y., et al., *Liver transplantation for hepatocellular carcinoma: validation of the UCSF-expanded criteria based on preoperative imaging*. Am J Transplant, 2007. **7**(11): pp. 2587–96.

[21] Mazzaferro, V., et al., *Predicting survival after liver transplantation in patients with hepatocellular carcinoma beyond the Milan criteria: a retrospective, exploratory analysis*. Lancet Oncol, 2009. **10**(1): pp. 35–43.

[22] Raj, A., J. McCall, and E. Gane, *Validation of the "Metroticket" predictor in a cohort of patients transplanted for predominantly HBV-related hepatocellular carcinoma*. J Hepatol, 2011. **55**(5): pp. 1063–8.

[23] Lencioni, R., *Loco-regional treatment of hepatocellular carcinoma*. Hepatology, 2010. **52**(2): pp. 762–73.

[24] Roskams, T. and M. Kojiro, *Pathology of early hepatocellular carcinoma: conventional and molecular diagnosis*. Semin Liver Dis, 2010. **30**(1): pp. 17–25.

[25] Lin, S.M., *Recent advances in radiofrequency ablation in the treatment of hepatocellular carcinoma and metastatic liver cancers*. Chang Gung Med J, 2009. **32**(1): pp. 22–32.

[26] Martin, R.C., C.R. Scoggins, and K.M. McMasters, *Safety and efficacy of microwave ablation of hepatic tumors: a prospective review of a 5-year experience*. Ann Surg Oncol, 2010. **17**(1): pp. 171–8.

[27] Tsochatzis, E.A., G. Germani, and A.K. Burroughs, *Transarterial chemoembolization, transarterial chemotherapy, and intra-arterial chemotherapy for hepatocellular carcinoma treatment*. Semin Oncol, 2010. **37**(2): pp. 89–93.

[28] Lin, S., K. Hoffmann, and P. Schemmer, *Treatment of hepatocellular carcinoma: a systematic review*. Liver Cancer, 2012. **1**(3–4): pp. 144–58.

[29] Yeo, W., et al., *A randomized phase III study of doxorubicin versus cisplatin/interferon alpha-2b/doxorubicin/fluorouracil (PIAF) combination chemotherapy for unresectable hepatocellular carcinoma*. J Natl Cancer Inst, 2005. **97**(20): pp. 1532–8.

[30] Fuchs, C.S., et al., *A phase II trial of gemcitabine in patients with advanced hepatocellular carcinoma*. Cancer, 2002. **94**(12): pp. 3186–91.

[31] Cervello, M., et al., *Targeted therapy for hepatocellular carcinoma: novel agents on the horizon*. Oncotarget, 2012. **3**(3): pp. 236–60.

[32] Forner, A., J.M. Llovet, and J. Bruix, *Chemoembolization for intermediate HCC: is there proof of survival benefit?* J Hepatol, 2012. **56**(4): pp. 984–6.

[33] Chang, Y.S., et al., *Sorafenib (BAY 43–9006) inhibits tumor growth and vascularization and induces tumor apoptosis and hypoxia in RCC xenograft models*. Cancer Chemother Pharmacol, 2007. **59**(5): pp. 561–74.

[34] Kudo, M., K. Ueshima, and T. Arizumi, *Real-life clinical practice with sorafenib in advanced hepatocellular carcinoma: a single-center experience*. Dig Dis, 2012. **30**(6): pp. 609–16.

[35] Zhu, A.X., et al., *SEARCH: a phase III, randomized, double-blind, placebo-controlled trial of sorafenib plus erlotinib in patients with advanced hepatocellular carcinoma*. J Clin Oncol, 2015. **33**(6): pp. 559–66.

[36] Llovet, J.M., et al., *Brivanib in patients with advanced hepatocellular carcinoma who were intolerant to sorafenib or for whom sorafenib failed: results from the randomized phase III BRISK-PS study*. J Clin Oncol, 2013. **31**(28): pp. 3509–16.

[37] Zhu, A., et al., *Ramucirumab (RAM) as second-line treatment in patients (pts) with advanced hepatocellular carcinoma (HCC) following first-line therapy with sorafenib: results from the randomized phase III REACH study*. Ann Oncol, 2014. **25**: pp. v1–v41.

[38] Zhu, A.X., et al., *Effect of everolimus on survival in advanced hepatocellular carcinoma after failure of sorafenib: the EVOLVE-1 randomized clinical trial*. JAMA, 2014. **312**(1): pp. 57–67.

Chapter 2

Intestinal Microbiota, Nonalcoholic Steatohepatitis and Hepatocellular Carcinoma: The Potential Role of Dysbiosis in the Hepatocarcinogenesis

Giovanni Brandi, Stefania De Lorenzo,
Marco Candela and Francesco Tovoli

Additional information is available at the end of the chapter

http://dx.doi.org/10.5772/67322

Abstract

Introduction: Hepatocellular carcinoma (HCC) accounts for the majority of primary liver cancers. Approximately 5–30% of HCC patients lack a readily identifiable risk factor for their cancer, and most of these cases are attributed to nonalcoholic fatty liver disease (NAFLD) and nonalcoholic steatohepatitis (NASH).

Body: Recent lines of evidence have suggested the role of intestinal microbiota, in particular the dysbiosis, in the pathogenesis of chronic liver diseases, such as NAFLD/NASH. Intestinal microbes produce a large array of bioactive molecules from mainly dietary compounds, establishing an intense microbiota-host transgenomic metabolism with a great impact on physiological and pathological conditions. A derangement of intestinal microbiota may lead to microbial translocation of bacteria or their products in the liver, where endotoxins trigger inflammation, and hepatocellular damage, which in turn plays a key role in the development of HCC. The following liver injury and hepatocellular necrosis can promote the activation of a secondary proliferative pathway involving the hepatic progenitor cells (HPCs), a bipotential cell compartment that seems to contribute to hepatocarcinogenesis.

Conclusion: The aim of this chapter is to summarize current knowledge on the potential role of intestinal microbiota in the pathogenesis of NAFLD and the subsequent development of HCC.

Keywords: dysbiosis, nonalcoholic steatohepatitis, hepatic progenitor cells, hepatocellular carcinoma

1. Introduction

Nonalcoholic fatty liver disease (NAFLD) is a common form of a chronic liver disorder worldwide, with an estimated global prevalence of 25% among adults and ~10% among children [1, 2]. NAFLD is traditionally regarded as hepatic manifestations of metabolic syndrome and encompasses the pathological spectrum ranging from simple hepatic steatosis (so-called "nonalcoholic fatty liver or NAFL") to the more aggressive form nonalcoholic steatohepatitis (NASH), which can progress to cirrhosis and its associated complications, including liver failure and hepatocellular carcinoma (HCC) [3, 4].

HCC accounts for the majority of primary cancers of the liver, representing the fifth most common cancer and the third leading cause of cancer death [5]. Many risk factors, including hepatitis B (HBV), hepatitis C (HCV), and alcohol, are well established, but 5–30% of HCC cases lack a readily identifiable risk factor. The majority of these cases of HCC is attributed to NAFLD, in particular in Western countries, and coincides with the growing epidemic of metabolic disorders. Diabetes mellitus and obesity are known to play a pivotal role in the development and progression of NAFLD [6–8]. An increase in the body-mass index and emergence of diabetes mellitus have been associated with progression to cirrhosis, whereas a reduction in body weight, and improved glycemic control promote resolution of liver fibrosis. The risk of progression to end-stage liver disease is influenced by the severity of the underlying liver histopathology. Although most patients with NAFLD remain asymptomatic, 20% of them progress to chronic hepatic inflammation, which in turn can lead to cirrhosis, portal hypertension, and HCC [9, 10].

Recent evidence points to a new factor involved in the development and progression of NAFLD: the intestinal microbiota [11, 12]. Many authors show that patients with NAFLD are characterized by dysbiosis, defined as any change in the composition of the microbiota that deviates from the composition commonly found in healthy people [13]. Intestinal microbes produce a large array of bioactive molecules mainly from dietary compounds, thus establishing intense microbiota-host transgenomic metabolism with a strong influence on physiological and pathological conditions [14]. In this regard, it is important to know the role of the various phyla, genera, or species of bacteria in maintaining the proper (healthy) metabolism or in inducing pathological changes predisposing to metabolic syndrome (or obesity, diabetes, or NASH).

Dysbiosis of the intestinal microbiota increases the ability of bacteria to harvest energy from the host diet and intestinal permeability and may lead to translocation of bacterial endotoxins into the liver [15]. These endogenous mediators can initiate hepatic inflammation and exacerbate hepatocyte damage through production of proinflammatory cytokines. The final result is lipid accumulation in (and death of) hepatocytes, causing steatosis, inflammation, and stimulation of hepatic stellate cells (HSCs) to produce collagen, resulting in fibrosis and cirrhosis [16, 17].

There is a broad consensus regarding the association between dysbiosis and colorectal cancer [18–21]. In contrast, the associations of microbiota with NAFLD and cancers other than colorectal are less proven [22, 23]. As suggested by the strong relation between the liver and gut, the microbiota seems to be also involved in the pathogenesis and development of HCC, although the exact molecular mechanisms integrating these events remain unclear (**Figure 1**) [24, 25].

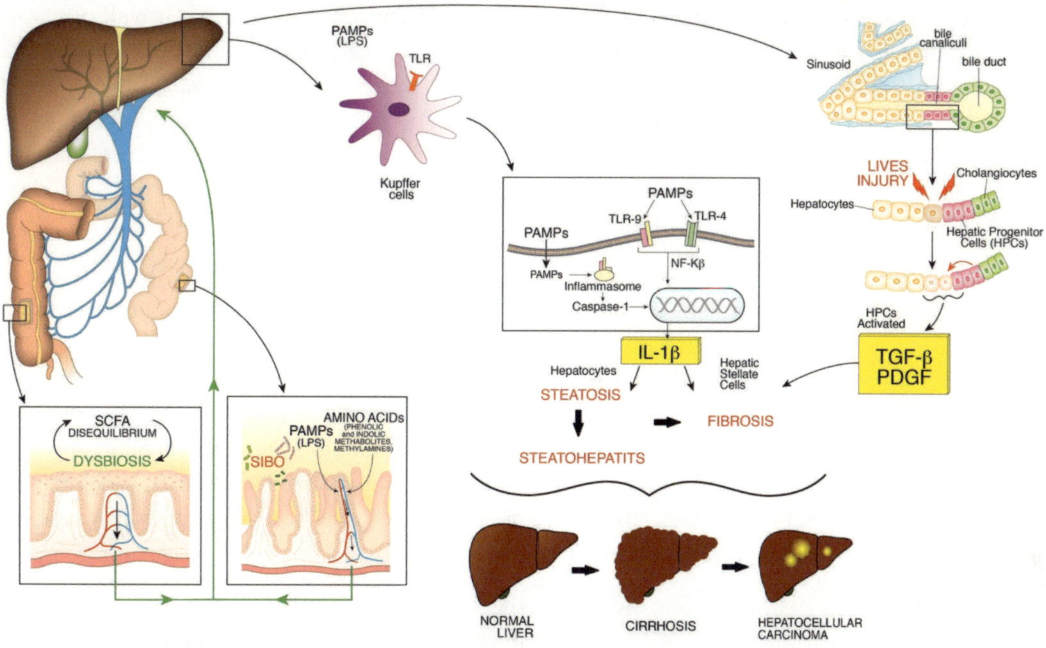

Figure 1. Role of intestinal microbiota and hepatic progenitor cells in the progression of liver injury from steatosis to steatohepatitis and cirrhosis.

Activation of hepatic progenitor cells (HPCs) is one of the factors likely promoting inflammation and hepatocarcinogenesis in NAFLD [26]. Chronic inflammation and DNA-damaging agents such as reactive oxygen species (ROS) induce replicative senescence of mature hepatocytes, and this inhibition can activate a secondary proliferative pathway involving HPCs [26, 27]. Activation of HPCs also leads to the production of several profibrogenic factors, such as transforming growth factor β (TGF-β) and platelet-derived growth factor (PDGF), which activate HSCs and boost the production of collagen [28].

The aim of this chapter is to summarize current knowledge on the potential role of the intestinal microbiota in the pathogenesis of NAFLD and in subsequent development of HCC.

2. Microbiota-host transgenomic metabolism of dietary compounds

Intestinal microbes produce a vast array of bioactive molecules from any dietary compounds, thus establishing intense microbiota-host transgenomic metabolism with a tremendous impact on our physiology and nutritional state [29]. In particular, fermentation of indigestible plant polysaccharides by the gut microbiota involves a remarkable interspecies metabolic network, where primary and secondary fermenters act in concert [30]. Plant cell wall polysaccharides—including hemicellulose, pectins, and xylans—reach the colon solubilized or trapped in the plant cellulose matrix. The latter is solubilized by specialized cellulolytic ruminococci, which produce acetate and propionate from cellulose. Furthermore, soluble cell wall polysaccharides are readily metabolized by butyrate producers of *Clostridium* clusters IV and XIVa (e.g., *Faecalibacterium prausnitzii, Butyrivibrio, Roseburia,* and *Eubacterium rectale*). On the other hand, soluble starches are preferentially fermented to propionate, acetate, and succinate by Bacteroidetes [31, 32]. These microorganisms are also capable of fermenting host mucus polysaccharides and plant cell wall polysaccharides, shifting from one carbon source to another depending on their bioavailability [33, 34].

Primary fermenters of polysaccharides produce both short-chain fatty acids (SCFAs: acetate, propionate, and butyrate) and molecular hydrogen (H_2). In turn, H_2 is the principal energy resource for secondary fermenters in the gut microbial community, and many of them compete for H_2 in the gut [35]. Indeed, acetogens such as *Blautia hydrogenotrophica,* sulfate-reducing bacteria such as *Bilophila wadsworthia,* and methanogen *Methanobrevibacter smithii* can all metabolize H_2, thereby producing different endpoint molecules, such as acetate, H_2S, and CH_4, respectively. Finally, acetate produced by primary and secondary fermenters can be metabolized to butyrate by members of *Clostridium* clusters IV and XIVa; this phenomenon establishes balanced syntrophy among members of intestinal microbial communities [32].

The metabolism of dietary amino acids by the intestinal microbiota involves proteolytic clostridia, such as members of *Clostridium* clusters I and XI [36, 37], Bacteroidetes, and some enterococci and enterobacteria [38]. The metabolism of amino acids involves production of a variety of bacterial metabolites, also depending on the type of amino acid being fermented [37]. In particular, in addition to SCFAs, fermentation of simple aliphatic amino acids results in the production of methylamines, whereas branched-chain amino acids lead to the production of branched-chain fatty acids. Microbiota-mediated metabolism of aromatic amino acids generates a variety of phenolic and indolic metabolites [39].

The microbial metabolites derived from the metabolism of dietary compounds modulate several traits of the host physiology [29, 40]. In particular, SCFAs perform a key multifactorial function in human physiology and homeostasis [41]. For instance, acetate, propionate, and butyrate modulate several parameters of our nutritional state. Although butyrate represents an important energy source for host colonocytes [40, 42], acetate and propionate regulate lipid synthesis in the liver [41] and intestinal gluconeogenesis [43]. Furthermore, by supporting insulin secretion, butyrate is also involved in the regulation of the host energy storage and is known to regulate appetite by enhancing the production of leptin and peptide YY [29].

SCFAs are also strategic modulators of immune function. Butyrate acts both locally, throughout regulatory mechanisms governing production of proinflammatory cytokines in the gut [44], and systemically, by modulating the extrathymic formation of regulatory T cells [45]. In contrast, propionate governs the de novo formation of peripheral regulatory T cells and, together with acetate, guides their homing in the colon. Moreover, propionate has been implicated in the enhancement of hematopoiesis of dendritic cells with impaired T helper 2 type of activation [45].

Certain microbial metabolites generated by amino acid fermentation in the gut have a detrimental effect on the host [39]. In particular, phenolic and indolic metabolites generated by the bacterial metabolism of aromatic amino acids in the gut have been linked with immune

http://dx.doi.org/10.5772/67322

activation and diabetes [39]. Similarly, production of methylamines from aliphatic amino acids is associated with diabetes, obesity, and NAFLD or NASH [46]. Finally, the endpoint metabolites produced by secondary fermenters in the microbiota are relevant to host health. Although acetate produced by acetogens supports butyrate producers in a feedback process, sulfate reducers are detrimental for host health because they support inflammation [47].

The microbiota-mediated metabolism of complex polysaccharides mainly results in the production of beneficial SCFAs, whereas protein fermentation involves production of a vast array of harmful metabolites. Therefore, we can hypothesize that the gut microbiota-host mutualism evolved in the context of a plant-based diet, with only occasional consumption of meat. In fact, according to the aforementioned observations, a plant-based diet should lead to massive production of SCFAs by a saccharolytic intestinal microbiota, preventing the accumulation of detrimental metabolites as a result of bacterial proteolytic fermentation processes [38]. Finally, recent studies support a direct connection between the intake of saturated fats and proinflammatory dysbioses of the intestinal microbiota [48]. High intake of saturated fats results in an increase of bile acid secretion, stimulating the growth of bile-resistant sulfate-reducing bacteria *B. wadsworthia* in the gut and forcing an inflammatory boost as a result of increased H_2S production.

Aside from the diet, there are some stressors that can influence the balance of a microbiota; in particular, antibiotics modify the microbiota, which, after this treatment, is characterized by a different equilibrium [49].

3. Microbiota and liver diseases

In the last two decades, there has been considerable growth in the number of publications evaluating the associations among NAFLD, NASH, and HCC. The progression from NAFLD or NASH to hepatic carcinogenesis represents another growing area of study [50]. A "two-hit" mechanism has been proposed for the NAFLD and NASH pathogenesis. The "first hit," hepatic steatosis, is closely associated with lipotoxicity-induced mitochondrial abnormalities that sensitize the liver to additional proinflammatory insults. The "second hit" includes enhanced lipid peroxidation and increased production of ROS [51]. Recently, some investigators proposed a multiple-hit process with successive liver injuries leading from fat accumulation to inflammation and fibrosis [52]. In particular, there is a report of a relation between the liver-gut correlation and the development of liver diseases [53].

Alteration of a microbiota seems to be involved in the induction and progression of liver damage, in addition to direct injury resulting from various casual agents [54].

Using a metagenomic approach, Turnbaugh et al. compared animals fed a low-fat diet or high-fat high-sugar "Western" diet and demonstrated a relative increase in the number of bacterial cells belonging to the Firmicutes phylum and a reduction in the number of bacterial cells belonging to Bacteroides during the Western diet [55]. The switch from a low-fat to the Western diet shifts composition of the microbiota and increases the ability of the bacteria to harvest energy from the host diet, with progressive development of obesity [56]. In mouse models, Ley et al. observed a similar difference: a rise of the ratio of Firmicutes/Bacteroides in the microbiota in obese humans and re-equilibrium in favor of Bacteroidetes in case of a fat-restricted diet [57].

Therefore, in obese subjects, there are several changes in composition of the intestinal microbiota, which are characterized by upregulation of Firmicutes and a decline of Bacteroidetes (resulting in the so-called "obese microbiota") and a reduction in gut bacterial richness [58, 59]. Small intestinal bacterial overgrowth (SIBO) by Gram-negative organisms may promote insulin resistance and induce choline deficiency: all of these factors are implicated in NAFLD [60]. The intestinal microbiota is the primary source of bacterial endotoxins (e.g., lipopolysaccharide; LPS) produced by Gram-negative bacteria. LPS normally crosses the mucosa only in trace amounts and enters portal blood to be cleared in the liver. LPS can initiate inflammation and insulin resistance associated with obesity [16, 61].

Quantitative and qualitative alterations of the gut microbiota may lead to increased intestinal permeability via several mechanisms, including regulation of tight junctions, and may favor microbial translocation defined as migration of bacteria or their products—also termed pathogen-associated molecular patterns (PAMPs)—from the gut to mesenteric lymph nodes or to other organs [62–64].

A link between bacterial overgrowth and NAFLD or NASH was first demonstrated by Wigg et al. [13]. In another study, Miele et al. [65] compared intestinal permeability in the three groups of human subjects (NAFLD, celiac disease, and healthy controls) and observed higher prevalence of SIBO and of leaky gut in the NAFLD group, thereby demonstrating the role of this increased permeability in the pathogenesis of hepatic fat deposition.

The gut-liver axis is the way bacteria and their possible hepatotoxic products (e.g., LPS, DNA, or RNA) can easily reach the liver. The final effect is activation of the signaling cascade triggered by a specific immune receptor resulting in the expression of proinflammatory cytokine genes, which may exacerbate the hepatocyte damage and contribute to the subsequent development of HCC [66, 67].

Bacterial components stimulate a toll-like receptor (TLR), which represents a highly conserved family of receptors that recognize specific PAMPs and are expressed on Kupffer cells, biliary epithelial cells, hepatocytes, HSCs, endothelial cells, and dendritic cells [68]. An interaction of a TLR with an endotoxin results in activation of nuclear transcription factors, leading to the release of numerous proinflammatory mediators, such as tumor necrosis factor α (TNF-α), which can induce liver injury, fibrosis, and insulin resistance [69, 70].

Miura and colleagues [71] showed that TLR9 ligands induce the production of IL-1β by Kupffer cells in a mouse model of NASH. IL-1β then promotes lipid accumulation in (and death of) hepatocytes, causing steatosis and inflammation and stimulates HSCs to produce fibrogenic mediators, such as collagen, resulting in fibrosis. In particular, TLR9-deficient mice ($TLR9^{-/-}$) show a significant reduction in hepatic lipid accumulation when compared with their wild-type counterparts [71]. In addition, TLR4 contributes to the development of inflammation and fibrosis by inducing production of proinflammatory cytokines (TNF-α, IL-1β) and cooperates with TLR9 to induce active IL-1β in Kupffer cells [72, 73].

The inflammasome is a cytoplasmic multiprotein complex that recognizes a diverse set of inflammation-inducing stimuli and directly activates caspase 1. Activated caspase 1 causes a release of strong proinflammatory cytokines, such as IL-1β and/or IL-18, which are involved in the pathogenesis of the majority of chronic liver diseases, such as NAFLD and NASH [74, 75]. In particular, the NLRP3 inflammasome is activated by microbial PAMPs (via a two-step process involving a TLR), and therefore, it is the principal inflammasome subtype involved in the NAFLD progression and promoting insulin resistance and β-cell death [11]. Csak et al. [76] described for the first time the role of NLRP3 inflammasome activation in NASH. In mice on a high-fat diet, those authors observed upregulation of the inflammasome, according to increased caspase 1 activity and higher serum levels of IL-1β, in comparison with controls. Another study confirmed these data, pointing to a contribution of the inflammasome to the pathogenesis of NAFLD or NASH [77].

Recent evidence revealed that dysbiosis can promote the development of NAFLD or NASH by modifying the bile acid metabolism. Bile acids can modulate glucose and lipid metabolism via their binding to and activation of G protein-coupled receptor TGR5 and farnesoid X receptor (FXR): nuclear hormone receptors expressed by hepatic Kupffer, stellate, and endothelial cells. In FXR-deficient mice, researchers have demonstrated glucose intolerance, insulin resistance, and elevated circulating levels of free fatty acids, which lead to the development of severe hepatic steatosis [78–80].

FXR regulates hepatic inflammation and fibrosis and is important for hepatocarcinogenesis. Fickert et al. [81] studied FXR knockout mice ($FXR^{-/-}$) and showed that the FXR loss alleviates fibrosis of the hepatic biliary tree. $FXR^{-/-}$ mice develop spontaneous HCC at age >12 months [82, 83]. Selective reactivation of intestinal FXR can restore bile acid enterohepatic circulation and protect $FXR^{-/-}$ mice from spontaneous development of HCC [84].

4. NAFLD and hepatic progenitor cells

Several lines of evidence suggest that another factor is implicated in the development and progression of chronic liver diseases. Namely, HPCs are a bipotent cell population that can differentiate into hepatocytes or into biliary epithelium cells and reside in the terminal biliary ductules and in the so-called "canals of Hering" [85, 86]. They represent a heterogeneous cell population expressing phenotypic markers of both immature hepatocytes (such as α-fetoprotein) and bile duct cells (such as bile duct-type cytokeratins) [26, 87].

HPCs have been studied regarding regeneration after severe hepatocellular necrosis [88], but recent studies revealed that this cellular compartment is also activated in chronic viral hepatitis, alcoholic liver disease, and NAFLD [89]: the most important hepatocarcinogenic conditions in the Western world. Activation of progenitor cells in these diseases suggests that they are a possible target cell population for hepatocarcinogens [67, 90].

In the healthy liver, replacement of necrotic and apoptotic hepatocytes involves proliferation of adjacent hepatocytes within the lobules [26]. Nonetheless, this primary pathway is often impaired by a variety of insults, including experimental toxins, viral infection, steatosis, oxidative stress, and alcohol. Chronic inflammation, the presence of growth factors, and DNA-damaging agents like ROS and reactive nitrogen species induce replicative senescence of hepatocytes, and this inhibition activates a secondary proliferative pathway involving HPCs [91–93].

The combination of oxidative liver damage and inhibited hepatocyte proliferation, as observed in NAFLD and NASH, seems to provide a strong stimulus for activation of HPCs and plays a key role in the pathogenesis of HCC. Roskams et al. [91] studied three murine models of fatty liver disease (genetically obese ob/ob mice and normal mice with fatty livers induced either by ethanol or methionine choline-deficient diets) and patients with nonalcoholic fatty liver disease or alcoholic liver disease. Mice with fatty liver show greater numbers of progenitor cells than controls do, and mitochondrial ROS production is significantly increased in all three groups. This increased oxidative stress promotes replicative senescence in mature hepatocytes and expansion of progenitor cells, in both mice and humans [91].

The magnitude of progenitor cell activation seems to correlate with the severity of liver disease [89, 91]. In a recent work, Richardson et al. showed that NASH with portal or linking fibrosis (disease stages 2–4) is associated with more frequent replicative arrest of hepatocytes and with expansion of HPC numbers as compared to steatosis alone [94].

Literature data are suggestive of the involvement of the inflammatory infiltrate in the activation of progenitor cells, through the secretion of inflammatory cytokines, in particular TNF-α [95, 96]. Expression of these cytokines is upregulated during hepatic injury and performs an important function in HPC activation [97, 98]. The result is production of some profibrogenic factors that activate HSCs and boost the production of collagen [28].

Other signaling pathways participate in the complex mechanism controlling the behavior of HPCs. *Must1*, *Must2*, and *Yap* genes are important for proliferative control and tumorigenesis in the liver. Defects in this signaling pathway lead to sustained liver overgrowth and eventual development of either HCC or cholangiocarcinoma in mice [99]. Studies in humans confirmed that a loss of regulation of Mst1 or Mst2 is a common aberration in HCC and may account for Yap activation in these tumors. In fact, approximately 30% of HCCs show reduced Yap phosphorylation and aberrant overexpression of Yap [100, 101].

Approximately, a half of human HCCs (28–50%) express one or more markers of progenitor cells that are not present in normal mature hepatocytes [102, 103]. When analyzing the precursor lesions of HCC, many authors detected HPCs and intermediate hepatocyte like cells in 50% of small cell dysplastic foci and in hepatocellular adenoma [90, 104]. These findings support the hypothesis that some human HCCs arise from HPCs. Moreover, HCCs expressing HPC markers have a worse prognosis than HPC marker-negative HCCs. Wu et al. observed significantly shorter survival of patients with HCCs expressing CK19 [105]. Similar findings were made by Uenishi et al. [106]. In a recent study, Durnez reported that CK19-positive HCC shows a higher rate of tumor recurrence after a liver transplant as compared with CK19-negative HCC [103].

The available data suggest that HPCs are involved in fibrogenesis and progression of NAFLD and that their activation during chronic liver disease may increase the risk of HCC. Nonetheless, further studies are necessary to better clarify the function of these cells in hepatocarcinogenesis and in the liver's response to NAFLD injury.

5. Conclusion

Recent pieces of evidence are indicative of the role of the intestinal microbiota—in particular its dysbiosis and activation of HPCs—in the clinical course of NAFLD and in the subsequent development of HCC. Intestinal microbes produce a large array of bioactive molecules mainly from dietary compounds, thus establishing intense microbiota-host transgenomic metabolism with a strong impact on pathological conditions. Derangement of the intestinal microbiota may lead to translocation of bacteria or their products to the liver, where endotoxins trigger inflammation and hepatocellular damage, which in turn is crucial for the development of HCC.

The subsequent liver injury and hepatocellular necrosis can activate a secondary proliferative pathway involving HPCs: a bipotential cell compartment that seems to contribute to hepatocarcinogenesis.

Better knowledge of these factors is necessary for understanding the HCC pathogenesis in NAFLD and for discovery of new therapies, but further research is necessary to identify the carcinogenesis process.

Abbreviations

Nonalcoholic fatty liver disease	NAFLD
Nonalcoholic fatty liver	NAFL
Nonalcoholic steatohepatitis	NASH
Hepatocellular carcinoma	HCC
Hepatitis B	HBV
Hepatitis C	HCV
Hepatic stellate cells	HSCs
Hepatic progenitor cells	HPCs
Reactive oxygen species	ROS
Transforming growth factor β	TGF-β
Platelet-derived growth factor	PDGF
Short-chain fatty acids	SCFAs
Molecular hydrogen	H_2

Small intestinal bacterial overgrowth	SIBO
lipopolysaccharide	LPS
Pathogen-associated molecular patterns	PAMPs
Toll-like receptor	TLR
Tumor necrosis factor	α (TNF-α)
Farnesoid X receptor	FXR

Author details

Giovanni Brandi[1,2]*, Stefania De Lorenzo[1], Marco Candela[3] and Francesco Tovoli[4]

*Address all correspondence to: giovanni.brandi@unibo.it

1 Department of Experimental, Diagnostic and Specialty Medicine, Sant'Orsola-Malpighi Hospital, Bologna University, Bologna, Italy

2 "G. Prodi" Interdepartmental Center for Cancer Research (C.I.R.C.), Bologna University, Bologna, Italy

3 Department of Pharmacy and Biotechnology, Bologna University, Bologna, Italy

4 Department of Medical and Surgical Sciences, University of Bologna, Bologna, Italy

References

[1] Younossi ZM, Koenig AB, Abdelatif D, Fazel Y, Henry L, Wymer M. Global epidemiology of non-alcoholic fatty liver disease-meta-analytic assessment of prevalence, incidence and outcomes. *Hepatology*, 2016; 64: 73–84.

[2] Abd El-Kader SM, El-Den Ashmawy EMS. Non-alcoholic fatty liver disease: the diagnosis and management. *World J Hepatol*, 2015; 7: 846–858.

[3] Starley BQ, Calcagno CJ, Harrison SA. Nonalcoholic fatty liver disease and hepatocellular carcinima; a weighty connection. *Hepatology*, 2010; 51: 1820–1832.

[4] Musso G, Gambino R, Cassader M, Pagano G. Meta-analysis: natural history of non-alcoholic fatty liver disease (NAFLD) and diagnostic accuracy of non-invasive tests for liver disease severity. *Ann Med*, 2011; 43: 617–649.

[5] Gomaa AI, Khan SA, Toledano MB, Waked I, Taylor-Robinson SD. Hepatocellular carcinoma: epidemiology, risk factors, and pathogenesis. *World J Gastroenterol*, 2008; 14: 4300–4308.

[6] Wong VW-S, Wong GL-H, Choi PC-L, Chan AW-H, Li MK-P, Chan H-Y, Chim AM, Yu J, Sung JJ, Chan HL. Disease progression of non-alcoholic fatty liver disease: a prospective study with paired liver biopsies at 3 years. *Gut*, 2010; 59: 969–974.

[7] Pais R, Charlotte F, Fedchuk L, Bedossa P, Lebray P, Poynard T, Ratziu V, LIDO Study Group. A systematic review of follow-up biopsies reveals disease progression in patients with non-alcoholic fatty liver, *J Hepatol*, 2013; 59: 550–556.

[8] McPherson S, Hardy T, Henderson E, Burt AD, Day CP, Anstee QM. Evidence of NAFLD progression from steatosis to fibrosing-steatohepatitis using paired biopsies: implications for prognosis and clinical management. *J Hepatol*, 2015; 62: 1148–1155.

[9] Shimada M, Hashimoto E, Taniai M, Hasegawa K, Okuda H, Hayashi N, Takasaki K, Ludwig J. Hepatocellular carcinoma in patients with nonalchololic steatohepatitis. *J Hepatol*, 2002; 37: 154–160.

[10] Matteoni CA, Younossi ZM, Gramlich T, Boparai N, Liu YC, McCullough AJ. Nonalcoholic fatty liver disease: a spectrum of clinical and pathological severity. *Gastroenterology*, 1999; 116: 1413–1419.

[11] Henao-Mejia J, Elinav E, Jin C, Hao L, Mehal WZ, Strowig T, Thaiss CA, Kau AL, Eisenbarth SC, Jurczak MJ, et al. Inflammasome-mediated dysbiosis regulates progression of NAFLD and obesity. *Nature*, 2012; 482: 179–185.

[12] Cani PD, Delzenne NM. The role of the gut microbiota in energy metabolism and metabolic disease. *Curr Pharm Design*, 2009; 13: 1546–1558.

[13] Wigg AJ, Roberts-Thomson IC, Dymock RB, McCarthy PJ, Grose RH, Cummins AG. The role of small intestinal bacterial overgrowth, intestinal permeability, endotoxaemia, and tumour necrosis factor α in the pathogenesis of non-alcoholic steatohepatitis. *Gut*, 2001; 48: 206–211.

[14] Huycke MM, Gaskius HR. Commensal bacteria, redox stress, and colorectal cancer: mechanisms and models. *Exp Biol Med (Maywood)*, 2004; 229: 586–597.

[15] Wiest R, Rath HC. Bacterial translocation in the gut. *Bailliere's Best Pract Res Clin Gastroenterol*, 2003; 17: 397–425.

[16] Cani P, Bibiloni R, Knauf C, Waget A, Neyrinck AM, Delzenne NM, Burcelin R. Changes in gut microbiota control metabolic endotoxemia-induced inflammation in high-fat diet-induced obesity and diabetes in mice. *Diabetes*, 2008; 57: 1470–1481.

[17] Wu WC, Zhao W, Li S. Small intestinal bacteria overgrowth decreases small intestinal motility in the NASH rats. *World J Gastroenterol*, 2008; 14: 313–317.

[18] Wong VW-S, Wong GL-H, Tsang SW-C, Fan T, Chu WC, Woo J, Chan AW, Choi PC, Chim AM, Lau JY, Chan FK, Sung JJ, Chan HL. High prevalence of colorectal neoplasm in patients with non-alcoholic steatohepatitis. *Gut*, 2011; 60: 829–836.

[19] Stadlmayr A, Aigner E, Steger B, Scharinger L, Lederer D, Mayr A, Strasser M, Brunner E, Heuberger A, Hohla F, Steinwendner J, Patsch W, Datz C. Nonalcoholic fatty liver disease: an independent risk factor for colorectal neoplasia. *J Intern Med*, 2011; 270: 41–49.

[20] Louis P, Hold GL, Flint HJ. The gut microbiota, bacterial metabolites and colorectal cancer. *Nat Rev Microbiol*, 2014; 12: 661–672.

[21] Brandi G, De Rosa F, Liguori G, Agostini V, Di Girolamo S, Gaboriau-Routhiau V, Raibaud P, Biasco G. Intestinal microbiota aruond colorectal canger genesis. In: *The research and biology of cancer II*, 2013; 59.

[22] Singh S, Sharma AN, Murad MH, Buttar NS, El-Serag HB, Katzka DA, Iyer PG. Central adiposity is associated within creased risk of esophageal inflammation, metaplasia, and adenocarcinoma: a systematic review and meta-analysis. *Clin Gastroenterol Hepatol*, 2013; 11: 1399–1412.

[23] Aune D, Greenwood DC, Chan DS, Vieira R, Vieira AR, Navarro Rosenblatt DA, Cade JE, Burley VJ, Norat T. Body mass index, abdominal fatness and pancreatic cancer risk: a systematic review and non-linear dose-response meta-analysis of prospective studies. *Ann Oncol*, 2012; 23: 843–852.

[24] Vongsuvanh R, George J, Qiao L, van der Poorten D. Visceral adiposity in gastrointestinal and hepatic carcinogenesis. *Cancer Lett*, 2013; 330: 1–10.

[25] Ohtani N, Yoshimoto S, Hara E. Obesity and cancer: a gut microbial connection. *Cancer Res*, 2014; 74: 1885–1889.

[26] Roskams T, Libbrecht L, Desmet V. Progenitors cells in diseased human liver. *Semin Liver Dis*, 2003; 23: 385–396.

[27] Roskams T. Liver stem cells and their implication in hepatocellular and cholangiocarcinoma. *Oncogene*, 2006; 225: 3818–3822.

[28] Carpino G, Renzi A, Onori P, Gaudio E. Role of hepatic progenitor cells in nonalcoholic fatty liver disease development: cellular cross-talks and molecular networks. *Int J Mol Sci*, 2013; 14: 20112–20130.

[29] Tremaroli V, Backhed F. Functional interactions between the gut microbiota and host metabolism. *Nature*, 2012; 489: 242–249.

[30] Flint HJ, Bayer EA, Rincon MT, Lamed R, White BA. Polysaccharide utilization by gut bacteria: potential for new insights from genomic analysis. *Nat Rev Microbiol*, 2008; 6: 121–131.

[31] Koropatkin NM, Cameron EA, Martens EC. How glycan metabolism shapes the human gut microbiota. *Nat Rev Microbiol*, 2012; 10: 323–335.

[32] Fischbach MA, Sonnenburg JL. Eating for two: how metabolism establishes interspecies interactions in the gut. *Cell Host Microbe*, 2011; 10: 336–347.

[33] Sonnenburg ED, Zheng H, Joglekar P, Higginbottom SK, Firbank SJ, Bolam DN, Sonnenburg JL. Specificity of polysaccharide use in intestinal Bacteroides species determines diet-induced microbiota alterations. *Cell*, 2010; 141: 1241–1252.

[34] Rakoff-Nahoum S, Coyne MJ, Comstock LE. An ecological network of polysaccharide utilization among human intestinal symbionts. *Curr Biol*, 2014; 24: 40–49.

[35] Miller TL, Wolin MJ. Enumeration of *Methanobrevibacter smithii* in human feces. *Arch Microbiol*, 1982; 131: 14–18.

[36] Schwab C, Cristescu B, Northrup JM, Stenhouse GB, Ganzie M. Diet and environment shape fecal bacterial microbiota composition and enteric pathogen load of grizzly bears. *PLoS One*, 2011; 6: e27905.

[37] Smith EA, Macfarlane GT. Dissimilatory amino-acid metabolism in human colonic bacteria. *Anaerobe*, 1997; 3: 327–337.

[38] David LA, Maurice CF, Carmody RN, Gootenberg DB, Button JE, Wolfe BE, Ling AV, Devlin AS, Varma Y, Fischbach MA, Biddinger SB, Dutton RJ, Turnbaugh PJ. Diet rapidly and reproducibly alters the human gut microbiome. *Nature*, 2014; 505: 559–563.

[39] Moco S, Candela M, Chuang E, Draper C, Cominetti O, Montoliu I, Barron D, Kussmann M, Brigidi P, Gionchetti P, Martin FP. Systems biology approaches for inflammatory bowel disease: emphasis on gut microbial metabolism. *Inflamm Bowel Dis*, 2014; 20: 2104–2114.

[40] Nichilson JK, Holmes E, Kinross J, Burcelin R, Gbson G, Jia W, Pettersson S. Host-gut microbiota metabolic interactions. *Science*, 2012; 336: 1262–1267.

[41] Besten DG, van Eunen K, Groen AK, Venema K, Reijngoud DJ, Bakker BM. The role of short-chain fatty acids in the interplay between diet, gut microbiota, and host energy metabolism. *J Lipid Res*, 2013; 54: 2325–2340.

[42] Neish AS. Microbes in gastrointestinal health and disease. *Gastroenterology*, 2009; 136: 65–80.

[43] De Vadder F, Kovatcheva-Datchary P, Goncalves D, Vinera J, Zitoun C, Duchampt A, Backhed F, Mithieux G. Microbiota-generated metabolites promote metabolic benefits via gut-brain neural circuits. *Cell*, 2014; 156: 84–96.

[44] Segain JP, Raingeard de la Blétière D, Bourreille A, Leray V, Gervois N, Rosales C, Ferrier L, Bonnet C, Blottière HM, Galmiche JP. Butyrate inhibits inflammatory responses through NF-kappa B inhibition: implications for Crohn's disease. *Gut*, 2000; 47: 397–403.

[45] Trompette A, Gollwitzer ES, Yadava K, Sichelstiel AK, Sprenger N, Ngom-Bru C, Blanchard C, Junt T, Nicod LP, Harris NL, Marsland BJ. Gut microbiota metabolism of dietary fiber influences allergic airway disease and hematopoiesis. *Nat Med*, 2014; 20: 159–166.

[46] Holmes E, Li JV, Marchesi JR, Nicholson JK. Gut microbiota composition and activity in relation to host metabolic phenotype and disease risk. *Cell Metab*, 2012; 16: 559–564.

[47] Devkota S, Wang Y, Musch MW, Leone V, Fehlner-Peach H, Nadimpalli A, Antonopoulos DA, Jabri B, Chang EB. Dietary-fat-induced taurocholic acid promotes pathobiot expansion and colitis in IL-$10^{-/-}$ mice. *Nature*, 2012; 5: 104–108.

[48] Cox LM, Yamanishi S, Sohn J, Alekseyenko AV, Leung JM, Cho I, Kim SG, Li H, Gao Z, Mahana D, Zárate Rodriguez JG, Rogers AB, Robine N, Loke P, Blaser MJ. Altering the intestinal microbiota during a critical developmental window has lasting metabolic consequences. *Cell*, 2014; 158: 705–721.

[49] Dethlefsen L, Relman DA. Incomplete recovery and individualized responses of the human distal gut microbiota to repeated antibiotic perturbation. *Proc Natl Acad Sci USA*, 2011; 108: 4554–4561.

[50] White DL, Kanwal F, El Serag HB. Association between nonalcoholic fatty liver disease and risk for hepatocellular cancer, based on systematic review. *Clinical Gastroenterol Hepatol*, 2012; 1: 1342–1359.

[51] Sanyal AJ, Campbell-Sargent C, Mirshahi F, Rizzo WB, Contos MJ, Sterling RK, Luketic VA, Shiffman ML, Clore JN. Nonalcoholic steatohepatitis: association of insulin resistance and mitochondrial abnormalities. *Gastroenterology*, 2001; 120: 1183–1192.

[52] Tilg H, Moschen AR. Evolution of inflammation in nonalcoholic fatty liver disease: the multiple parallel hits hypothesis. *Hepatology*, 2010; 52: 1836–1846.

[53] Musso G, Gambino R, Cassader M. Gut microbiota as a regulator of energy homeostasis and ectopic fat deposition: mechanisms and implications for metabolic disorders. *Curr Opin Lipidol*, 2010; 21: 76–83.

[54] Loguercio C, De Simone T, Federico A, Terracciano F, Tuccillo C, Di Chicco M, Cartenì M. Gut-liver axis: a new point of attack to treat chronic liver damage? *Am J Gastroenterol*, 2002; 97: 2144–2146.

[55] Turnbaugh PJ, Backhed F, Fulton L, Gordon JI. Diet-induced obesity is linked to marked but reversible alterations in the mouse distal gut microbiome. *Cell Host Microbe*, 2008; 17: 213–223.

[56] Turnbaugh PJ, Ley RE, Mahowald MA, Magrini ER, Gordon JI. An obesity-associated gut microbiome with increased capacity for energy harvest. *Nature*, 2006; 21: 1027–1031.

[57] Ley RE, Turnbaugh PJ, Klein S, Gordon JI. Microbial ecology: human gut microbes associated with obesity. *Nature*, 2006; 21: 1022–1023.

[58] Tilg H, Moschen AR, Kaser A. Obesity and the microbiota. *Gastroenterology*, 2009; 136: 1476–1483.

[59] Le Chatelier E, Nielsen T, Qin J, Prifti E, Hildebrand F, Falony G, Almeida M, Arumugam M, Batto JM, Kennedy S, Leonard P, Li J, Burgdorf K, Grarup N, Jørgensen T, Brandslund I, Nielsen HB, Juncker AS, Bertalan M, Levenez F, Pons N, Rasmussen S, Sunagawa S, Tap J, Tims S, Zoetendal EG, Brunak S, Clément K, Doré J, Kleerebezem M, Kristiansen K, Renault P, Sicheritz-Ponten T, de Vos WM, Zucker JD, Raes J, Hansen T, MetaHIT consortium, Bork P, Wang J, Ehrlich SD, Pedersen O. Richness of human gut microbiome correlates with metabolic markers. *Nature*, 2013; 500: 541–546.

[60] Abu-Shanab A, Quigley EMM. The role of the gut microbiota in nonalcoholic fatty liver disease. *Nature Reviews Gastroenterol Hepatol*, 2010; 27: 691–701.

[61] Cani PD, Amar J, Iglesias MA, Poggi M, Knauf C, Bastelica D, Neyrinck AM, Fava F, Tuohy KM, Chabo C, Waget A, Delmée E, Cousin B, Sulpice T,Chamontin B, Ferrières J, Tanti JF, Gibson GR, Casteilla L, Delzenne NM, Alessi MC, Burcelin R. Metabolic endotoxemia initiates obesity and insulin resistance. *Diabetes*, 2007; 56: 1761–1772.

[62] Compare D, Coccoli P, Rocco A, Nardone OM, De Maria S, Cartenì M, et al. Gut–liver axis: the impact of gut microbiota on nonalcoholic fatty liver disease. *Nut Metab Cardiovasc Dis*, 2012; 22: 471–476.

[63] Vanni E, Marengo A, Mezzabotta L, Bugianesi E. Systemic complications of nonalcoholic fatty liver disease: when the liver is not an innocent bystander. *Semin Liver Dis*, 2015; 35: 236–249.

[64] Mehal WZ. The Gordian Knot of dysbiosis, obesity and NAFLD. *Nat Rev Gastroenterol Hepatol*, 2013; 10: 637–644.

[65] Miele L, Valenza V, La Torre G, Montalto M, Cammarota G, Ricci R, Mascianà R, Forgione A, Gabrieli ML, Perotti G, Vecchio FM, Rapaccini G, Gasbarrini G,Day CP, Grieco A. Increased intestinal permeability and tight junction alterations in nonalcoholic fatty liver disease. *Hepatology*, 2009; 49: 1877–1887.

[66] Alisi A, Ceccarelli S, Panera N, Nobili V. Causative role of gut microbiota in non-alcoholic fatty liver disease pathogenesis. *Front Cell Infect Microbiol* (*opinion article*), 2012; 2: 132. doi:10.3389/fcimb.2012.00132.

[67] Lade A, Noon LA, Friedman SL. Contributions of metabolic dysregulation and inflammation of nonalcoholic steatohepatitis, hepatic fibrosis and cancer. *Curr Opin*, 2014; 26: 100–107.

[68] Miyake Y, Yamamoto K. Role of gut microbiota in liver diseases. *Hepatol Res*, 2013; 43: 139–146.

[69] Nagata K, Suzuki H, Sakaguchi S. Common pathogenic mechanism in development progression of liver injury caused by nn-alcoholic or alcoholic steatohepatitis. *J Toxicol Sci*, 2007; 32: 453–468.

[70] Nagy LE. Recent insights into the role of innate immune system in the development of alcoholic liver disease. *Exp Biol Med* (*Maywood*), 2003; 228: 882–890.

[71] Miura K, Kodama Y, Inokuchi S, Schnabl B, Aoyama T, Ohnishi H, Olefsky JM, Brenner DA, Seki E. Toll-like receptor-9 promotes steatohepatitis by induction of interleukin-1beta in mice. *Gastoenterology*, 2010; 139: 323–334.

[72] Rivera CA, Adegboyega P, van Rooijen N, Tagalicud A, Allman M, Wallace M. Toll-like receptor-4 signaling and Kupffer cells play pivotal roles in the pathogenesis of nonalcoholic steatohepatitis. *J Hepatol*, 2007; 47: 571–579.

[73] Spruss A, Kanuri G, Wagnerberger S, Haub S, Bischoff SC, Bergheim I. Toll-like receptor 4 is involved in the development of fructose-induced hepatic steatosis in mice. *Hepatology*, 2009; 50: 1094–1104.

[74] Strowing T, Henao-Mejia J, Elivian E, Flavell R. Inflammasome in health and disease. *Nature*, 2012; 481: 133–144.

[75] Szabo G, Csak T. Inflammasome in liver diseases. *J Hepatol*, 2012; 57: 642–654.

[76] Csak T, Ganz M, Pespisa J, Kodys K, Dolganiuc A, Szabo G. Fatty acid and endotoxin activate inflammasomes in mouse hepatocytes that release danger signals to stimulate immune cells. *Hepatology*, 2011; 54: 133–144.

[77] Vandanmagsar B, Youm YH, Ravussin A, Galgani JE, Stadler K, Mynatt RL, Ravussin E, Stephens JM, Dixit VD. The NALP3/NLRP3 inflammasome instigates obesity-induced autoinflammation and insuline resistance. *Nat Med*, 2011; 17: 179–188.

[78] Claudel T, Staels B, Kuipers F. The Farnesoid X receptor: a molecular link between bile acid and lipid and glucose metabolism. *Arterioscler Thromb Vasc Biol*, 2005; 25: 2020–2030.

[79] Schreuder TC, Marsman HA, Lenicek M, van Werven JR, Nederveen AJ, Jansen PL, Schaap FG. The hepatic response to FGF19 is impaired in patients with nonalcoholic fatty liver disease and insulin resistance. *Am J Physiol Gastrointest Liver Physiol*, 2010; 298: G440–G445.

[80] Miyata M, Sakaida Y, Matsuzawa H, Yoshinari K, Yamazoe Y. Fibroblast growth factor 19 treatment ameliorates disruption of hepatic lipid metabolism in farnesoid X receptor (Fxr)-null mice. *Biol Pharm Bull*, 2011; 34: 1885–1889.

[81] Fickert P, Fuchsbichler A, Moustafa T, Wagner M, Zollner G, Halilbasic E, Stöger U, Arrese M, Pizarro M, Solís N, Carrasco G, Caligiuri A, Sombetzki M, Reisinger E, Tsybrovskyy O, Zatloukal K, Denk H, Jaeschke H, Pinzani M, Trauner M. Farnesoid X receptor critically determines the fibrotic response in mice but is expressed to a low extent in human hepatic stellate cells and periductal myofibroblasts. *Am J Pathol*, 2009; 175: 2392–2405.

[82] Zhang Y, Ge X, Heemstra LA, Chen WD, Xu J, Smith JL, Ma H, Kasim N, Edwards PA, Novak CM. Loss of FXR protects against diet-induced obesity and accelerates liver carcinogenesis in ob/ob mice. *Mol Endocrinol*, 2012; 26: 272–280.

[83] Kim I, Morimura K, Shah Y, Yang Q, Ward JM, Gonzalez FJ. Spontaneous hepatocarcinogenesis in farnesoid X receptor-null mice. *Carcinogenesis*, 2007; 28: 940–946.

[84] Degirolamo C, Modica S, Vacca M, Di Tullio G, Morgano A, D'Orazio A, Kannisto K, Parini P, Moschetta A. Prevention of spontaneous hepatocarcinogenesis in farnesoid X receptor-null mice by intestinal-specific farnesoid X receptor reactivation. *Hepatology*, 2015; 61: 161–170.

[85] Haque S, Haruna Y, Saito K, Nalesnik MA, Atillasoy E, Thung SN, Gerber MA. Identification of bipotential progenitor cells in human liver regeneration. *Lab Invest*, 1996; 75: 699–705.

[86] Theise ND, Saxena R, Portmann BC, Thung SN, Yee H, Chiriboga L, Kumar A, Crawford JM. The canals of Hering and hepatic stem cells in humans. *Hepatology*, 1999; 30: 1425–1433.

[87] Germain L, Goyette R, Marceau N. Differential cytokeratin and alpha-fetoprotein expression in morphologically distinct epithelial cells emerging at the early stage of rat hepatocarcinogenesis. *Cancer Res*, 1985; 45: 673–681.

[88] Fujita M, Furukawa H, Hattori M, Todo S, Ishida Y, Nagashima K. Sequential observation of liver cell regeneration after massive hepatic necrosis in auxiliary partial orthotopic liver transplantation. *Mod Pathol*, 2000; 13: 152–157.

[89] Libbrecht L, Desmet V, Van Damme B, Roskams T. Deep intralobular extension of human hepatic "progenitor cells" correlates with parenchymal inflammation in chronic viral hepatitis can "progenitor cells" migrate? *J Pathol*, 2000; 192: 373–378.

[90] Libbrecht L, Desmet V, Van Damme B, Roskams T. The immunohistochemical phenotype of dysplastic foci in human liver: correlation with putative progenitor cells. *J Hepatol*, 2000; 33: 76–84.

[91] Roskams T, Yang SQ, Koteish A, Durnez A, De Vos R, Huang X, Achten R, Verslype C, Diehl AM. Oxidative stress and oval cell accumulation in mice and humans with alcoholic and nonalcoholic fatty liver disease. *Am J Pathol*, 2003; 163: 1301–1311.

[92] Marshall A, Rushbrook S, Davies SE, Morris LS, Scott IS, Vawel SL, Coleman N, Alexander G. Relation between hepatocyte G1 arrest, impaired hepatic regeneration, and fibrosis in chronic hepatitis C virus infection. *Gastroenterology*, 2005; 128: 33–42.

[93] Yang S, Koteish A, Liu H, Huang J, Roskams T, Dawson V, Diehl AM. Oval cells compensate for damage and replicative senescence of mature hepatocytes in mice with fatty liver disease. *Hepatology*, 2004; 39: 403–411.

[94] Richardson MM, Jonsson JR, Powell EE, Brunt EM, Neuschwander-Tetri BA, Bhathal PS, Dixon JB, Weltman MD, Tilg H, Moschen AR, Purdie DM, Demetris AJ, Clouston AD. Progressive fibrosis in nonalcoholic steatohepatitis: association with altered regeneration and a ductular reaction. *Gastroenterology*, 2007; 133: 80–90.

[95] Knight B, Matthews VB, Akhurst B, Croager EJ, Klinken E, Abraham LJ, Olynyk JK, Yeoh G. Liver inflammation and cytokine production, but not acute phase protein synthesis, accompany the adult liver progenitor (oval) cell response to chronic liver injury. *Immunol Cell Biol*, 2005; 83: 364–374.

[96] Akhurst B, Matthews V, Husk K, Smyth MJ, Abraham LJ, Yeoh GC. Differential lymphotoxin-beta and interferon gamma signaling during mouse liver regeneration induced by chronic and acute liver injury. *Hepatology*, 2005; 41: 327–335.

[97] Knight B, Yeoh GC, Husk KL, Ly T, Abraham LJ, Yu C, Rhim JA, Fausto N. Impaired preneoplastic changes and liver tumor formation in tumor necrosis factor receptor type 1 knockout mice. *J Exp Med*, 2000; 192: 1809–1818.

[98] Jakubowski A, Ambrose C, Parr M, Lincecum JM, Wang MZ, Zheng S, Browning B, Michaelson JS, Baetscher M, Wang B, Bissell DM, Burkly LC. TWEAK induces liver progenitor cell proliferation. *J Clin Invest*, 2005; 115: 2330–2340.

[99] Avruch J, Zhou D, Fitamant J, Bardeesy N. Mst1/2 signalling to Yap: gatekeeper for liver size and tumour development. *Br J Cancer*, 2011; 104: 24–32.

[100] Zhao B, Wei X, Li W, Udan RS, Yang Q, Kim J, Xie J, Ikenoue T, Yu J, Li L, Zheng P, Ye K, Chinnaiyan A, Halder G, Lai ZC, Guan KL. Inactivation of Yap oncoproteins by the Hippo pathway is involved in cell contact inhibition and tissue growth control. *Genes Dev*, 2007; 21: 2747–2761.

[101] Zhou D, Conrad C, Xia F, Park JS, Payer B, Yin Y, Lauwers GY, Thasler W, Lee JT, Avruch J, Bardeesy N. Mst1 and Mst2 maintain hepatocyte quiescence and suppress hepatocellular carcinoma development through inactivation of the Yap1 oncogene. *Cancer Cell*, 2009; 16: 425–438.

[102] Yoon DS, Jeong J, Park YN, Kim KS, Kwon SW, Chi HS, Park C, Kim BR. Expression of biliary antigen and its clinical significance in hepatocellular carcinoma. *Yonsei Med J*, 1999; 40: 472–477.

[103] Durnez A, Verslype C, Nevens F, Fevery J, Aerts R, Pirenne J, Lesaffre E, Libbrecht L, Desmet V, Roskams T. The clinicopathological and prognostic relevance of cytokeratin 7 and 19 expression in hepatocellular carcinoma. A possible progenitor cell origin. *Histopathology*, 2006; 49: 138–151.

[104] Libbrecht L, De Vos R, van den Oord JJ, Desmet V, Aerts R, Roskams T. Hepatic progenitor cells in hepatocellular adenomas. *Am J Surg Pathol*, 2001; 25: 1388–1396.

[105] Wu PC, Lai VCH, Fang JWS, Gerber M, Lai CL, Lau JYN. Hepatocellular carcinoma expressing both hepatocellular and biliary markers also express cytokeratin 14, a marker of bipotential progenitor cells. *J Hepatol*, 1999; 31: 965–966.

[106] Uenishi T, Kubo S, Yamamoto T, Shuto T, Ogawa M, Tanaka H, Tanaka S, Kaneda K, Hirohashi K. Cytokeratin 19 expression in hepatocellular carcinoma predicts early postoperative recurrence. *Cancer Sci*, 2003; 94: 851–857.

Chapter 3

Cancer Stem Cells and Aldehyde Dehydrogenase 1 in Liver Cancers

Hiroyuki Tomita, Tomohiro Kanayama, Ayumi Niwa,
Kei Noguchi, Kazuhisa Ishida, Masayuki Niwa and
Akira Hara

Additional information is available at the end of the chapter

http://dx.doi.org/10.5772/66454

Abstract

The cancer stem cell (CSC) theory posits that a small population of cells with stem cell-like features is responsible for tumor growth, resistance, and recurrence in many malignancies. This theory could be a useful paradigm for designing innovative targeted drug therapies. Liver cancer is the fifth most common cancer worldwide, with hepatocellular carcinoma (HCC) and cholangiocarcinoma (CCA) as the predominant forms. Hepatic stem/progenitor cells are believed to be the origin of HCCs and CCAs; however, this remains a controversial topic. Aldehyde dehydrogenase (ALDH) is the main enzymatic system responsible for the clearance of acetaldehyde from the hepatocytes in the liver tissue. Therefore, ALDH1 has been suggested to be a potential, biological and CSC marker in liver cancers. We here provide an overview of the current state of knowledge of CSCs in liver and the role of ALDH1 in the development and progression of liver cancers and discuss its potential value as a prognostic and diagnostic biomarker.

Keywords: aldehyde dehydrogenase, stem cell, cancer stem cell, hepatocellular carcinoma, cholangiocarcinoma, liver cancer

1. Introduction

Liver cancer is the second most common cause of death from cancer and is the fifth most commonly diagnosed cancer worldwide [1]. Given that the incidence of liver cancer has been on the rise globally and its poor prognosis, the overall mortality rate has also been increased [1, 2]. Some hepatic stem/progenitor markers are currently available for identifying a subset of cells with stem cell-like features known as cancer stem cells (CSCs). Identifying CSC-specific genes and understanding their mechanisms in liver cancers are important issues in the development of cancer therapy. Aldehyde dehydrogenase 1 (ALDH1) has been reported to indicate the therapeutic drug resistance of many malignancies, and shows potential to be widely used as a marker to identify cells with stem cell-like features, including those in primary liver cancers. We describe an overview of CSCs in liver and the role of ALDH1 in liver cancers.

2. The concept of CSCs

The CSC concept derives from the fact that cancer cells are dysregulated clones whose continued propagation occurs in a biologically distinct subset of rare cells. This concept is not novel but has gained prominence in recent years owing to advances in gaining a greater appreciation of the multistep nature of oncogenesis [3]. This concept has important therapeutic implications and may explain why it is possible to treat many malignancies until the tumor can no longer be detected, and yet the cancer returns [4]. Although radiation therapy and chemotherapy have been the mainstay of cancer treatment, these modalities do not show a substantial effect on CSCs [5]. Furthermore, it may be tough to create conditions that assist the production of all the mature cell types of the tissue as well as the survival and self-renewal of the stem cells (SCs) from which the mature cell types derive. Very few phenotypic markers have proven to be reliable surrogates for enumerating SCs, particularly when they have been physiologically or experimentally perturbed [3].

3. SCs in the normal liver

3.1. Liver function and architecture

The liver is the largest parenchymatous organ in the body. It carries out a wide variety of functions for maintaining homeostasis, such as metabolism, glycogen storage, drug detoxification, production of various serum proteins, and bile secretion. Most of the metabolic and synthetic functions of the liver are carried out by hepatocytes. The bile duct is formed by cholangiocytes, a type of epithelial cell. Other cell types that compose the liver are hepatic sinusoidal endothelial cells, Kupffer cells located at the luminal side of the sinusoid, and stellate cells at the space of Disse.

3.2. Liver stem/progenitor cells

In addition to self-renewability, liver stem/progenitor cells have another specific characteristic: the bipotential to differentiate into hepatocytes and cholangiocytes. Liver stem/progenitor cells play important roles in development, homeostasis, and regeneration. Thus, the liver comprises two stem/progenitor cell systems: fetal liver stem/progenitor cells relating to development and adult liver stem/progenitor cells associated with homeostasis and regeneration.

3.3. Fetal liver stem/progenitor cells

The onset of mouse liver development begins at embryonic day (E) 8.5 from the foregut endoderm [6]. The foregut endoderm cells destined for a hepatic fate begin to express the transcription factors HEX and HNF4α as well as the liver-specific genes α-fetoprotein (*Afp*) and albumin (*Alb*) and migrate as cords into the surrounding septum transversum mesenchyme. These cells are common progenitor cells, which give rise to both hepatocytes and cholangiocytes and are called "hepatoblasts" during liver development. Recently, the combination of specific cell-surface markers has been used to isolate fetal liver stem/progenitor cells. The CD45$^-$ TER119$^-$ c-Kit$^-$ CD29$^+$ CD49f$^+$ fraction of the E13.5 mouse liver was shown to include colony-forming cells with the potential to differentiate into hepatocytic and cholangiocytic lineages [7]. Other reported cell-sorting markers that are useful to define fetal liver stem/progenitor cells are c-Kit^{low} [8], c-Kit$^-$ c-Met$^+$ CD49f$^{+/low}$ [9], CD13$^+$ [10], or CD13$^+$ c-Kit$^-$ CD49f$^{-/low}$ CD133$^+$ [11] in combination with CD45$^-$ and TER119$^-$. Delta-like 1 homolog (DLK1) is expressed in the liver buds as early as E9.0 in the mouse embryo, and DLK1$^+$ cells isolated from E14.5 mouse livers have the capacity to form proliferative colonies *in vitro*, consisting of the hepatocyte and cholangiocyte lineages [12]. E-cadherin and LIV2 are also useful epithelial-specific markers to isolate epithelial cells expressed in the E12.5 mouse liver [13–16]. CD24a and neighbor of Punc E11 (NOPE) were also identified as sorting markers [17]. HNF4α+ liver stem/progenitor cells express epithelial cell adhesion molecule (EpCAM) in mice as early as E9.5. The EpCAM$^+$ DLK1$^+$ cells from the E11.5 mouse liver include cells that form colonies *in vitro* [18]. The EpCAM$^+$ cells isolated from the human fetal liver were shown to contain multipotent precursors of liver stem/progenitor cells [19].

3.4. Adult liver stem/progenitor cells

The liver has a remarkable capacity to regenerate. Liver regeneration depends primarily on the proliferation of adult hepatocytes. In the course of liver generation, hypertrophy of hepatocytes is also observed. In contrast to the regeneration induced by acute liver damage, severe and chronic liver damage induces a defect in the proliferation of mature hepatocytes. Adult liver stem/progenitor cells are thought to be involved in the regeneration induced by such chronic liver damage. During serious liver injury in rodents, the number of characteristic nonparenchymal oval cells increases in the periportal regions. These cells express both cholangiocellular (*Ck7* and *Ck19*) and hepatocellular (*Afp* and *Alb*) marker genes and differentiate into both hepatocytic and cholangiocytic cells, suggesting that oval cells are candidate hepatic progenitors [20–23].

There are several specific markers for sorting cells containing postnatal stem/progenitor cells. Some of them are the same as fetal stem/progenitor cell surface markers such as EpCAM and CD133. Other reported markers are LGR5 [24], CD13$^+$ CD133$^+$ [11], and CD133$^+$ MIC1-1C3$^+$ [25].

3.5. Transdifferentiation between hepatocytes and cholangiocytes

Hepatocytes and cholangiocytes are considered to be derived from single stem/progenitor cells, and they show potential to transdifferentiate into other liver epithelial cell types. Tarlow et al. [26] labeled SOX9-positive cells in mice, analyzed the formation of organoids in culture, monitored the responses of cells in mice on a choline-deficient ethionine diet or diets containing 3,5-diethoxycarbonyl-1,4-dihydrocollidine, and tracked cells transferred into fumarylacetoacetate hydrolase (*Fah*)-deficient mice. Hepatocytes from normal, immune-compatible donors could be transplanted and successfully recolonized the livers of these mice; <1% of the hepatocytes were derived from SOX9-positive precursors [27]. The hepatocyte-derived cholangiocytes continued to express some hepatocyte-specific genes such as *Hnf4* and showed low EpCAM expression [28]. Lu et al. [29] reported the conversion of cholangiocytes to hepatocytes when hepatocyte *Mdm2* (an E3 ubiquitin ligase gene) was deleted. Huch et al. [27] isolated cholangiocytes from the human liver based on the expression of EpCAM. The cells were grown into organoids, induced to transdifferentiate in culture, and expressed hepatocyte-specific genes. Cholangiocytes isolated from liver biopsies of patients with liver diseases also differentiated into hepatocytes in the organoid cultures, but still carried markers of the patients' diseases. However, it is important to note that in these previous studies, the transdifferentiation of cholangiocytes to hepatocytes was observed in culture, and the hepatocyte phenotype detected after transplantation of the cells into mice was observed before the cells were transplanted. It seems therefore fair to conclude that under most conditions of chronic toxic injury or normal liver regeneration, hepatocytes and cholangiocytes proliferate and retain their phenotype. This phenomenon is strongly supported by both rat and mouse studies.

4. CSCs in hepatocellular carcinoma (HCC)

4.1. The characteristics of HCC

HCC represents the major histological subtype of liver cancers, accounting for approximately 85% of primary cancers in the liver [30]. HCC derives from hepatocytes constituting the liver parenchyma, and liver cirrhosis is a precursor in about 80% of all cases. As the precursor lesion of HCC, liver cirrhosis is caused by chronic liver injury, leading to the consecutive liver regeneration and aberrant nodule formation with neighboring fibrosis.

The liver cirrhosis is known to be caused by chronic viral hepatitis B and C infections; metabolic liver diseases, such as nonalcoholic fatty liver disease, nonalcoholic steatohepatitis, hemochromatosis, a1-antitrypsin deficiency, and Wilson's disease; alcoholic liver disease; and autoimmune diseases [2].

4.2. CSC markers in HCC

Recently, cell aggregates with stronger proliferation potency than other tissues comprising HCCs have been discovered. The cell markers of these aggressive tissues have also been identified and classified as SC markers [31]. CD133 (prominin-1), CD90 (THY-1), CD44, CD326 (EpCAM), CD24, and CD13 are the most common cell-surface markers used to detect the CSCs of HCC [32]. Furthermore, several functional markers are available to classify cells according to CSC potency, such as ALDH1, side population, and high green fluorescent molecule fused to the degron of ornithine decarboxylase, associated with low reactive oxygen species (ROS) levels [33].

4.3. Prognosis of HCC

According to the CSC theory, CSCs could influence a patient's prognosis by promoting metastasis and recurrence. Consistent with this hypothesis, recent findings have shown that the presence of CSCs could be associated with patient survival. For example, overexpression of CD90 in HCC is associated with a poor diagnosis. An immunohistochemical study demonstrated the association between CD90 expression and clinical factors, in which CD90 was overexpressed in approximately 70% of the HCC cases. Furthermore, CD90 overexpression was associated with hepatitis B virus infection, age, and histological grade [34]. CD133 overexpression is an independent prognostic factor for survival and tumor recurrence in HCC patients, however, CD133 expression is not shown in normal liver cells. The other report [35] described that the cytoplasmic CD133 expression in HCC patients is associated with high-serum AFP levels, histological high-grade, and invasion. Other studies [36, 37] have demonstrated that CD133 expression is associated with clinical and pathological factors, including poorly differentiated tumors. Furthermore, a significant association was observed between the cytoplasmic expression of CD133 and overall survival of patients with HCC, which was due to multicentric carcinogenicity and hematogenous metastasis to the liver and remote organs. Consequently, positive cytoplasmic expression of CD133 has been proposed to indicate a risk of poor prognosis, especially in patients with HCC at an advanced stage. Chan et al. [36] showed that CD133 is a highly effective prognostic factor for overall survival in patients affected by disease at stage I. In contrast, EpCAM is associated with lower histological differentiation and the invasion of vessel [37]. CK19 expression in HCC is also associated with poor prognosis. Particularly, the increase of CK19-positive cells in HCC was correlated with upregulation of epithelial-mesenchymal transition-related genes. CD44 expression in HCC is related to a higher frequency of extrahepatic metastasis and a shortened survival rate [38] and is correlated with more aggressive tumor behavior and poor clinical outcomes [39].

4.4. Therapy for HCC

Although chemotherapy and ionizing radiation can eliminate tumor cells in proliferating cell cycles, CSCs are intrinsically resistant to these treatments. Therefore, interference with the self-renewal, survival, and niche properties of CSCs is a possible strategy for targeted therapy.

The CSC-specific signal is expected to be a therapeutic target. The self-renewal of CSCs in colorectal cancers is functionally dependent on BMI1, which is one of the polycomb proteins [40]. Furthermore, inhibition of EZH2, a major component of polycomb repressive complex 2 (PRC2), has been demonstrated to dysfunction the self-renewal and tumor-initiating capabilities in some cancers [41], including HCC. Disruption of epigenetic regulations, such as DNA methylation and histone modification, is associated with the initiation and progression of tumors. The efficacy of epigenetic drugs has been proposed to eliminate CSCs in HCC [42]. Zebularine, a DNA methyltransferase (DNMT) inhibitor, declined CSC properties such as self-renewal and tumor-initiating capacities in HCC cells [43]. Histone deacetylase (HDAC) inhibitors such as trichostatin A and vorinostat have been shown to preferentially suppress the cell growth of SALL4-overexpressing HCC cell lines compared with that of $SALL4^-$ HCC cell lines [44, 45]. These findings suggest that epigenetic therapy using DNMT inhibitors and/or HDAC inhibitors may be a promising approach for the eradication of CSCs in HCC.

Another approach for eliminating CSCs has been suggested to be monoclonal antibodies targeting CSC-specific antigens [46], such as CD13, EpCAM, and CD133 antibodies, against hepatic CSCs [47–49]. However, these markers express in not only CSCs but also normal liver cells and tissue SCs. Thus, preclinical experiments and clinical trials will be needed for ensuring safety and efficacy.

On the other hand, hepatocyte nuclear factor-4a (HNF4A), a hepatocyte differentiation factor, decreases the number of CD90+ and CD133+ tumor-initiating cells [50] while simultaneously causing the cells to lose their tumorigenicity by inducing differentiation of the subpopulations. Similarly, oncostatin M (OSM) has been shown to induce the differentiation of EpCAM+ liver CSCs through the OSM receptor signaling pathway [51].

Both CSCs and normal tissue SCs are thought to reside in specialized microenvironments called niches. Brain tumor CSCs have been reported to exist in vascular niches where they are maintained in an undifferentiated state by endothelial cells [52]. An oral multikinase inhibitor, sorafenib, is the sole molecular target drug clinically approved to treat advanced HCC. This drug blocks tumor cell proliferation by targeting Raf/mitogen-activated protein kinase/extracellular signal-regulated kinase signaling and exerts an antiangiogenic effect by targeting tyrosine kinase receptors such as vascular endothelial growth factor receptor and platelet-derived growth factor receptor [53]. Although its role in the CSC niche in HCC has not been investigated, sorafenib may contribute to the eradication of CSCs in HCC.

5. CSCs in cholangiocarcinoma (CCA)

5.1. The characteristics of CCA

CCA is an epithelial cell malignancy arising from varying locations within the biliary tree showing markers of cholangiocyte differentiation. CCA is classified by the anatomical location, including intrahepatic, perihilar, and distal CCA. Intrahepatic CCA is defined by the location from proximally to the second-degree bile ducts in the liver. Perihilar CCA is defined by the location from the second-degree bile ducts to the insertion of the cystic duct into the common bile duct. Distal CCA is defined by the location from the origin of the cystic duct to ampulla of Vater.

Perihilar, distal, and intrahepatic disease represent about 50%, 40%, and <10% of CCA cases, respectively [54]. Mixed hepatocellular CCA was only recently acknowledged and accounts for about 1% of CCA cases. The incidence of intrahepatic CCA increases in western countries [55, 56]. The age-matched rate of CCA has been reported to be the highest in Hispanic and Asian populations (approximately 3 per 100,000) and the lowest in non-Hispanic white and black populations [57–59].

The mortality rate in intrahepatic CCA is largest in American Indian, Alaska Native groups, and Asian populations and is lowest in white and black populations [56]. Increases in both the recognition and incidence have contributed to the rising interest in this type of cancer. Most cases of CCA arise *de novo*, and no risk factors have yet been identified.

Cirrhosis and hepatitis C and B virus infections have been implicated as risk factors for CCA, in particular intrahepatic CCA. In the USA and European studies, viral hepatitis C was shown to be a risk factor for CCA with the strongest association observed for intrahepatic CCA [60], and a Japanese study subsequently confirmed these findings [61]. However, studies from South Korea and China have shown that hepatitis B is a more consistent risk factor for intrahepatic CCA [62–64]. A meta-analysis of several case-control studies on risk factors for intrahepatic CCA showed that the combined odds ratios (ORs) (95% confidence interval [CI]) of cirrhosis, hepatitis C, and hepatitis B were 22.92 (18.24–28.79), 4.84 (2.41–9.71), and 5.10 (2.91–8.95), respectively [65].

Southeast Asia has a very high incidence of CCA due to the high prevalence of the hepatobiliary flukes *Opisthorchis viverrini* and *Clonorchissinensis*, which are risk factors for CCA [65]. This risk is probably increased by environmental and genetic factors. Several genetic polymorphisms have been reported to increase the risk of CCA. The genes have been indicated as risk factors associated with DNA repair, cellular protection against toxins, or immunological surveillance [57].

Hepatolithiasis and biliary enteric drainage, predisposing patients to enteric bacteria bile duct colonization and infections, are additional risk factors for CCA [66]. The results from the studies on the role of alcohol and smoking exposure have been inconsistent [57]. Furthermore, metabolic syndrome was associated with an increased risk of intrahepatic CCA in the Surveillance and Epidemiology Results database analysis (OR: 1.6, 95% CI: 1.32–1.83, $p < 0.0001$). Consistent with these observations, a meta-analysis of the US and Danish studies identified an association of intrahepatic CCA with diabetes (OR: 1.89, 95% CI: 1.74–2.07) and obesity (OR: 1.56, 95% CI: 1.26–1.94). Although obesity is a biologically plausible risk factor for CCA development, the data are too scarce to definitively establish an association at this time.

5.2. The molecular pathway in CCA

The genetic pathways contributing to the selective growth advantage of cancer cells can be organized into those governing cell fate and differentiation, proliferation, cell survival, and maintenance of genome integrity. Several studies identifying genetic changes in CCA have been published, but most of the data generated from these single studies need further validation.

The Ras/mitogen-activated protein kinase pathway is one of the main signaling networks in CCA biology and was reported in several studies. Sia et al. described two distinct gene signature classes: a proliferation class and an inflammatory class. The proliferation class (62% of cases) was associated with copy number variations in several oncogenes, whereas the inflammatory class showed activation of inflammatory pathways causing overexpression of cytokines and the transcriptional factor STAT3, which modulates cell growth and survival and has been implicated in carcinogenesis [67, 68]. The Hedgehog survival signaling pathway in CCA has been identified to have tumor-suppressive activity in several studies [69, 70]. Hotspot mutations of genes encoding IDH1 and IDH2 were recently reported by several groups to be fairly specific to intrahepatic CCA among various gastrointestinal and biliary cancers (10–23%) [71, 72].

5.3. CSC markers in CCA

In CCA, chemotherapy adding surgery is usually needed for improving patient survival. The CSCs in CCA involves cell-surface markers, such as CD24, CD133, CD44, and EpCAM. CD133, known as prominin-1, is an important CSC marker, and has been also found in normal epithelial SCs [73]. CD133 also is an important CSC marker in CCA [74]. CD133-positive cells showed higher invasiveness compared with CD133-negative cells. Shimada et al. [75] analyzed CD133 expression in 29 patients with intrahepatic CCA and found that the 5-year survival rate in the CD133-positive group (8%) was worse than that in the CD133-negative group [76]. However, Fan et al. [77] reported contrasting results, in which CD133 expression was correlated with a higher tumor differentiation status in 54 consecutively analyzed CCA specimens. Moreover, positive CD133 expression significantly correlated with a better prognosis.

CD24 is expressed in cellular adhesion processes, cell motility, and invasive cell growth in cancers [78]. The median survival for patients with high CD24 expression was shorter than that for patients with low expression [79]. CD24 expression is also associated with a poor response to chemotherapy and radiation therapy [80]. However, CD24 is not detected in either the normal or inflamed epithelium, indicating that it may be a useful marker for early CCA carcinogenesis.

EpCAM is a hemophilic, Ca^{2+}-independent cell-cell adhesion molecule that is expressed in many human epithelial tissues while the expression in CCA remains unclear. There is just one report that EpCAM is much expressed in CCA cells compared with HCCs cells [81].

CD44 glycoprotein is expressed on epithelial cells and cancer cells. Wang et al. demonstrated that $CD24^{+}$ $CD44^{+}$ $EpCAM^{high}$ cells isolated from CCA xenografts had high tumorigenic potential compared with $CD24^{-}$ $CD44^{-}$ $EpCAM^{low/-}$ cells. Cells with high EpCAM expression exhibited the characteristic SC properties of self-renewal and heterogenous progeny [82]. The other markers, CD49f, CD117, and SCA-1, have been only scarcely investigated.

5.4. Therapy for CCA

Surgical treatment is the main therapy for improving patient survival in CCA [83]. The 5-year survival rate after radical surgical resection is approximately 35% in intrahepatic CCA and about 40% in perihilar CCA [83–85]. Regarding liver transplantation, the experience of liver transplantation for CCA is still limited, having performed in only a few selective centers, and it is mainly limited to early-stage perihilar CCA [86]. The first line of the chemotherapy in advanced and metastatic CCAs has been proposed to use the gemcitabine with cisplatin [87, 88]. The role of radiation or chemoradiation in CCA remains to be defined. The patterns of recurrence following resection of hilar or distal CCA play an important role in defining the appropriate strategy for adjuvant therapy [89].

The CSC-target therapy has been challenged *in vivo* experiments. CD133 inhibits cell growth of Hep3B human hepatoma cell line and abrogated tumor growth *in vivo* [49]. The EpCAM inhibition by small-interfering RNA (siRNA) in hepatic progenitor cells decreased tumorigenicity [90]. Further, CCA cell lines were inhibited by CD44 siRNA on invasiveness and migration [91]. CD24 suppression decreased the invasive ability of CCA cells [79]. These data suggest that the therapy associated with the surface markers is a new candidate for a CSC-target therapy for CCA.

6. ALDH1 in liver cancers

The *ALDH* gene superfamily contains 19 putatively human functional genes, which encode enzymes that are critical for detoxification through the NAD(P)+-dependent oxidation of aldehyde substrates. Among the 19 genes, *ALDH1* has been reported to encode the key ALDH isozyme linked to SC and CSC populations. In the liver SCs and CSCs, retinoic acid (RA), ROS, and aldehyde metabolism are likely to be deeply associated with the functional roles of ALDH1 (**Figure 1**).

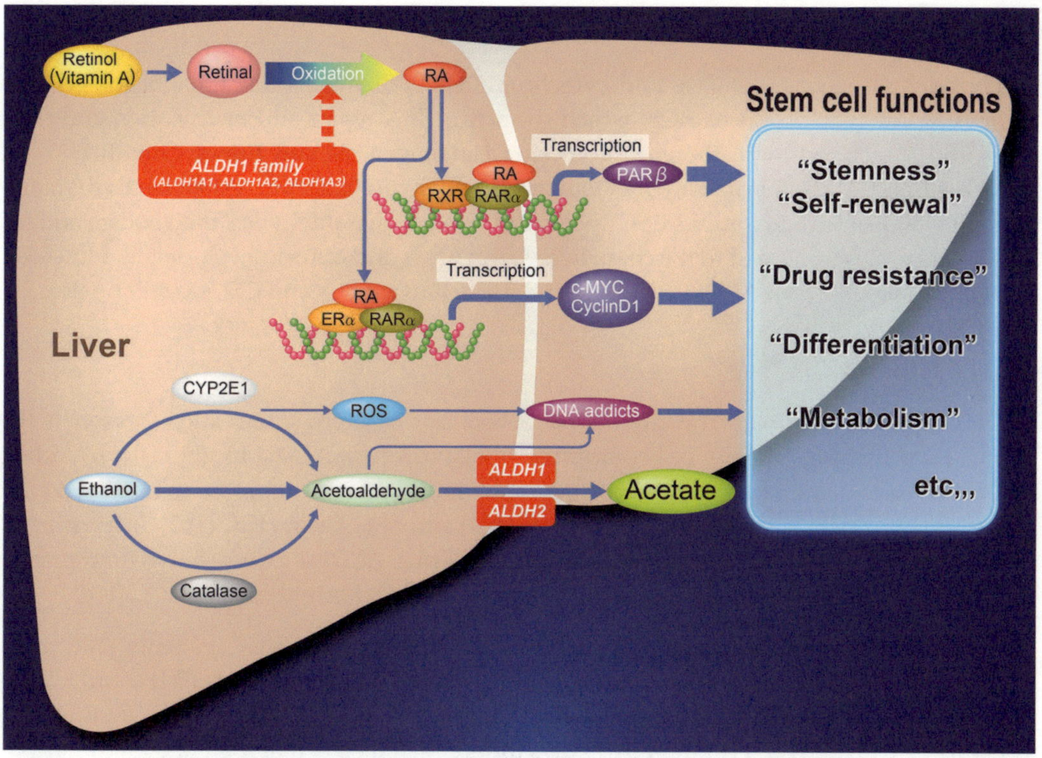

Figure 1. Regulation and function of ALDH1 in normal SCs and CSCs in the liver. Members of the ALDH1 family metabolize RA, regulating the self-renewal, differentiation, and drug resistance of SCs and CSCs. Retinol absorbed by cells is oxidized to retinal, which in turn is oxidized to RA by ALDH1 enzymes. RA binds to RARα and RXRs to induce the transcription of downstream target genes. RA can bind to dimers of RXRs and ERα and induces the expression c-MYC and cyclin D1. Furthermore, ALDH1 and ALDH2 reduce the levels of ROS and reactive aldehydes, thereby promoting tumor growth and initiating carcinogenesis in CSCs. SC, stem cell; CSC, cancer stem cell; RA, retinoic acid; RAR, retinoic acid receptor; RXR, retinoid X receptors; ER, estrogen receptor; and ROS, reactive oxygen species.

6.1. ALDH1 in retinoid signaling

Retinoid signaling has important roles in SCs and CSCs [92]. In retinoid signaling, retinol dehydrogenases oxidize the retinol absorbed by cells to retinal [93]. Retinal is then oxidized to RA in a reaction catalyzed by ALDH1 family members such as ALDH1A1, ALDH1A2, and ALDH1A3. The metabolized product RA includes all-*trans* RA, 9-*cis* RA, and 13-*cis* RA. RA enters the nucleus and induces the transcription of downstream genes through the activation of retinoic acid receptors (RARs) and retinoid X receptors (RXRs). Finally, increased ALDH1 contributes to not only RA synthesis but also cellular protection against cytotoxic drugs.

ALDH1 has been reported to regulate CSCs in breast cancer by promoting the metabolism of retinoid [94]. RA binds to RARs and RXRs and activates the expression of genes associated with differentiation, cell cycle arrest, and morphological variation [95]. Increasing RAR and RXR levels creates a positive feedback loop for retinoid signaling. RA formation by the oxidation of all-*trans*-retinal and 9-*cis*-retinal in retinoid signaling is closely associated with the function of SCs and CSCs [96].

6.2. ALDH1 in acetaldehyde metabolism

Alcohol dehydrogenase catalase and cytochrome P4502E1 metabolize ethanol to acetaldehyde. Acetaldehyde produces ROS, which suppress DNA repair and methylation and form DNA and protein adducts, thereby promoting carcinogenesis and tumor growth [97, 98]. ALDH1A1 and ALDH2 primarily metabolize acetaldehyde to acetate. ALDH activity maintains a low ROS level and inhibits CSC apoptosis [99]. Reactive aldehydes' metabolism and the ROS level are closely related to the characteristics of CSCs and cancer development. However, the relationship between ALDH and ROS in the functions of SCs and CSCs is still unclear.

6.3. ALDH1 in HCC

ALDH1 expression evaluated by immunohistochemistry is heterogenous and is present in the normal liver tissue, especially in hepatocytes [100]. However, ALDH bright cells, including ALDH1 isoforms, evaluated using the Aldefluor assay, have been reported to be a marker of liver progenitor cells in the normal liver tissue [101] and of CSCs in HCC [102]. Interestingly, ALDH bright cells are attributed to ALDH1 activity. Thus, ALDH1 expression in immunohistochemistry is considered to be slightly different from ALDH bright cells in HCC [93].

ALDH1 expression is associated with a favorable outcome for HCC patients [100, 103]. Furthermore, putative CSC markers such as CD24, CD13, CD90, EpCAM, BMI1, and CD133 were not colocalized with ALDH1-expressing cells in HCC [100]. Consequently, immunohistochemistry with an ALDH1 antibody shows differentiated cells that look like mature hepatocytes but not CSCs.

Taken together, these findings suggest that increased ALDH1 expression is associated with a factor indicative of a well-differentiated morphology and favorable prognosis in HCC. Furthermore, ALDH1-expressing cells may serve as a useful differentiation biological marker for HCC rather than as a CSC marker.

http://dx.doi.org/10.5772/66454

6.4. ALDH1 in CCA

Shuang et al. [104] demonstrated that ALDH1 is a valuable marker of CSCs in CCA. Further, patients with high ALDH1 expression had a poor prognosis in the cases of both intrahepatic and extrahepatic CCA. ALDH1 and CD133 are two other molecular markers of putative CSCs in extrahepatic CCA [105]. ALDH1 has been reported to play a crucial role in the identification of CSCs and/or tumor-initiating cells in various types of cancers [106]. In breast cancer, ALDH1+ seems to be a more significant predictive marker than other markers for the identification of breast CSCs. However, the identification of putative CSCs using a single marker such as ALDH1 is controversial. Nevertheless, ALDH1 has been shown to be a very important molecular marker for CSCs. To clarify the correlation among ALDH1 and other putative CSC markers, i.e., CD133, CD24, CD44, and EpCAM, and to identify cells with multiple CSC phenotypes might improve the selection of CSCs, and further studies are needed in this regard.

Recently, HCC and CCA have been shown to share the same origin. Hepatic progenitor cells can differentiate into hepatocytes and cholangiocytes and give rise to HCC as well as CCA [107]. ALDH1 expression has been reported to be specific to the liver CSCs' population [102] and can be assessed to reliably identify CCA cells with stem-like properties. With respect to other ALDH isoforms, only one study has described that ALDH1A3 was a poor prognostic factor and a good biomarker of gemcitabine resistance in intrahepatic CCA [108].

7. Conclusions

CSCs represent key cell populations among the heterogenous malignant cells of liver cancers, and their biological characteristics highlight them as a major target for cancer research. In particular, they provide reliable biomarkers for prognosis, such as ALDH1. Discovery of the mechanisms and molecules associated with CSCs offers great potential to accelerate the development of novel therapeutic options and improve the treatment outcome and quality of life of patients with liver cancers.

Conflicting interest

The authors declare no conflicts of interest.

Acknowledgements

We thank all the members of our laboratory and our collaborators for their research work and helpful discussions. This work was partly supported by grants from the Ministry of Education, Culture, Sports, Science, and Technology of Japan (#15K11289 and #26430111).

Author details

Hiroyuki Tomita[1,*], Tomohiro Kanayama[1], Ayumi Niwa[1], Kei Noguchi[1], Kazuhisa Ishida[1], Masayuki Niwa[2] and Akira Hara[1]

*Address all correspondence to: h_tomita@gifu-u.ac.jp

1 Department of Tumor Pathology, Gifu University Graduate School of Medicine, Gifu, Japan

2 Medical Science Division, United Graduate School of Drug Discovery and Medical Information Sciences, Gifu, Japan

References

[1] Ferlay J, Soerjomataram I, Dikshit R, Eser S, Mathers C, Rebelo M, et al. Cancer incidence and mortality worldwide: sources, methods and major patterns in GLOBOCAN 2012. Int J Cancer. 2015;136(5):E359–E386.

[2] Grandhi MS, Kim AK, Ronnekleiv-Kelly SM, Kamel IR, Ghasebeh MA, Pawlik TM. Hepatocellular carcinoma: from diagnosis to treatment. Surg Oncol. 2016;25(2):74–85.

[3] Nguyen LV, Vanner R, Dirks P, Eaves CJ. Cancer stem cells: an evolving concept. Nat Rev Cancer. 2012;12(2):133–143.

[4] Vescovi AL, Galli R, Reynolds BA. Brain tumour stem cells. Nat Rev Cancer. 2006;6(6):425–436.

[5] Bao S, Wu Q, McLendon RE, Hao Y, Shi Q, Hjelmeland AB, et al. Glioma stem cells promote radioresistance by preferential activation of the DNA damage response. Nature. 2006;444(7120):756–760.

[6] Tremblay KD, Zaret KS. Distinct populations of endoderm cells converge to generate the embryonic liver bud and ventral foregut tissues. Dev Biol. 2005;280(1):87–99.

[7] Suzuki A, Zheng Y, Kondo R, Kusakabe M, Takada Y, Fukao K, et al. Flow-cytometric separation and enrichment of hepatic progenitor cells in the developing mouse liver. Hepatology. 2000;32(6):1230–1239.

[8] Minguet S, Cortegano I, Gonzalo P, Martinez-Marin JA, de Andres B, Salas C, et al. A population of c-Kit(low)(CD45/TER119)- hepatic cell progenitors of 11-day postcoitus mouse embryo liver reconstitutes cell-depleted liver organoids. J Clin Invest. 2003;112(8):1152–1163.

[9] Suzuki A, Iwama A, Miyashita H, Nakauchi H, Taniguchi H. Role for growth factors and extracellular matrix in controlling differentiation of prospectively isolated hepatic stem cells. Development. 2003;130(11):2513–2524.

[10] Kakinuma S, Ohta H, Kamiya A, Yamazaki Y, Oikawa T, Okada K, et al. Analyses of cell surface molecules on hepatic stem/progenitor cells in mouse fetal liver. J Hepatol. 2009;51(1):127–138.

[11] Kamiya A, Kakinuma S, Yamazaki Y, Nakauchi H. Enrichment and clonal culture of progenitor cells during mouse postnatal liver development in mice. Gastroenterology. 2009;137(3):1114–1126, 1126e1–14.

[12] Tanimizu N, Nishikawa M, Saito H, Tsujimura T, Miyajima A. Isolation of hepatoblasts based on the expression of Dlk/Pref-1. J Cell Sci. 2003;116(Pt 9):1775–1786.

[13] Miyajima A, Tanaka M, Itoh T. Stem/progenitor cells in liver development, homeostasis, regeneration, and reprogramming. Cell Stem Cell. 2014;14(5):561–574.

[14] Nierhoff D, Ogawa A, Oertel M, Chen YQ, Shafritz DA. Purification and characterization of mouse fetal liver epithelial cells with high in vivo repopulation capacity. Hepatology. 2005;42(1):130–139.

[15] Watanabe T, Nakagawa K, Ohata S, Kitagawa D, Nishitai G, Seo J, et al. SEK1/MKK4-mediated SAPK/JNK signaling participates in embryonic hepatoblast proliferation via a pathway different from NF-kappaB-induced anti-apoptosis. Dev Biol. 2002;250(2):332–347.

[16] Nitou M, Sugiyama Y, Ishikawa K, Shiojiri N. Purification of fetal mouse hepatoblasts by magnetic beads coated with monoclonal anti-e-cadherin antibodies and their in vitro culture. Exp Cell Res. 2002;279(2):330–343.

[17] Nierhoff D, Levoci L, Schulte S, Goeser T, Rogler LE, Shafritz DA. New cell surface markers for murine fetal hepatic stem cells identified through high density complementary DNA microarrays. Hepatology. 2007;46(2):535–547.

[18] Tanaka M, Okabe M, Suzuki K, Kamiya Y, Tsukahara Y, Saito S, et al. Mouse hepatoblasts at distinct developmental stages are characterized by expression of EpCAM and DLK1: drastic change of EpCAM expression during liver development. Mech Dev. 2009;126(8–9):665–676.

[19] Schmelzer E, Zhang L, Bruce A, Wauthier E, Ludlow J, Yao HL, et al. Human hepatic stem cells from fetal and postnatal donors. J Exp Med. 2007;204(8):1973–1987.

[20] Okabe M, Tsukahara Y, Tanaka M, Suzuki K, Saito S, Kamiya Y, et al. Potential hepatic stem cells reside in EpCAM+ cells of normal and injured mouse liver. Development. 2009;136(11):1951–1960.

[21] Yovchev MI, Grozdanov PN, Zhou H, Racherla H, Guha C, Dabeva MD. Identification of adult hepatic progenitor cells capable of repopulating injured rat liver. Hepatology. 2008;47(2):636–647.

[22] Suzuki A, Sekiya S, Onishi M, Oshima N, Kiyonari H, Nakauchi H, et al. Flow cytometric isolation and clonal identification of self-renewing bipotent hepatic progenitor cells in adult mouse liver. Hepatology. 2008;48(6):1964–1978.

[23] Rountree CB, Barsky L, Ge S, Zhu J, Senadheera S, Crooks GM. A CD133-expressing murine liver oval cell population with bilineage potential. Stem Cells. 2007;25(10):2419–2429.

[24] Huch M, Dorrell C, Boj SF, van Es JH, Li VS, van de Wetering M, et al. In vitro expansion of single Lgr5+ liver stem cells induced by Wnt-driven regeneration. Nature. 2013;494(7436):247–250.

[25] Dorrell C, Erker L, Schug J, Kopp JL, Canaday PS, Fox AJ, et al. Prospective isolation of a bipotential clonogenic liver progenitor cell in adult mice. Genes Dev. 2011;25(11):1193–1203.

[26] Tarlow BD, Finegold MJ, Grompe M. Clonal tracing of Sox9+ liver progenitors in mouse oval cell injury. Hepatology. 2014;60(1):278–289.

[27] Huch M, Gehart H, van Boxtel R, Hamer K, Blokzijl F, Verstegen MM, et al. Long-term culture of genome-stable bipotent stem cells from adult human liver. Cell. 2015;160(1–2):299–312.

[28] Tarlow BD, Pelz C, Naugler WE, Wakefield L, Wilson EM, Finegold MJ, et al. Bipotential adult liver progenitors are derived from chronically injured mature hepatocytes. Cell Stem Cell. 2014;15(5):605–618.

[29] Lu WY, Bird TG, Boulter L, Tsuchiya A, Cole AM, Hay T, et al. Hepatic progenitor cells of biliary origin with liver repopulation capacity. Nat Cell Biol. 2015;17(8):971–983.

[30] Janevska D, Chaloska-Ivanova V, Janevski V. Hepatocellular carcinoma: risk factors, diagnosis and treatment. Open Access Maced J Med Sci. 2015;3(4):732–736.

[31] Romano M, De Francesco F, Pirozzi G, Gringeri E, Boetto R, Di Domenico M, et al. Expression of cancer stem cell biomarkers as a tool for a correct therapeutic approach to hepatocellular carcinoma. Oncoscience. 2015;2(5):443–456.

[32] Anfuso B, Tiribelli C, Sukowati CH. Recent insights into hepatic cancer stem cells. Hepatol Int 2014;8 Suppl 2:458–463.

[33] Chiba T, Iwama A, Yokosuka O. Cancer stem cells in hepatocellular carcinoma: therapeutic implications based on stem cell biology. Hepatol Res. 2016;46(1):50–57.

[34] Lu JW, Chang JG, Yeh KT, Chen RM, Tsai JJ, Hu RM. Overexpression of Thy1/CD90 in human hepatocellular carcinoma is associated with HBV infection and poor prognosis. Acta Histochem. 2011;113(8):833–838.

[35] Sasaki A, Kamiyama T, Yokoo H, Nakanishi K, Kubota K, Haga H, et al. Cytoplasmic expression of CD133 is an important risk factor for overall survival in hepatocellular carcinoma. Oncol Rep. 2010;24(2):537–546.

[36] Chan AW, Tong JH, Chan SL, Lai PB, To KF. Expression of stemness markers (CD133 and EpCAM) in prognostication of hepatocellular carcinoma. Histopathology. 2014;64(7):935–950.

[37] Song W, Li H, Tao K, Li R, Song Z, Zhao Q, et al. Expression and clinical significance of the stem cell marker CD133 in hepatocellular carcinoma. Int J Clin Pract. 2008;62(8):1212–1218.

[38] Hirohashi K, Tanaka H, Kanazawa A, Kubo S, Ohno K, Tsukamoto T, et al. Living-related liver transplantation in a patient with end-stage hepatolithiasis and a biliary-bronchial fistula. Hepatogastroenterology. 2004;51(57):822–824.

[39] Yang XR, Xu Y, Yu B, Zhou J, Li JC, Qiu SJ, et al. CD24 is a novel predictor for poor prognosis of hepatocellular carcinoma after surgery. Clin Cancer Res. 2009;15(17):5518–5527.

[40] Kreso A, van Galen P, Pedley NM, Lima-Fernandes E, Frelin C, Davis T, et al. Self-renewal as a therapeutic target in human colorectal cancer. Nat Med. 2014;20(1):29–36.

[41] Suva ML, Riggi N, Janiszewska M, Radovanovic I, Provero P, Stehle JC, et al. EZH2 is essential for glioblastoma cancer stem cell maintenance. Cancer Res. 2009;69(24):9211–9218.

[42] Marquardt JU, Thorgeirsson SS. SnapShot: hepatocellular carcinoma. Cancer Cell. 2014;25(4):550e1.

[43] Raggi C, Factor VM, Seo D, Holczbauer A, Gillen MC, Marquardt JU, et al. Epigenetic reprogramming modulates malignant properties of human liver cancer. Hepatology. 2014;59(6):2251–2262.

[44] Zeng SS, Yamashita T, Kondo M, Nio K, Hayashi T, Hara Y, et al. The transcription factor SALL4 regulates stemness of EpCAM-positive hepatocellular carcinoma. J Hepatol. 2014;60(1):127–134.

[45] Yong KJ, Gao C, Lim JS, Yan B, Yang H, Dimitrov T, et al. Oncofetal gene SALL4 in aggressive hepatocellular carcinoma. N Engl J Med. 2013;368(24):2266–2276.

[46] Deonarain MP, Kousparou CA, Epenetos AA. Antibodies targeting cancer stem cells: a new paradigm in immunotherapy? MAbs. 2009;1(1):12–25.

[47] Ogawa K, Tanaka S, Matsumura S, Murakata A, Ban D, Ochiai T, et al. EpCAM-targeted therapy for human hepatocellular carcinoma. Ann Surg Oncol. 2014;21(4):1314–1322.

[48] Haraguchi N, Ishii H, Mimori K, Tanaka F, Ohkuma M, Kim HM, et al. CD13 is a therapeutic target in human liver cancer stem cells. J Clin Invest. 2010;120(9):3326–3339.

[49] Smith LM, Nesterova A, Ryan MC, Duniho S, Jonas M, Anderson M, et al. CD133/prominin-1 is a potential therapeutic target for antibody-drug conjugates in hepatocellular and gastric cancers. Br J Cancer. 2008;99(1):100–109.

[50] Yin C, Lin Y, Zhang X, Chen YX, Zeng X, Yue HY, et al. Differentiation therapy of hepatocellular carcinoma in mice with recombinant adenovirus carrying hepatocyte nuclear factor-4alpha gene. Hepatology. 2008;48(5):1528–1539.

[51] Yamashita T, Honda M, Nio K, Nakamoto Y, Yamashita T, Takamura H, et al. Oncostatin M renders epithelial cell adhesion molecule-positive liver cancer stem cells sensitive to 5-fluorouracil by inducing hepatocytic differentiation. Cancer Res. 2010;70(11):4687–4697.

[52] Gilbertson RJ, Rich JN. Making a tumour's bed: glioblastoma stem cells and the vascular niche. Nat Rev Cancer. 2007;7(10):733–736.

[53] Wilhelm SM, Carter C, Tang L, Wilkie D, McNabola A, Rong H, et al. BAY 43-9006 exhibits broad spectrum oral antitumor activity and targets the RAF/MEK/ERK pathway and receptor tyrosine kinases involved in tumor progression and angiogenesis. Cancer Res. 2004;64(19):7099–7109.

[54] DeOliveira ML, Cunningham SC, Cameron JL, Kamangar F, Winter JM, Lillemoe KD, et al. Cholangiocarcinoma: thirty-one-year experience with 564 patients at a single institution. Ann Surg. 2007;245(5):755–762.

[55] Khan SA, Emadossadaty S, Ladep NG, Thomas HC, Elliott P, Taylor-Robinson SD, et al. Rising trends in cholangiocarcinoma: is the ICD classification system misleading us? J Hepatol. 2012;56(4):848–854.

[56] McLean L, Patel T. Racial and ethnic variations in the epidemiology of intrahepatic cholangiocarcinoma in the United States. Liver Int. 2006;26(9):1047–1053.

[57] Tyson GL, El-Serag HB. Risk factors for cholangiocarcinoma. Hepatology. 2011;54(1):173–184.

[58] Everhart JE, Ruhl CE. Burden of digestive diseases in the United States part I: overall and upper gastrointestinal diseases. Gastroenterology. 2009;136(2):376–386.

[59] Shaib Y, El-Serag HB. The epidemiology of cholangiocarcinoma. Semin Liver Dis. 2004;24(2):115–125.

[60] Welzel TM, Mellemkjaer L, Gloria G, Sakoda LC, Hsing AW, El Ghormli L, et al. Risk factors for intrahepatic cholangiocarcinoma in a low-risk population: a nationwide case–control study. Int J Cancer. 2007;120(3):638–641.

[61] Yamamoto S, Kubo S, Hai S, Uenishi T, Yamamoto T, Shuto T, et al. Hepatitis C virus infection as a likely etiology of intrahepatic cholangiocarcinoma. Cancer Sci. 2004;95(7):592–595.

[62] Sekiya S, Suzuki A. Intrahepatic cholangiocarcinoma can arise from Notch-mediated conversion of hepatocytes. J Clin Invest. 2012;122(11):3914–3918.

[63] Zhou HB, Chen JM, Cai JT, Du Q, Wu CN. Anticancer activity of genistein on implanted tumor of human SG7901 cells in nude mice. World J Gastroenterol. 2008; 14(4):627–631.

[64] Lee TY, Lee SS, Jung SW, Jeon SH, Yun SC, Oh HC, et al. Hepatitis B virus infection and intrahepatic cholangiocarcinoma in Korea: a case–control study. Am J Gastroenterol. 2008;103(7):1716–1720.

[65] Palmer WC, Patel T. Are common factors involved in the pathogenesis of primary liver cancers? A meta-analysis of risk factors for intrahepatic cholangiocarcinoma. J Hepatol. 2012;57(1):69–76.

[66] Tocchi A, Mazzoni G, Liotta G, Lepre L, Cassini D, Miccini M. Late development of bile duct cancer in patients who had biliary-enteric drainage for benign disease: a follow-up study of more than 1,000 patients. Ann Surg. 2001;234(2):210–214.

[67] Sia D, Hoshida Y, Villanueva A, Roayaie S, Ferrer J, Tabak B, et al. Integrative molecular analysis of intrahepatic cholangiocarcinoma reveals 2 classes that have different outcomes. Gastroenterology. 2013;144(4):829–840.

[68] Sansone P, Bromberg J. Targeting the interleukin-6/Jak/stat pathway in human malignancies. J Clin Oncol. 2012;30(9):1005–1014.

[69] Jinawath A, Akiyama Y, Sripa B, Yuasa Y. Dual blockade of the Hedgehog and ERK1/2 pathways coordinately decreases proliferation and survival of cholangiocarcinoma cells. J Cancer Res Clin Oncol. 2007;133(4):271–278.

[70] Berman DM, Karhadkar SS, Maitra A, Montes De Oca R, Gerstenblith MR, Briggs K, et al. Widespread requirement for Hedgehog ligand stimulation in growth of digestive tract tumours. Nature. 2003;425(6960):846–851.

[71] Wang P, Dong Q, Zhang C, Kuan PF, Liu Y, Jeck WR, et al. Mutations in isocitrate dehydrogenase 1 and 2 occur frequently in intrahepatic cholangiocarcinomas and share hypermethylation targets with glioblastomas. Oncogene. 2013;32(25):3091–3100.

[72] Borger DR, Tanabe KK, Fan KC, Lopez HU, Fantin VR, Straley KS, et al. Frequent mutation of isocitrate dehydrogenase (IDH)1 and IDH2 in cholangiocarcinoma identified through broad-based tumor genotyping. Oncologist. 2012;17(1):72–79.

[73] Mizrak D, Brittan M, Alison M. CD133: molecule of the moment. J Pathol. 2008;214(1):3–9.

[74] Wang M, Xiao J, Shen M, Yahong Y, Tian R, Zhu F, et al. Isolation and characterization of tumorigenic extrahepatic cholangiocarcinoma cells with stem cell-like properties. Int J Cancer. 2011;128(1):72–81.

[75] Shimada M, Sugimoto K, Iwahashi S, Utsunomiya T, Morine Y, Imura S, et al. CD133 expression is a potential prognostic indicator in intrahepatic cholangiocarcinoma. J Gastroenterol. 2010;45(8):896–902.

[76] Leelawat K, Thongtawee T, Narong S, Subwongcharoen S, Treepongkaruna SA. Strong expression of CD133 is associated with increased cholangiocarcinoma progression. World J Gastroenterol. 2011;17(9):1192–1198.

[77] Fan L, He F, Liu H, Zhu J, Liu Y, Yin Z, et al. CD133: a potential indicator for differentiation and prognosis of human cholangiocarcinoma. BMC Cancer. 2011;11:320.

[78] Riener MO, Vogetseder A, Pestalozzi BC, Clavien PA, Probst-Hensch N, Kristiansen G, et al. Cell adhesion molecules P-cadherin and CD24 are markers for carcinoma and dysplasia in the biliary tract. Hum Pathol. 2010;41(11):1558–1565.

[79] Keeratichamroen S, Leelawat K, Thongtawee T, Narong S, Aegem U, Tujinda S, et al. Expression of CD24 in cholangiocarcinoma cells is associated with disease progression and reduced patient survival. Int J Oncol. 2011;39(4):873–881.

[80] Agrawal S, Kuvshinoff BW, Khoury T, Yu J, Javle MM, LeVea C, et al. CD24 expression is an independent prognostic marker in cholangiocarcinoma. J Gastrointest Surg. 2007;11(4):445–451.

[81] de Boer CJ, van Krieken JH, Janssen-van Rhijn CM, Litvinov SV. Expression of Ep-CAM in normal, regenerating, metaplastic, and neoplastic liver. J Pathol. 1999;188(2):201–206.

[82] Zhu Z, Hao X, Yan M, Yao M, Ge C, Gu J, et al. Cancer stem/progenitor cells are highly enriched in CD133+CD44+ population in hepatocellular carcinoma. Int J Cancer. 2010;126(9):2067–2078.

[83] de Jong MC, Nathan H, Sotiropoulos GC, Paul A, Alexandrescu S, Marques H, et al. Intrahepatic cholangiocarcinoma: an international multi-institutional analysis of prognostic factors and lymph node assessment. J Clin Oncol. 2011;29(23):3140–3145.

[84] Zaydfudim VM, Rosen CB, Nagorney DM. Hilar cholangiocarcinoma. Surg Oncol Clin N Am. 2014;23(2):247–263.

[85] Fendrich V, Langer P, Celik I, Bartsch DK, Zielke A, Ramaswamy A, et al. An aggressive surgical approach leads to long-term survival in patients with pancreatic endocrine tumors. Ann Surg. 2006;244(6):845–851; discussion 52–53.

[86] Darwish Murad S, Kim WR, Harnois DM, Douglas DD, Burton J, Kulik LM, et al. Efficacy of neoadjuvant chemoradiation, followed by liver transplantation, for perihilar cholangiocarcinoma at 12 US centers. Gastroenterology. 2012;143(1):88–98 e3; quiz e14.

[87] Valle J, Wasan H, Palmer DH, Cunningham D, Anthoney A, Maraveyas A, et al. Cisplatin plus gemcitabine versus gemcitabine for biliary tract cancer. N Engl J Med. 2010;362(14):1273–1281.

[88] Okusaka T, Nakachi K, Fukutomi A, Mizuno N, Ohkawa S, Funakoshi A, et al. Gemcitabine alone or in combination with cisplatin in patients with biliary tract cancer: a comparative multicentre study in Japan. Br J Cancer. 2010;103(4):469–474.

[89] Jarnagin WR, Ruo L, Little SA, Klimstra D, D'Angelica M, DeMatteo RP, et al. Patterns of initial disease recurrence after resection of gallbladder carcinoma and hilar cholangiocarcinoma: implications for adjuvant therapeutic strategies. Cancer. 2003;98(8):1689–1700.

[90] Yamashita T, Ji J, Budhu A, Forgues M, Yang W, Wang HY, et al. EpCAM-positive hepatocellular carcinoma cells are tumor-initiating cells with stem/progenitor cell features. Gastroenterology. 2009;136(3):1012–1024.

[91] Nathan H, Pawlik TM, Wolfgang CL, Choti MA, Cameron JL, Schulick RD. Trends in survival after surgery for cholangiocarcinoma: a 30-year population-based SEER database analysis. J Gastrointest Surg. 2007;11(11):1488–1496; discussion 96–97.

[92] Chanda B, Ditadi A, Iscove NN, Keller G. Retinoic acid signaling is essential for embryonic hematopoietic stem cell development. Cell. 2013;155(1):215–227.

[93] Tomita H, Tanaka K, Tanaka T, Hara A. Aldehyde dehydrogenase 1A1 in stem cells and cancer. Oncotarget. 2016;7(10):11018–11032.

[94] Ginestier C, Wicinski J, Cervera N, Monville F, Finetti P, Bertucci F, et al. Retinoid signaling regulates breast cancer stem cell differentiation. Cell Cycle. 2009;8(20):3297–3302.

[95] Ying M, Wang S, Sang Y, Sun P, Lal B, Goodwin CR, et al. Regulation of glioblastoma stem cells by retinoic acid: role for Notch pathway inhibition. Oncogene. 2011;30(31):3454–3467.

[96] Marcato P, Dean CA, Giacomantonio CA, Lee PW. Aldehyde dehydrogenase: its role as a cancer stem cell marker comes down to the specific isoform. Cell Cycle. 2011;10(9):1378–1384.

[97] Seitz HK, Stickel F. Molecular mechanisms of alcohol-mediated carcinogenesis. Nat Rev Cancer. 2007;7(8):599–612.

[98] Brennan P, Boffetta P. Mechanistic considerations in the molecular epidemiology of head and neck cancer. IARC Sci Publ. 2004(157):393–414.

[99] Xu X, Chai S, Wang P, Zhang C, Yang Y, Yang Y, et al. Aldehyde dehydrogenases and cancer stem cells. Cancer Lett. 2015;369(1):50–57.

[100] Tanaka K, Tomita H, Hisamatsu K, Nakashima T, Hatano Y, Sasaki Y, et al. ALDH1A1-overexpressing cells are differentiated cells but not cancer stem or progenitor cells in human hepatocellular carcinoma. Oncotarget. 2015;6(28):24722–24732.

[101] Dolle L, Best J, Empsen C, Mei J, Van Rossen E, Roelandt P, et al. Successful isolation of liver progenitor cells by aldehyde dehydrogenase activity in naive mice. Hepatology. 2012;55(2):540–552.

[102] Ma S, Chan KW, Lee TK, Tang KH, Wo JY, Zheng BJ, et al. Aldehyde dehydrogenase discriminates the CD133 liver cancer stem cell populations. Mol Cancer Res. 2008;6(7):1146–1153.

[103] Suzuki E, Chiba T, Zen Y, Miyagi S, Tada M, Kanai F, et al. Aldehyde dehydrogenase 1 is associated with recurrence-free survival but not stem cell-like properties in hepatocellular carcinoma. Hepatol Res. 2012;42(11):1100–1111.

[104] Shuang ZY, Wu WC, Xu J, Lin G, Liu YC, Lao XM, et al. Transforming growth factor-beta1-induced epithelial-mesenchymal transition generates ALDH-positive cells with stem cell properties in cholangiocarcinoma. Cancer Lett. 2014;354(2):320–328.

[105] Wang M, Xiao J, Jiang J, Qin R. CD133 and ALDH may be the molecular markers of cholangiocarcinoma stem cells. Int J Cancer. 2011;128(8):1996–1997.

[106] Moreb JS. Aldehyde dehydrogenase as a marker for stem cells. Curr Stem Cell Res Ther. 2008;3(4):237–246.

[107] Roskams T. Liver stem cells and their implication in hepatocellular and cholangiocarcinoma. Oncogene. 2006;25(27):3818–3822.

[108] Chen MH, Weng JJ, Cheng CT, Wu RC, Huang SC, Wu CE, et al. ALDH1A3, the major aldehyde dehydrogenase isoform in human cholangiocarcinoma cells, affects prognosis and gemcitabine resistance in cholangiocarcinoma patients. Clin Cancer Res. 2016;22(16)4225–4235.

Chapter 4

Lipid Metabolism in Liver Cancer

Guo-Dong Lu and Shing Chuan Hooi

Additional information is available at the end of the chapter

http://dx.doi.org/10.5772/64993

Abstract

Hepatocellular carcinoma (HCC) represents 90% cases of liver cancer that is the second leading cause of cancer death in the world. With the pandemic of obesity and other metabolic syndromes in both adults and children, the incidences of fatty liver diseases and the derived HCC are on their upward track. Emerging metabolomic studies have revealed the perturbation of lipid profiles and other metabolites in fatty liver diseases and HCC. Two common metabolic features including enforced fatty acid oxidation and glycolysis could distinguish HCC from healthy liver and chronic non-tumor liver diseases. The potential translational impacts of fatty acid oxidation are gaining great interests, because many recent investigations have demonstrated that tumor cells were dependent on fatty acid oxidation for cell survival and tumor growth. Blockage of fatty acid oxidation could sensitize to metabolic stress-induced cell death and tumor growth inhibition. Thus, lipid catabolism, in terms of fatty oxidation, is tuned for tumor maintenance but vulnerable to pharmacological disruption. The therapeutic potentials of blocking fatty acid oxidation are yet to be further carefully examined.

Keywords: liver cancer, lipid metabolism, metabolomics, fatty liver diseases, nonalcoholic fatty liver disease, nonalcoholic steatohepatitis, cirrhosis

1. Introduction

Liver cancer is the second leading cause of cancer death worldwide [1]. Hepatocellular carcinoma (HCC) represents 90% of primary liver cancer. The incidence of HCC has been successfully improved in China and Southeast Asia, owing to several decades' endeavor in controlling viral hepatitis B and environmental toxicants, for example, aflatoxin in contaminated food and microcystin in pond water [1–3]. By contrast, HCC incidence has been increased in the United States and other Western countries in the last three decades. The fast-growing fraction of the cases was reported to result from chronic fatty liver diseases: nonalcoholic fatty liver disease (NAFLD) and nonalcoholic steatohepatitis (NASH) [4].

Epidemiologic studies lend the credence to the importance of NAFLD as the most common cause of liver disease in the world [4]. The prevalence of NAFLD can reach as high as 25–45% [4–6], when image scanning is applied into diagnostic decision. This heavy disease burden of NAFLD may mirror the epidemic of obesity, diabetes, and other metabolic syndromes, which are still on their upward trend in the world [7]. These metabolic disorders are well characterized with the disruption of glucose and lipid homeostasis, accumulated deposition of systemic and hepatic fat, and insulin resistance. As a consequence, these metabolic alterations may predispose liver to chronic inflammation and fibrogenesis, and finally cancerous transformation into HCC, no matter whether liver cirrhosis ensues. Furthermore, the coexistence of NAFLD with viral hepatitis and environmental toxicants may drive the disease progression in a more complicated manner.

The emerging metabolomic technologies enable hepatologists and biologists to have a panorama view of a highly complex and dynamic flux of small metabolites in liver diseases [8]. This methodology includes high-throughput analytical mass spectrometry, nuclear magnetic resonance spectroscopy, and multivariate data analysis, permitting unbiased comparison of "global" profiles of hundreds to thousands of metabolites between samples from two or more liver disease status. As same as the other omics technologies, the metabolomic investigations have provided new insights into liver disease mechanisms and identified novel biomarkers involved in liver diseases and oncogenesis. Recent findings, comparing different phases of liver diseases from healthy liver to NAFLD/NASH, cirrhosis, and eventually HCC, revealed that both Warburg shift (from mitochondrial oxidative phosphorylation to enforced cytosolic glycolysis) and the up-regulation of lipid catabolism occurred as early as in NAFLD/NASH, and throughout the whole oncogenic processes [9].

Different from the well-studied lipogenesis and fat deposition in the liver, the emerging roles of lipid catabolism in cancer maintenance and progression have been unveiled recently [10]. Mechanically, lipid catabolism in terms of fatty acid oxidation and its upstream autophagy pathway may promote cancer cell survival and tumor growth, especially during stringent nutrient deprivation. The aforementioned nutrient deprivation and the metabolic stress ensued usually occur during rapid solid tumor development and during clinical embolization intervention. These recent findings brought to light the translational significance of lipid catabolism in cancer therapeutics.

2. Lipid metabolism in liver physiology: a brief introduction

Liver is the central organ for lipid metabolism and fat deposition in the body [11]. Through well-tuned coordination with adipose, muscle, and other tissues, liver plays an essential role in the maintenance of lipid homeostasis and energy balance. Whenever an excess of calories is ingested, fatty acids are synthesized primarily in the liver, and to a lesser extent in the adipose tissue [12]. Dietary carbohydrate, which is digested into two-carbon units acetyl-CoA, is the major source of carbon for the synthesis of fatty acids. The process is termed as lipogenesis. An excess of dietary protein also can promote lipogenesis through conversion to acetyl-CoA and other intermediates of tricarboxylic acid cycle (also known as citric acid cycle). After elongation and desaturation, three fatty acids join together by one glycerol molecule to form triacylglycerols. Subsequently, triacylglycerols are packaged into very long low-density lipoprotein (VLDL) particles with cholesterol, phospholipids, and proteins. VLDL particles are then released into blood and then transported to major organs including adipose tissues for storage in the form of triacylglycerols, and muscle for energy metabolism. The aforementioned process is briefly summarized in **Figure 1**.

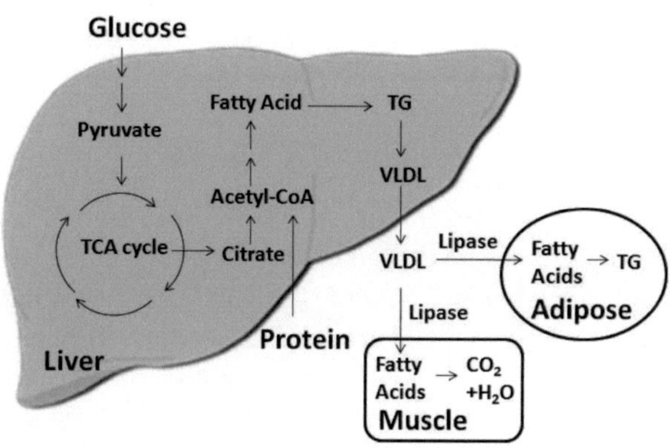

Figure 1. Schematic diagram of lipogenesis in the liver. Fatty acids are synthesized from glucose and excess protein in the liver after meals. After conversion into triacylglycerol, fatty acids are packaged in VLDL particles and then transported to adipose for storage and muscle for energy metabolism. TCA cycle: tricarboxylic acid cycle; TG: triacylglycerol; VLDL: very long low-density lipoprotein.

When the serum level of glucose runs low before next meal or during short-term fasting, the body can mobilize energy deposits sequentially from glycogen to triacylglycerols. This process is tightly regulated by hormones, in a coordination of decrease in insulin and increase in glucagon. The hormone-sensitive lipase breaks down triacylglycerols into glycerol and fatty acids, and the latter are released into the blood. The fatty acids are then transported to muscle and other tissues to meet immediate energy demands, where fatty acids are oxidized to CO_2 and water to produce energy. During extended fasting, the body mainly mobilizes lipids through fatty acid beta-oxidation, and even digests unnecessary protein and organelles through a catabolic process called autophagy.

Therefore, lipid metabolism is important for normal liver physiology. Triacylglycerols are the predominant form to store fat energy, mainly in adipose tissue and also in liver. However, unhealthy lifestyles of nutrition overload and physical inactivity may tilt the balance of lipid homeostasis and disrupt the body sensitivity to insulin [7]. In the long run, fat accumulates systemically in the adipose tissues and locally in the liver, contributing to inflammation and fibrogenesis, and consequently obesity and fatty liver diseases [12].

3. A heavy burden of fatty liver diseases for liver carcinogenesis

NAFLD is a well-recognized common liver disease in the world [4, 13, 14]. Most individuals with NAFLD are restricted to benign and dormant liver steatosis. Up to 25–30% NAFLD patients progress to NASH [14], an aggressive form of NAFLD with combined complications of steatosis, inflammation, and fibrosis. NAFLD is a growing etiological cause of HCC, especially in those regions with low incidence of viral hepatitis, for example, USA, UK, and other Western countries [13, 14]. The incidence of HCC has tripled from 1.5 to 4.9 per 100,000 individuals in the past three decades in the United States alone [15]. It has been suggested that NAFLD will become the leading cause of HCC in the coming decade [16, 17], due to not only the epidemics of obesity and type 2 diabetes but the successful control of risk factors including hepatitis B virus (HBV) by at-birth vaccination, hepatitis C virus (HCV) by novel antiviral treatments, aflatoxin contamination by food hygiene, and microcystin in pond water by the change of drinking water source.

NAFLD coincides with or occurs on the basis of preexisting metabolic conditions, accounting for up to 90% of obese patients [18, 19] and up to 70% of type 2 diabetic patients [20, 21], which were confirmed by large cohort studies based on examinations using ultrasound examination and liver biopsy. The high prevalence of NAFLD (25–45% for all ages and 10–20% for children) is not surprising [14, 22], if the pandemic background of overweight and obesity in the world is considered. The proportion of adults with overweight or obesity, whose BMI (body mass index) was more than 25 kg/m^2, increased between 1980 and 2013 from 28.8 to 36.9% in male and from 29.8 to 38.0% in female globally [7]. Note that there were 23.8% boys (younger than 20) and 22.6% girls suffering from overweight or obesity in 2013. In China, the biggest developing country in the world, the prevalence of adult overweight (30.1%, BMI between 25 and 30) and obesity (11.9%, BMI of >30) in 2012 was catching up with those of Western countries. Thus, obesity has become and will remain a major public health challenge in both developed and developing countries. Undoubtedly, the prevalence of NAFLD is also on its upward track in the foreseeable future.

Meta-analysis of large prospective population-based cohorts demonstrated that overweight or obese persons had relatively 17 or 89% higher risks, respectively, to develop HCC, compared to their normal-weight peers [23]. The risk in male was much higher than that in female. According to a large Swedish cohort study, obese males had 3.1-fold higher risk than the normal-weight control [24]. Another US study reported a 4.5-fold increase in HCC risks in overweight and obese males [25]. Similar trends have been found in diabetic patients. El-Serag and colleagues reported that the risk of males with type 2 diabetes to develop HCC was 2.5 times of those without, according to a systematic review and meta-analysis of case-control and cohort studies [26]. Although yet unproven in large cross-section populations, some case-control studies have shown that the active treatment of obesity (by Statins) and/or diabetes (by Metformin) may be beneficial for HCC reduction with odds ratio of 0.74 (95% confidence interval (CI): 0.64–0.87) and 0.38 (95% CI: 0.24–0.59), respectively [27, 28].

NAFLD may coexist with other chronic liver disease and synergistically promote liver oncogenesis [13, 14]. A large Taiwan cohort study observed that obesity and hepatitis C combined had a higher HCC risk than obesity alone or obesity and hepatitis B combined (odds ratio 4.13 vs. 2.36 and vs. 1.36, respectively) [29]. Furthermore, according to another study based on 23,712 Taiwan residents, obesity and alcohol use had a synergistic effect in HCC incidence with an unadjusted odds ratio of 7.19 (95% CI: 3.69–14.00), compared to obesity alone (odds ratio 1.47, 95% CI: 0.95–2.30) and alcohol use alone (odds ratio 2.56, 95% CI: 1.96–3.35) [30]. After multivariate adjustment, the combined effect was still significant with an odds ratio of 3.82 (95% CI: 1.94–7.52). NAFLD may also contribute to cryptogenic cirrhosis, which represents 30–40% of HCC cases in developed countries [31]. The relationship between NAFLD and cryptogenic HCC could only be verified through medical history taking. Cryptogenic HCC may account for more advanced stage HCC through a complicated process from initial NAFLD/NASH-based hepatosteatosis to subsequent extensive lipid catabolism [32–34], so that the original steatosis was not observable at diagnosis. Although cirrhosis usually precedes HCC, increasing studies showed that NAFLD might induce HCC independent of cirrhosis [34–36]. It has been reported that NAFLD may account for 59% of non-cirrhotic HCC, compared to diabetes (36%) and chronic hepatitis C (22%), according to a recent study based on US health-care claims database [17].

It is worth noting that the risk of NAFLD to develop HCC may not be as high as those of hepatic virus and aflatoxin. The relative risk of NAFLD/NASH alone in the absence of cirrhosis for HCC mortality was found to be as weak as 0–3% for a follow-up period up to 20 years [37]. The cumulative incidence for NAFLD with cirrhosis increased to a range between 2.4 and 11.3%, which was yet comparatively lower than that of hepatitis C with cirrhosis (17–30% for a 5-year cumulative incidence) [34, 35, 38]. By contrast, the relative risks for HBV and HCV to develop HCC are 15–20 folds, according to large case-control and cross-sectional studies [3, 39, 40]. A nested case-control study of 18,000 male residents in Shanghai, China, found that exposure to HBV alone caused an increased HCC risk by 7.3, exposure to aflatoxin alone 3.4, and exposure to both remarkably 59.4 [41]. The public health impact of NAFLD on HCC development, however, could not be overlooked, if considering the higher prevalence of NAFLD than that of viral hepatitis (20–40% for NAFLD vs. 6.3% for viral hepatitis in the Western countries, and 15–30% for NAFLD vs. 11–14% for viral hepatitis in China) [3, 4, 13, 40].

The underlying molecular mechanisms involving how NAFLD promote HCC are yet unclear. Several hypotheses have been suggested. First, chronic inflammation, the increased release of adipokine, and insulin resistance may affect cell proliferation and responsiveness [42, 43]. Second, enhanced lipogenesis and fat deposition may induce extensive lipotoxicity, oxidative stress, and subsequent DNA damages [44, 45]. Third, oncogenic insulin-like growth factor (IGF)-1/PI3K/mTOR, tumor necrosis factor (TNF)-alpha/mitogen-activated protein kinase (MAPK), and/or interleukin (IL)-6/STAT3 pathways were actively involved in HCC [46, 47]. Fourth, hepatosteatosis may influence the hepatic stellate cells and alter microenvironment, causing irreversible fibrosis and cirrhosis [48]. Lastly, the alteration of gut microbiota may influence HCC through bacterial metabolites [49].

Taken together, the growing contribution of NAFLD to HCC development is acknowledged globally. Although the risk of NAFLD alone is comparatively low, the public health impact of

NAFLD and its synergistic effects with other chronic liver diseases on HCC development may pose a huge threat in the coming decades.

4. Lipid metabolism in liver oncogenesis: insights from metabolomic studies

Emerging metabolomic technologies represent a powerful platform to dissect global metabolite profiles in an unbiased manner and to discover novel biomarkers and pathways in liver oncogenesis [8]. This high-throughput strategy may complement the other omics technologies (genomics, proteomics, and others) to improve diagnosis, prognostication, and tumor therapy in HCC. Recent metabolomic investigations have shed light on the importance of lipid metabolism on the liver oncogenic processes.

Dr. Beyoglu and Idle in the University of Bern, Switzerland [9], recently well summarized the metabolomic findings conducted in chronic liver diseases and HCC, and proposed a three-stage biochemical progression from healthy liver to carcinoma through intermediate phases of chronic liver diseases including NAFLD/NASH and cirrhosis, according to the alterations of major metabolites and the involved metabolic pathways. A common alteration of "core metabolic phenotype [9]" was found between liver diseases and healthy liver. Deregulation of bile acid and phospholipid occurred in the early phase of NAFLD/NASH, and maintained in cirrhosis and HCC. In HCC, Warburg effect (enforced cytosolic glycolysis over mitochondrial oxygen respiration) and induction of lipid catabolism were commonly observed phenotypes, and could be detected as early as in a few NAFLD/NASH cases. The NAFLD-derived HCC also demonstrated the up-regulation of metabolites from triglycerides that were originally stored in adipose. These alterations observed in HCC (also termed as metabolic reprogramming), as summarized in **Figure 2**, were regarded as one of common hallmarks of tumor [50].

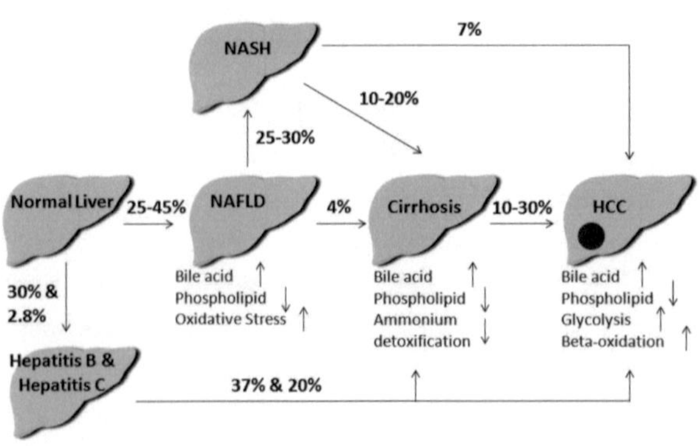

Figure 2. The metabolomic alterations during liver oncogenesis. Liver oncogenesis progresses from healthy liver to HCC through several intermediate chronic liver diseases including NAFLD/NASH, cirrhosis, and viral hepatitis. The percentages of early-stage or intermediate liver diseases progress to the next advanced stage were shown as indicated. The major metabolomic alterations were summarized.

Metabolomic investigations of NAFLD utilized serum and tissue specimens from animal models and human. As a manifestation of steatosis, the lipogenesis (triacylglycerols, diacylglycerol, and phospholipids) [51–53] and bile acid biosynthesis (cholesterol esters, choline, and bile acids) [54, 55] pathways were found to be up-regulated. The hepatic lipids were found to be rearranged and repartitioned from adipose to liver, rather than *de novo* lipogenesis and deposition in the liver, possibly through increased turnover of phosphatidylcholine and phosphatidylethanolamine [9]. This conclusion was supported by a mouse starvation experiment that TG(44:2) and TG(48:3), the most abundant triacylglycerols in adipose, were significantly deposited in the liver after 24-h starvation [52]. Similar increase in glycolysis was also demonstrated by the common elevation of lactate and reduction of glucose in mouse obesity models and human NAFLD specimens [56, 57], which is consistent with the inductive role of insulin resistance on pyruvate kinase M2 [58]. On the other hand, the sustained hyperactivation of hepatic lipid metabolism subsequently aroused extensive oxidative stress and competitively repressed antioxidant biochemical species such as glutathione and cysteine-glutathione disulfide [54, 56]. As an advanced stage of NAFLD, NASH has a similar demonstration of increased lipogenesis (triacylglycerols) and bile acid biosynthesis [53, 56], but differs in the decreased lysophosphatidylcholine [59]. The decrease of lysophosphatidylcholine and increase of bile acids were indicative of inflammation in NASH.

Cirrhosis is characterized by extensive liver fibrosis/regeneration and liver dysfunction, attributable directly to liver cell damages and indirectly to portal hypertension. It has been estimated that 10–20% of NASH cases eventually progressed to cirrhosis over a follow-up period of 10 years [4]. Metabolomic studies examined the alterations of metabolite profiles comparing serum or biopsies from healthy liver and from cirrhotic liver in human, but the results varied possibly due to the different etiologies. As same as NASH, the cirrhotic liver had attenuated lysophosphatidylcholine [60]. But cirrhosis differed from NASH in liver dysfunctions of several metabolic pathways. First, amino acids metabolism was impaired, as exemplified by the increase of serum nonessential amino acids and aromatic amino acids but the decrease of essential amino acids particularly branched-chain amino acids valine and isoleucine [61, 62]. Second, ammonium detoxication was found to be reduced, as evidenced by the increase of glutamate but the decrease of glutamine and glucose [63]. Therefore, these metabolic dysfunctions of amino acid metabolism and ammonium detoxification may collectively mirror the pathological damages in cirrhosis.

The metabolic reprogramming in HCC has been investigated by a greatest number of metabolomic studies. Accumulated data suggested that glycolysis and beta-oxidation were commonly elevated in HCC. On one hand, the enforced glycolysis over mitochondrial oxygen respiration (also called Warburg effect), although comparatively lower in reaction rates (fourfold increase) than the other types of tumor, was a common metabolic phenotype in tumor. This phonotype was evidenced by the following metabolic changes including the decrease in glucose, citrate, and glycerol 3-phosphate but the increase in lactic acid and pyruvate [64–69]. On the other hand, the common induction of beta-oxidation was exemplified by the elevation of 2-oxoglutarate and reduction of free fatty acids, carnitine and carnitine esters [61, 64, 66, 68, 70–73]. This theme will be further explored in the next section. As same as the intermediate liver diseases, HCC maintained the aforementioned "core metabolic phenotype" of bile acid and phospholipid perturbation [66, 71, 73–75]. Some findings also demonstrated similar liver impairments of ammonium detoxication and amino acid metabolism in HCC as in cirrhosis [66, 72, 73, 76].

Other chronic liver diseases, for example, alcoholic liver disease and viral hepatitis, share some similar metabolic alterations to NASH, such as increased lipogenesis and reduction in lysophosphatidylcholine [77, 78]. Metabolomic profiling of a hepatitis B virus X (HBx) transgenic mouse model confirmed the involvement of lipid metabolism (triacylglycerol, cholesterol, saturated, and monounsaturated fatty acids) in HBV-induced liver oncogenesis [79]. This similarity indicated that chronic liver diseases may share some common biochemical and mechanical pathways particularly lipid metabolism, in spite of the differences in etiologies.

A recent nested case-control study from a large European prospective cohort compared serums collected before diagnosis in 114 HCC with 222 matched controls and carefully controlled possible confounders such as tobacco usage, alcohol consumption, and so on [80]. Sixteen metabolites involved in amino acid metabolism, choline metabolism, polyunsaturated lipid metabolism, and ammonium detoxication were selected for potential biomarkers. These metabolomic changes are actually reflective of the underlying precancer liver dysfunctions before HCC occurrence (as discussed above). And these data are pivotal for understanding the process of HCC oncogenesis. The results also demonstrated that the pre-diagnostic metabolic profiles between HCC cases and respective control were different, which was dependent on hepatitis infection status, liver function, and the length of time from blood collection to HCC diagnosis.

Many recent investigations applied metabolomics technologies in biomarker discovery to advance HCC diagnosis. One Chinese study using a panel of metabolic markers (formate, phytosphingosine, and $3\alpha,6\alpha,7\alpha,12\alpha$-tetrahydroxy-$5\beta$-cholan-24-oleic acid) achieved high accuracy (area under curve (AUC): 0.995–1.000, sensitivity: 100%, and specificity: 94.7–100%) in diagnosing HCC patients with low alpha-fetoprotein (a commonly accepted but mediocre biomarker to differentiate HCC from non-tumor liver at a cut-off value of 20 ng/ml) [73]. Another Chinese study, which used tryptophan, glutamine, and 2-hydroxybutyric acid as biomarkers in 183 human serum, also achieved high accuracy (AUC: 0.969–0.990) in both training and validation dataset [69]. Furthermore, the aforementioned European study [80] also demonstrated better diagnostic performance of metabolites than alpha-fetoprotein and liver enzymes.

Taken together, metabolomic investigations have suggested many useful biomarkers and potential biochemical pathways in chronic liver diseases and HCC. Some of them such as bile acid and lysophosphatidylcholine may belong to the "core metabolic phenotype" of background chronic liver diseases and are not necessarily indicative of the tumor status of HCC. Some other alterations, for example, those of ammonium detoxication or amino acid metabolism, may suggest the impaired liver functions. In HCC, there are common findings of enforced glycolysis and enhanced lipid catabolism. These two changes are consistent with the high demand of energy and intermediate metabolites in HCC cells for protein and membrane synthesis during fast tumor growth.

5. Lipid catabolism in liver cancer: a potential therapeutic target

As same as the enforced glycolysis, hyperactivation of lipid catabolism is commonly observed in HCC and other types of cancer. In tumor cells, lipid catabolism and glycolysis may share a few common oncogenic functions. First, both of them are important energy resources physically and pathologically. Second, their metabolisms support cell survival and tumor growth during stringent metabolic stress. Third, they can donor essential metabolic intermediates for protein and membrane anabolic biosynthesis in the fast growing tumor.

The body stores two types of major energy resources: triacylglycerol and glycogen. After a meal, the liver synthesizes both triacylglycerol and glycogen. Comparatively, triacylglycerol can provide six times as much ATP as glycogen, so that triacylglycerol is the preferred resource for storage. Lipid catabolism in terms of fatty acid oxidation is physically performed in heart and skeletal muscle, the highest energy-demanding tissues in the body. But the high activity of fatty acid oxidation in HCC and other types of cancer tissues, as revealed above by metabolomic studies, may provide excess ATP generation when needed.

During fast proliferation, tumor cells, especially those in the core of solid tumor nodules, may experience limited nutrient and oxygen availability because of insufficient tumor neoangiogenesis. This type of nutrient deprivation and the metabolic stress ensued may drive the tumor cells to programmed cell death. However, active fatty acid oxidation in the resistant HCC cells can protect cells with necessary ATP generation even if the exogenous glucose is unavailable and the endogenous glycogen is depleted. The author recently confirmed this hypothesis by comparing the starvation-sensitive with -resistant HCC cells [81]. The results demonstrated that the sensitive HCC cells, lack of an important transcription factor C/EBPalpha, could not initiate fatty acid oxidation and died within 12 h during enforced glucose deprivation *in vitro*. By contrast, the resistant C/EBPalpha-expressing HCC cells could activate autophagy-mediated lipid catabolism and survive as long as 8 days. But blockage of autophagy and the downstream fatty acid beta-oxidation by either pharmacological inhibitors or genetic shRNA intervention could significantly abolish the protective effect. Furthermore, this phenotype could be reproduced *in vivo* in a mice xenograft experiment that the C/EBPalpha-silenced HCC cells failed to develop tumor nodules due to extensive necrosis within a few days after inoculation of the tumor cells into the flank of mice. More importantly, we observed an inverse association of the expression level of C/EBPalpha with tumor necrosis in human HCC tissues. The higher C/EBPalpha expressed in human HCC, the less tumor necrosis observed. Consistently, these results shed the light on the importance of fatty acid oxidation on cell survival and tumor maintenance.

The involvement of fatty acid oxidation in cell survival was also observed during cell detachment from tumor matrix. Cells derived from solid tumor are dependent on fatty acid oxidation to survive when the cell experiences loss of attachment (LOA) to the extracellular matrix [82].

Otherwise, the cell will die in anoikis, a specific form of apoptotic cell death induced by inadequate cell-matrix interactions. Accumulating data have shown that antioxidants and oncogenes (e.g., promyelocytic leukemic protein, carnitine palmitoyltransferase isoform 1C) could activate fatty acid oxidation to support cell survival during LOA and other types of metabolic stresses [82–84]. Promyelocytic leukemic protein was found to be overexpressed in a subset of aggressive breast cancer [83], while the brain-isoform carnitine palmitoyltransferase 1C was abnormally up-regulated in human lung cancer [84]. With the aid of fatty acid oxidation, the survived cancer cells could migrate to distant locations and settle down in possible metastatic sites. Second, during metabolic stress, fatty acid oxidation could sustain NADPH level and consequently counteract harmful oxidative stress. In glioma cells, inhibition of fatty acid oxidation caused significant reduction of NADPH, accumulation of redox oxygen species, and eventually cell death [85]. The involved mechanisms of NADPH production by fatty acid oxidation were later found to be mediated by LKB1-AMPK pathway [86, 87]. Lastly, one study demonstrated that leukemia progenitor cells required fatty acid oxidation to maintain stem cell property [88].

The translational impact of fatty acid oxidation on cell survival and tumor growth has been tested recently. Dr. Samuduio and colleagues initially showed that pharmacological inhibitors (etomoxir and ranolazine) of fatty acid beta-oxidation could sensitize leukemia cells to chemotherapeutic drugs-induced cell death *in vitro* [89]. Later, the antitumor effects of a novel inhibitor ST1326 were confirmed in patients-derived leukemia primary cells *in vitro* [90] and in an *in vivo* mice model of Burkitt's lymphoma [91]. Furthermore, the synergistic effects of fatty acid oxidation inhibitors (etomoxir or CVT-4325) were reproduced in L-asparaginase-treated childhood acute lymphoblastic leukemia cells [92] and in dexamethasone-treated lymphocytic leukemia cells [93], respectively. Recently, etomoxir was applied to MYC-overexpressing triple-negative breast cancer [94]. The results showed that the inhibition of fatty acid oxidation significantly abolished tumor growth in both an MYC-driven transgenic mice model of breast cancer and patient-derived xenografts.

Nutrient deprivation may occur not only in pathological solid tumor growth but during clinical intervention. Embolization treatment, especially transarterial chemoembolization, is applied to intermediate-stage HCC (BCLC B), which may account for 20% HCC patients [95]. By blocking the main arterial of blood supply to tumor nodules, this clinical intervention aims to starve and suffocate tumor cells. Whether fatty acid oxidation helps HCC cells escape cell death induced by embolization and whether this survival advantage contributes to HCC recurrence are yet to be determined. It will be also interesting to learn whether the addition of pharmacological inhibitors of fatty acid beta-oxidation is beneficial for the efficacy and safety of transarterial chemoembolization therapy.

Taken together, lipid catabolism (especially fatty acid oxidation) is important for tumor cell survival and tumor growth during nutrient deprivation-induced metabolic stress. Several investigations have confirmed the antitumor effects of the inhibitors of fatty acid oxidation *in vitro* and *in vivo*. The therapeutic potentials of this target need to be further explored.

6. Conclusion and perspective

Lipid metabolisms are essential for both healthy and diseased liver. It is apparent that with the pandemic of obesity, diabetes, and other metabolic syndromes, the incidence of NAFLD-, NASH-, and NAFLD-derived HCC will be on the upward trend in the foreseeable future. The *de novo* lipogenesis induced by nutrition overload dominates in the liver. Excess lipids deposit in the adipose and liver, causing lipotoxicity, oxidative stress, and inflammatory reactions. The metabolomic investigations have analyzed the perturbed metabolite profiles in the fatty liver diseases and identified several novel biomarkers and biochemical pathways. At this precancer stage, enhancement of lipid catabolism, together with dietary control, will be beneficial for the health. This goal can be achieved by regular physical exercises, medical intervention (e.g., administration of Statins or Metformin), and other preventive countermeasures. It has been reported that the consumption of coffee or tea could reduce HCC risks, according to large epidemiological studies [96]. Mechanically, the main components of coffee (caffeine) and tea (epigallocatechin-3-gallate) were found to promote autophagy and fatty acid oxidation [97, 98].

The induction of fatty acid beta-oxidation in HCC may reflect the high-energy demand for rapid tumor growth and cell survival. Accumulating metabolomic studies have confirmed this change. The oncogenic drivers for the metabolic reprogramming from the original net lipid gain in fatty liver diseases to the increased lipid loss in HCC, however, are yet to be unveiled. The translational impacts and therapeutic potentials of fatty acid oxidation are gaining growing interests. Oriented inhibition of fatty acid oxidation in the tumor cells may be useful for cancer treatment, especially if applied with the strictly localized application of transarterial chemoembolization. However, this hypothesis has not been carefully tested. It is of particular importance to examine the safety of systemic administration of fatty acid oxidation inhibitors in the non-tumor tissues.

Author details

Guo-Dong Lu[1,2*] and Shing Chuan Hooi[3]

*Address all correspondence to: golden_lu@hotmail.com

1 School of Public Health, Guangxi Medical University, Nanning, Guangxi Province, China

2 The Key Laboratory of High-Incidence Diseases Prevention and Control, Guangxi Medical University, Nanning, Guangxi Province, China

3 Department of Physiology, Yong Loo Lin School of Medicine, National University of Singapore, Singapore

References

[1] Stewart B, Wild C. International Agency for Research on Cancer. World Cancer Report 2014. Lyon: IARC Press; 2015.

[2] de Martel C, Maucort-Boulch D, Plummer M, Franceschi S. World-wide relative contribution of hepatitis B and C viruses in hepatocellular carcinoma. Hepatology 2015;62:1190–1200.

[3] El-Serag HB. Epidemiology of viral hepatitis and hepatocellular carcinoma. Gastroenterology 2012;142:1264–1273 e1261.

[4] Baffy G, Brunt EM, Caldwell SH. Hepatocellular carcinoma in non-alcoholic fatty liver disease: an emerging menace. Journal of Hepatology 2012;56:1384–1391.

[5] Younossi ZM, Stepanova M, Afendy M, Fang Y, Younossi Y, Mir H, et al. Changes in the prevalence of the most common causes of chronic liver diseases in the United States from 1988 to 2008. Clinical gastroenterology and hepatology : the official clinical practice. Journal of the American Gastroenterological Association 2011;9:524–530 e521; quiz e560.

[6] Blachier M, Leleu H, Peck-Radosavljevic M, Valla DC, Roudot-Thoraval F. The burden of liver disease in Europe: a review of available epidemiological data. Journal of Hepatology 2013;58:593–608.

[7] Ng M, Fleming T, Robinson M, Thomson B, Graetz N, Margono C, et al. Global, regional, and national prevalence of overweight and obesity in children and adults during 1980-2013: a systematic analysis for the Global Burden of Disease Study 2013. Lancet 2014;384:766–781.

[8] Wang X, Zhang A, Sun H. Power of metabolomics in diagnosis and biomarker discovery of hepatocellular carcinoma. Hepatology 2013;57:2072–2077.

[9] Beyoglu D, Idle JR. The metabolomic window into hepatobiliary disease. Journal of Hepatology 2013;59:842–858.

[10] Carracedo A, Cantley LC, Pandolfi PP. Cancer metabolism: fatty acid oxidation in the limelight. Nature Reviews Cancer 2013;13:227–232.

[11] Lieberman M, Marks AD, Peet A. Marks' Basic Medical Biochemistry: A Clinical Approach, 4th ed. Philadelphia: Wolter Kluwer Health/Lippincott Williams & Wilkins; 2013.

[12] Wang Y, Viscarra J, Kim SJ, Sul HS. Transcriptional regulation of hepatic lipogenesis. Nature Reviews Molecular Cell Biology 2015;16:678–689.

[13] Michelotti GA, Machado MV, Diehl AM. NAFLD, NASH and liver cancer. Nature Reviews Gastroenterology & Hepatology 2013;10:656–665.

[14] Rinella ME. Nonalcoholic fatty liver disease: a systematic review. JAMA 2015;313:2263–2273.

[15] Altekruse SF, McGlynn KA, Reichman ME. Hepatocellular carcinoma incidence, mortality, and survival trends in the United States from 1975 to 2005. Journal of Clinical Oncology: Official Journal of the American Society of Clinical Oncology 2009;27:1485–1491.

[16] Dyson J, Jaques B, Chattopadyhay D, Lochan R, Graham J, Das D, et al. Hepatocellular cancer: the impact of obesity, type 2 diabetes and a multidisciplinary team. Journal of Hepatology 2014;60:110–117.

[17] Sanyal A, Poklepovic A, Moyneur E, Barghout V. Population-based risk factors and resource utilization for HCC: US perspective. Current Medical Research and Opinion 2010;26:2183–2191.

[18] Bellentani S, Tiribelli C. The spectrum of liver disease in the general population: lesson from the Dionysos study. Journal of Hepatology 2001;35:531–537.

[19] Browning JD, Szczepaniak LS, Dobbins R, Nuremberg P, Horton JD, Cohen JC, et al. Prevalence of hepatic steatosis in an urban population in the United States: impact of ethnicity. Hepatology 2004;40:1387–1395.

[20] Byrne CD, Olufadi R, Bruce KD, Cagampang FR, Ahmed MH. Metabolic disturbances in non-alcoholic fatty liver disease. Clinical Science 2009;116:539–564.

[21] Williams CD, Stengel J, Asike MI, Torres DM, Shaw J, Contreras M, et al. Prevalence of nonalcoholic fatty liver disease and nonalcoholic steatohepatitis among a largely middle-aged population utilizing ultrasound and liver biopsy: a prospective study. Gastroenterology 2011;140:124–131.

[22] Patton HM, Yates K, Unalp-Arida A, Behling CA, Huang TT, Rosenthal P, et al. Association between metabolic syndrome and liver histology among children with nonalcoholic fatty liver disease. The American Journal of Gastroenterology 2010;105:2093–2102.

[23] Larsson SC, Wolk A. Overweight, obesity and risk of liver cancer: a meta-analysis of cohort studies. British Journal of Cancer 2007;97:1005–1008.

[24] Samanic C, Chow WH, Gridley G, Jarvholm B, Fraumeni JF, Jr. Relation of body mass index to cancer risk in 362,552 Swedish men. Cancer Causes & Control: CCC 2006;17:901–909.

[25] Calle EE, Rodriguez C, Walker-Thurmond K, Thun MJ. Overweight, obesity, and mortality from cancer in a prospectively studied cohort of U.S. adults. The New England Journal of Medicine 2003;348:1625–1638.

[26] El-Serag HB, Hampel H, Javadi F. The association between diabetes and hepatocellular carcinoma: a systematic review of epidemiologic evidence. Clinical Gastroenterology

and Hepatology: The Official Clinical Practice Journal of the American Gastroenterological Association 2006;4:369–380.

[27] El-Serag HB, Johnson ML, Hachem C, Morgana RO. Statins are associated with a reduced risk of hepatocellular carcinoma in a large cohort of patients with diabetes. Gastroenterology 2009;136:1601–1608.

[28] Zhang ZJ, Zheng ZJ, Shi R, Su Q, Jiang Q, Kip KE. Metformin for liver cancer prevention in patients with type 2 diabetes: a systematic review and meta-analysis. The Journal of Clinical Endocrinology and Metabolism 2012;97:2347–2353.

[29] Chen CL, Yang HI, Yang WS, Liu CJ, Chen PJ, You SL, et al. Metabolic factors and risk of hepatocellular carcinoma by chronic hepatitis B/C infection: a follow-up study in Taiwan. Gastroenterology 2008;135:111–121.

[30] Loomba R, Yang HI, Su J, Brenner D, Barrett-Connor E, Iloeje U, et al. Synergism between obesity and alcohol in increasing the risk of hepatocellular carcinoma: a prospective cohort study. American Journal of Epidemiology 2013;177:333–342.

[31] El-Serag HB, Rudolph KL. Hepatocellular carcinoma: epidemiology and molecular carcinogenesis. Gastroenterology 2007;132:2557–2576.

[32] Caldwell SH, Oelsner DH, Iezzoni JC, Hespenheide EE, Battle EH, Driscoll CJ. Cryptogenic cirrhosis: clinical characterization and risk factors for underlying disease. Hepatology 1999;29:664–669.

[33] Bugianesi E, Leone N, Vanni E, Marchesini G, Brunello F, Carucci P, et al. Expanding the natural history of nonalcoholic steatohepatitis: from cryptogenic cirrhosis to hepatocellular carcinoma. Gastroenterology 2002;123:134–140.

[34] Lee SS, Jeong SH, Byoun YS, Chung SM, Seong MH, Sohn HR, et al. Clinical features and outcome of cryptogenic hepatocellular carcinoma compared to those of viral and alcoholic hepatocellular carcinoma. BMC Cancer 2013;13:335.

[35] Ascha MS, Hanouneh IA, Lopez R, Tamimi TA, Feldstein AF, Zein NN. The incidence and risk factors of hepatocellular carcinoma in patients with nonalcoholic steatohepatitis. Hepatology 2010;51:1972–1978.

[36] Marrero JA, Fontana RJ, Su GL, Conjeevaram HS, Emick DM, Lok AS. NAFLD may be a common underlying liver disease in patients with hepatocellular carcinoma in the United States. Hepatology 2002;36:1349–1354.

[37] White DL, Kanwal F, El-Serag HB. Association between nonalcoholic fatty liver disease and risk for hepatocellular cancer, based on systematic review. Clinical Gastroenterology and Hepatology: The Official Clinical Practice Journal of the American Gastroenterological Association 2012;10:1342–1359 e1342.

[38] Sanyal AJ, Banas C, Sargeant C, Luketic VA, Sterling RK, Stravitz RT, et al. Similarities and differences in outcomes of cirrhosis due to nonalcoholic steatohepatitis and hepatitis C. Hepatology 2006;43:682–689.

[39] Xiang W, Shi JF, Li P, Wang JB, Xu LN, Wei WQ, et al. Estimation of cancer cases and deaths attributable to infection in China. Cancer Causes & Control: CCC 2011;22:1153–1161.

[40] Fattovich G, Bortolotti F, Donato F. Natural history of chronic hepatitis B: special emphasis on disease progression and prognostic factors. Journal of Hepatology 2008;48:335–352.

[41] Qian GS, Ross RK, Yu MC, Yuan JM, Gao YT, Henderson BE, et al. A follow-up study of urinary markers of aflatoxin exposure and liver cancer risk in Shanghai, People's Republic of China. Cancer Epidemiology, Biomarkers & Prevention: A Publication of the American Association for Cancer Research, co-sponsored by the American Society of Preventive Oncology 1994;3:3–10.

[42] Marra F, Bertolani C. Adipokines in liver diseases. Hepatology 2009;50:957–969.

[43] Angulo P, Alba LM, Petrovic LM, Adams LA, Lindor KD, Jensen MD. Leptin, insulin resistance, and liver fibrosis in human nonalcoholic fatty liver disease. Journal of Hepatology 2004;41:943–949.

[44] Mota M, Banini BA, Cazanave SC, Sanyal AJ. Molecular mechanisms of lipotoxicity and glucotoxicity in nonalcoholic fatty liver disease. Metabolism: Clinical and Experimental 2016;65:1049–1061.

[45] Vinciguerra M, Carrozzino F, Peyrou M, Carlone S, Montesano R, Benelli R, et al. Unsaturated fatty acids promote hepatoma proliferation and progression through downregulation of the tumor suppressor PTEN. Journal of Hepatology 2009;50:1132–1141.

[46] Stickel F, Hellerbrand C. Non-alcoholic fatty liver disease as a risk factor for hepatocellular carcinoma: mechanisms and implications. Gut 2010;59:1303–1307.

[47] Shen J, Tsoi H, Liang Q, Chu ES, Liu D, Yu AC, et al. Oncogenic mutations and dysregulated pathways in obesity-associated hepatocellular carcinoma. Oncogene. 2016 May 2. doi: 10.1038/onc.2016.162.

[48] Wright JH, Johnson MM, Shimizu-Albergine M, Bauer RL, Hayes BJ, Surapisitchat J, et al. Paracrine activation of hepatic stellate cells in platelet-derived growth factor C transgenic mice: evidence for stromal induction of hepatocellular carcinoma. International Journal of Cancer 2014;134:778–788.

[49] Yoshimoto S, Loo TM, Atarashi K, Kanda H, Sato S, Oyadomari S, et al. Obesity-induced gut microbial metabolite promotes liver cancer through senescence secretome. Nature 2013;499:97–101.

[50] Hanahan D, Weinberg RA. Hallmarks of cancer: the next generation. Cell 2011;144:646–674.

[51] Vinaixa M, Rodriguez MA, Rull A, Beltran R, Blade C, Brezmes J, et al. Metabolomic assessment of the effect of dietary cholesterol in the progressive development of fatty liver disease. Journal of Proteome Research 2010;9:2527–2538.

[52] van Ginneken V, Verhey E, Poelmann R, Ramakers R, van Dijk KW, Ham L, et al. Metabolomics (liver and blood profiling) in a mouse model in response to fasting: a study of hepatic steatosis. Biochimica et Biophysica Acta 2007;1771:1263–1270.

[53] Puri P, Wiest MM, Cheung O, Mirshahi F, Sargeant C, Min HK, et al. The plasma lipidomic signature of nonalcoholic steatohepatitis. Hepatology 2009;50:1827–1838.

[54] Garcia-Canaveras JC, Donato MT, Castell JV, Lahoz A. A comprehensive untargeted metabonomic analysis of human steatotic liver tissue by RP and HILIC chromatography coupled to mass spectrometry reveals important metabolic alterations. Journal of Proteome Research 2011;10:4825–4834.

[55] Barr J, Vazquez-Chantada M, Alonso C, Perez-Cormenzana M, Mayo R, Galan A, et al. Liquid chromatography-mass spectrometry-based parallel metabolic profiling of human and mouse model serum reveals putative biomarkers associated with the progression of nonalcoholic fatty liver disease. Journal of Proteome Research 2010;9:4501–4512.

[56] Kalhan SC, Guo L, Edmison J, Dasarathy S, McCullough AJ, Hanson RW, et al. Plasma metabolomic profile in nonalcoholic fatty liver disease. Metabolism: Clinical and Experimental 2011;60:404–413.

[57] Li H, Wang L, Yan X, Liu Q, Yu C, Wei H, et al. A proton nuclear magnetic resonance metabonomics approach for biomarker discovery in nonalcoholic fatty liver disease. Journal of Proteome Research 2011;10:2797–2806.

[58] Hines IN, Hartwell HJ, Feng Y, Theve EJ, Hall GA, Hashway S, et al. Insulin resistance and metabolic hepatocarcinogenesis with parent-of-origin effects in AxB mice. The American Journal of Pathology 2011;179:2855–2865.

[59] Tanaka N, Matsubara T, Krausz KW, Patterson AD, Gonzalez FJ. Disruption of phospholipid and bile acid homeostasis in mice with nonalcoholic steatohepatitis. Hepatology 2012;56:118–129.

[60] Lian JS, Liu W, Hao SR, Guo YZ, Huang HJ, Chen DY, et al. A serum metabonomic study on the difference between alcohol- and HBV-induced liver cirrhosis by ultraperformance liquid chromatography coupled to mass spectrometry plus quadrupole time-of-flight mass spectrometry. Chinese Medical Journal 2011;124:1367–1373.

[61] Gao H, Lu Q, Liu X, Cong H, Zhao L, Wang H, et al. Application of 1H NMR-based metabonomics in the study of metabolic profiling of human hepatocellular carcinoma and liver cirrhosis. Cancer Science 2009;100:782–785.

[62] Waldhier MC, Almstetter MF, Nurnberger N, Gruber MA, Dettmer K, Oefner PJ. Improved enantiomer resolution and quantification of free D-amino acids in serum and urine by comprehensive two-dimensional gas chromatography-time-of-flight mass spectrometry. Journal of Chromatography A 2011;1218:4537–4544.

[63] Martinez-Granados B, Morales JM, Rodrigo JM, Del Olmo J, Serra MA, Ferrandez A, et al. Metabolic profile of chronic liver disease by NMR spectroscopy of human biopsies. International Journal of Molecular Medicine 2011;27:111–117.

[64] Beyoglu D, Imbeaud S, Maurhofer O, Bioulac-Sage P, Zucman-Rossi J, Dufour JF, et al. Tissue metabolomics of hepatocellular carcinoma: tumor energy metabolism and the role of transcriptomic classification. Hepatology 2013;58:229–238.

[65] Budhu A, Roessler S, Zhao X, Yu Z, Forgues M, Ji J, et al. Integrated metabolite and gene expression profiles identify lipid biomarkers associated with progression of hepatocellular carcinoma and patient outcomes. Gastroenterology 2013;144:1066–1075 e1061.

[66] Chen T, Xie G, Wang X, Fan J, Qiu Y, Zheng X, et al. Serum and urine metabolite profiling reveals potential biomarkers of human hepatocellular carcinoma. Molecular & Cellular Proteomics: MCP 2011;10:M110 004945.

[67] Yang Y, Li C, Nie X, Feng X, Chen W, Yue Y, et al. Metabonomic studies of human hepatocellular carcinoma using high-resolution magic-angle spinning 1H NMR spectroscopy in conjunction with multivariate data analysis. Journal of Proteome Research 2007;6:2605–2614.

[68] Huang Q, Tan Y, Yin P, Ye G, Gao P, Lu X, et al. Metabolic characterization of hepatocellular carcinoma using nontargeted tissue metabolomics. Cancer Research 2013;73:4992–5002.

[69] Zeng J, Yin P, Tan Y, Dong L, Hu C, Huang Q, et al. Metabolomics study of hepatocellular carcinoma: discovery and validation of serum potential biomarkers by using capillary electrophoresis-mass spectrometry. Journal of Proteome Research 2014;13:3420–3431.

[70] Zhou L, Wang Q, Yin P, Xing W, Wu Z, Chen S, et al. Serum metabolomics reveals the deregulation of fatty acids metabolism in hepatocellular carcinoma and chronic liver diseases. Analytical and Bioanalytical Chemistry 2012;403:203–213.

[71] Xiao JF, Varghese RS, Zhou B, Nezami Ranjbar MR, Zhao Y, Tsai TH, et al. LC-MS based serum metabolomics for identification of hepatocellular carcinoma biomarkers in Egyptian cohort. Journal of Proteome Research 2012;11:5914–5923.

[72] Nahon P, Amathieu R, Triba MN, Bouchemal N, Nault JC, Ziol M, et al. Identification of serum proton NMR metabolomic fingerprints associated with hepatocellular carcinoma in patients with alcoholic cirrhosis. Clinical Cancer Research: An Official Journal of the American Association for Cancer Research 2012;18:6714–6722.

[73] Liu Y, Hong Z, Tan G, Dong X, Yang G, Zhao L, et al. NMR and LC/MS-based global metabolomics to identify serum biomarkers differentiating hepatocellular carcinoma from liver cirrhosis. International Journal of Cancer 2014;135:658–668.

[74] Patterson AD, Maurhofer O, Beyoglu D, Lanz C, Krausz KW, Pabst T, et al. Aberrant lipid metabolism in hepatocellular carcinoma revealed by plasma metabolomics and lipid profiling. Cancer Research 2011;71:6590–6600.

[75] Ressom HW, Xiao JF, Tuli L, Varghese RS, Zhou B, Tsai TH, et al. Utilization of metabolomics to identify serum biomarkers for hepatocellular carcinoma in patients with liver cirrhosis. Analytica Chimica Acta 2012;743:90–100.

[76] Stepien M, Duarte-Salles T, Fedirko V, Floegel A, Barupal DK, Rinaldi S, et al. Alteration of amino acid and biogenic amine metabolism in hepatobiliary cancers: Findings from a prospective cohort study. International Journal of Cancer 2016;138:348–360.

[77] Zivkovic AM, Bruce German J, Esfandiari F, Halsted CH. Quantitative lipid metabolomic changes in alcoholic micropigs with fatty liver disease. Alcoholism, Clinical and Experimental Research 2009;33:751–758.

[78] Yin P, Wan D, Zhao C, Chen J, Zhao X, Wang W, et al. A metabonomic study of hepatitis B-induced liver cirrhosis and hepatocellular carcinoma by using RP-LC and HILIC coupled with mass spectrometry. Molecular BioSystems 2009;5:868–876.

[79] Teng CF, Hsieh WC, Yang CW, Su HM, Tsai TF, Sung WC, et al. A biphasic response pattern of lipid metabolomics in the stage progression of hepatitis B virus X tumorigenesis. Molecular Carcinogenesis 2016;55:105–114.

[80] Fages A, Duarte-Salles T, Stepien M, Ferrari P, Fedirko V, Pontoizeau C, et al. Metabolomic profiles of hepatocellular carcinoma in a European prospective cohort. BMC Medicine 2015;13:242.

[81] Lu GD, Ang YH, Zhou J, Tamilarasi J, Yan B, Lim YC, et al. CCAAT/enhancer binding protein alpha predicts poorer prognosis and prevents energy starvation-induced cell death in hepatocellular carcinoma. Hepatology 2015;61:965–978.

[82] Schafer ZT, Grassian AR, Song L, Jiang Z, Gerhart-Hines Z, Irie HY, et al. Antioxidant and oncogene rescue of metabolic defects caused by loss of matrix attachment. Nature 2009;461:109–113.

[83] Carracedo A, Weiss D, Leliaert AK, Bhasin M, de Boer VC, Laurent G, et al. A metabolic prosurvival role for PML in breast cancer. The Journal of Clinical Investigation 2012;122:3088–3100.

[84] Zaugg K, Yao Y, Reilly PT, Kannan K, Kiarash R, Mason J, et al. Carnitine palmitoyltransferase 1C promotes cell survival and tumor growth under conditions of metabolic stress. Genes & Development 2011;25:1041–1051.

[85] Pike LS, Smift AL, Croteau NJ, Ferrick DA, Wu M. Inhibition of fatty acid oxidation by etomoxir impairs NADPH production and increases reactive oxygen species resulting in ATP depletion and cell death in human glioblastoma cells. Biochimica et Biophysica Acta 2011;1807:726–734.

[86] Jeon SM, Chandel NS, Hay N. AMPK regulates NADPH homeostasis to promote tumour cell survival during energy stress. Nature 2012;485:661–665.

[87] Herms A, Bosch M, Reddy BJ, Schieber NL, Fajardo A, Ruperez C, et al. AMPK activation promotes lipid droplet dispersion on detyrosinated microtubules to increase mitochondrial fatty acid oxidation. Nature Communications 2015;6:7176.

[88] Ito K, Carracedo A, Weiss D, Arai F, Ala U, Avigan DE, et al. A PML-PPAR-delta pathway for fatty acid oxidation regulates hematopoietic stem cell maintenance. Nature Medicine 2012;18:1350–1358.

[89] Samudio I, Harmancey R, Fiegl M, Kantarjian H, Konopleva M, Korchin B, et al. Pharmacologic inhibition of fatty acid oxidation sensitizes human leukemia cells to apoptosis induction. The Journal of Clinical Investigation 2010;120:142–156.

[90] Ricciardi MR, Mirabilii S, Allegretti M, Licchetta R, Calarco A, Torrisi MR, et al. Targeting the leukemia cell metabolism by the CPT1a inhibition: functional preclinical effects in leukemias. Blood 2015;126:1925–1929.

[91] Pacilli A, Calienni M, Margarucci S, D'Apolito M, Petillo O, Rocchi L, et al. Carnitine-acyltransferase system inhibition, cancer cell death, and prevention of myc-induced lymphomagenesis. Journal of the National Cancer Institute 2013;105:489–498.

[92] Hermanova I, Arruabarrena-Aristorena A, Valis K, Nuskova H, Alberich-Jorda M, Fiser K, et al. Pharmacological inhibition of fatty-acid oxidation synergistically enhances the effect of l-asparaginase in childhood ALL cells. Leukemia 2016;30:209–218.

[93] Tung S, Shi Y, Wong K, Zhu F, Gorczynski R, Laister RC, et al. PPARalpha and fatty acid oxidation mediate glucocorticoid resistance in chronic lymphocytic leukemia. Blood 2013;122:969–980.

[94] Camarda R, Zhou AY, Kohnz RA, Balakrishnan S, Mahieu C, Anderton B, et al. Inhibition of fatty acid oxidation as a therapy for MYC-overexpressing triple-negative breast cancer. Nature Medicine 2016;22:427–432.

[95] Villanueva A, Hernandez-Gea V, Llovet JM. Medical therapies for hepatocellular carcinoma: a critical view of the evidence. Nature Reviews Gastroenterology & Hepatology 2013;10:34–42.

[96] Bamia C, Lagiou P, Jenab M, Trichopoulou A, Fedirko V, Aleksandrova K, et al. Coffee, tea and decaffeinated coffee in relation to hepatocellular carcinoma in a European population: multicentre, prospective cohort study. International Journal of Cancer 2015;136:1899–1908.

[97] Sinha RA, Farah BL, Singh BK, Siddique MM, Li Y, Wu Y, et al. Caffeine stimulates hepatic lipid metabolism by the autophagy-lysosomal pathway in mice. Hepatology 2014;59:1366–1380.

[98] Zhou J, Farah BL, Sinha RA, Wu Y, Singh BK, Bay BH, et al. Epigallocatechin-3-gallate (EGCG), a green tea polyphenol, stimulates hepatic autophagy and lipid clearance. PloS One 2014;9:e87161.

Chapter 5

Hepatitis B Virus–Related Hepatocellular Carcinoma: Carcinogenesis, Prevention, and Treatment

Bolin Niu and Hie-Won Hann

Additional information is available at the end of the chapter

http://dx.doi.org/10.5772/65424

Abstract

Hepatocellular carcinoma (HCC) is the sixth most common cancer in the world and the second leading cause of cancer death. Hepatitis B virus (HBV) infection is one of the major risk factors for the development of HCC in the world. Most of the burden of disease (85%) is observed in the HBV endemic regions. Chronic infection with HBV predisposes patients with or without cirrhosis to HCC. Patients with high HBV DNA levels are at an increased risk for HCC. Studies have shown that the suppression of HBV with anti-viral therapy (nucleos(t)ide analogs) (NAs) decreases the incidence of HCC but does not eliminate the risk entirely. Chronic viral suppression alone is not sufficient treatment to prevent HCC development. Therefore, along with NAs, treatment may need to include targeting the cccDNA and inhibiting the viral entry into the newly formed hepatocytes and T-cell vaccine which specifically targets HBV and enhancing innate immunity with Toll-like receptor agonist. With all of these working together, we may achieve the goal of HBV cure.

Keywords: HBV, HCC, nucleos(t)ide analogs, antiviral treatment, prevention of HCC, HBV cure, hepatocarcinogenesis

1. Hepatitis B virus (HBV)

1.1. The discovery of HBV

Following the "icteric epidemic" in the 1880s, viral hepatitis was recognized as infectious in nature [1]. The discovery of HBV did not occur until 1965 when Baruch Blumberg, an American physician and geneticist, found a unique antigen in the serum of Australian aborigines (Australia Antigen, AuAg) that reacted with the serum of hemophiliacs [2, 3]. This antigen AuAg is now recognized as the hepatitis B surface antigen (HBsAg). Later, the link between viral hepatitis and this newly discovered antigen was firmly established when a technician in Blumberg's laboratory developed acute hepatitis [4]. Blumberg was awarded the Nobel Prize in Medicine in 1976 for his discovery of HBV.

Dane et al. identified the entire viral particle using electron microscopy in the 1970s [5]. Subsequently, in 1971, Blumberg and Millman developed a blood test to start screening blood donations for HBV [6]. In 1980, the FDA approved the first commercially available HBV vaccine once the genome of HBV was sequenced [7, 8]. While this first generation vaccine is no longer available in the United States, a recombinant HBV vaccine has been in use since 1986. A strong association between HBV and hepatocellular carcinoma (HCC) was described by Beasley et al. in their landmark study of 22,707 men in Taiwan [9]. Therefore, this vaccine has been designated by the World Health Organization as a bonafide "cancer vaccine".

1.2. HBV epidemiology

From a global view, a recent meta-analysis shows that the worldwide HBsAg prevalence is 3.61% [10]. There are over 248 million people currently living with chronic hepatitis B (CHB). Africa has the highest endemicity, with an HBsAg prevalence of 8.83%. However, the country with the largest number of people living with CHB is China with 95 million people, with an HBsAg prevalence of 5.49%. India and Nigeria have the second and third highest population of HBsAg (+) individuals, respectively, at 17 and 15 million people.

Chronic hepatitis B is a major risk factor for the development of hepatocellular carcinoma. A study in New York City found that Korean males had the highest rate of liver cancer–related mortality compared with all racial/ethnic groups. In fact, liver cancer was the second and third cause of cancer-related deaths in NYC Chinese and Korean men, respectively [11]. The Asian American Hepatitis B Program (AAHBP), a large community-based program in New York City, has found 13.3% HBsAg positivity among over 4000 newly screened individuals born in Asia [12].

2. HBV carcinogenesis

2.1. Risk of HCC from HBV infection

In a landmark paper in 1981, Beasley et al. established the association between HBV and HCC in 22,000 HBsAg (+) Taiwanese men. Compared to uninfected controls, their relative risk for HCC was found to be 63 [9]. Since then, co-infection with HCV [13], family history of HCC [14], alcohol intake [15], HBV genotype C greater than B [16, 17], and core promoter mutations [18, 19] have all been identified as risk factors for HCC development.

In highly endemic areas, HBV transmission is nearly all from mother to newborn and as many as 90% of infected babies develop chronic infections [20]. This differs from areas that have a low prevalence of HBV, where transmission is horizontal through sexual and parenteral routes in adulthood. More than 90% of these cases of acute HBV infection resolve spontaneously and

http://dx.doi.org/10.5772/65424

do not lead to chronic infections. Longer periods of chronic HBV infection contribute to a higher risk for HCC; therefore, endemic areas have a higher incidence of HCC.

Approximately 25% of those chronically infected people with HBV will develop HCC [21]. In addition to the earlier report by Beasley et al. [9], Franceschi et al. also reported a 30-fold increased risk of HCC in chronic HBV carriers [22]. A systematic review estimated the incidence rates of HCC in subjects with chronic HBV infection in East Asian countries to be 0.2 per 100 person-years in inactive carriers (HBsAg-positive but with normal levels of ALT), 0.6 person-years for those with chronic HBV infection without cirrhosis, and 3.7 person-years for those with compensated cirrhosis [23]. HBV can cause HCC in the absence of cirrhosis though 70–90% of HBV-related HCC occur in patients with cirrhosis [24].

The risk of HCC is increased in patients with higher levels of HBV replication. One large study followed 11,893 Taiwanese men for a mean of 8.5 years to evaluate the effect of HBV replication on the risk of HCC. The incidence rate of HCC was 1169 per 100,000 person-years among men who were positive for both HBsAg and HBeAg, 324 per 100,000 person-years for those who were only HBsAg-positive, and 39 per 100,000 person-years for those who were HBsAg-negative [25]. The relative risks of HCC among men who were positive for both HBsAg and HBeAg were increased 60-fold compared to 10-fold among those who were only HBsAg positive [25]. Another prospective study from Taiwan reported that in a cohort of 3653 HBsAg-positive participants, the incidence of cirrhosis and HCC increased in proportion to the HBV DNA level, from <300 copies/mL at 0.74% incidence to ≥1,000,000 copies/mL at 13.50% incidence over 13 years of follow up [26]. Furthermore, inactive carriers of HBV (HBeAg negative, HBV DNA <10,000 copies/mL, normal liver enzyme levels, no cirrhosis) are still at a 5-fold greater risk for HCC than HBsAg-negative controls [27].

2.2. Entry of HBV DNA into host cells

Hepatitis B virus is an enveloped DNA virus belonging to the *Hepadnaviridae* family. HBV contains a partially double-stranded circular DNA genome (rcDNA) [28]. HBV recognizes highly sulfated heparin sulfate proteoglycans (HSPGs) on the surface of liver cells, allowing the virus to be highly hepatotropic [29]. When HBsAg binds a liver-specific receptor named sodium taurocholate cotransporting polypeptide (NTCP or SLC10A1) during an infection, the virus gains entry into its host cell [30].

Upon entering the human hepatocyte, rcDNA becomes a covalently closed circular DNA (cccDNA) in the nucleus. This cccDNA functions as a template for transcription of all four viral mRNAs, which then translate all seven HBV proteins [28]. The largest viral mRNA transcript encodes the viral polymerase and is a template for DNA [31]. Current HBV antiviral medications thwart this step of the viral replication [32].

2.3. HBV X protein

The HBV X protein (HBx) is a 154 amino acid polypeptide with a mass of 17 kDa. Its role in the development of HCC is critical. HBx regulates cellular transcription, protein degradation, and cellular proliferation and apoptosis. HBx acts on cellular promoters by protein-protein interactions instead of binding directly to DNA. HBx can downregulate Wnt/β-catenin expression and suppress cell growth by not only repressing cell proliferation but also triggering cell apoptosis [33]. HBx protein also interacts with the tumor suppressor adenomatous polyposis coli to activate Wnt/β-catenin signaling, which upregulates the epithelial cell adhesion molecule in HCC cells to promote tumor initiation [34, 35]. Therefore, HBx activation of Wnt/β-catenin may directly promote the transformation of hepatocytes into cancer initiating cells [36]. Overall, the seemingly contradictory roles of HBx in regulating apoptosis demonstrate the complexity of hepatocarcinogenesis.

There are numerous ways in which HBx may induce anti-apoptotic effects. The most salient is its ability to inhibit p-53-mediated apoptosis. HBx may increase the expression of telomerase reverse transcriptase and telomerase activity, thus prolonging the lifespan of hepatocytes and leading to malignant transformation [36]. In addition, carboxyl-terminal (C-terminal) truncated HBx protein loses its proapoptotic properties and may enhance the protein's ability to transform oncogenes [36].

2.4. Integration of HBV DNA into host DNA

HBx truncation occurs with HBV integration into host DNA. The 3′-end of HBx is the preferred region of HBV genome involved in integration. When HBV integrates, the 3′-end of HBx is often deleted. Therefore, HBV integration is an important step in HCC development [37]. The C-terminal region produced by HBx truncation also contributes to HCC development. The C-terminal region has been suggested to be required for ROS production and 8-oxoguanine formation, biomarkers of oxidative stress [38]. The 24 amino acids truncated at the C-terminal end play a role in increasing cell invasiveness and metastasis in HCC through activation of MMP10 by C-Jun signaling [39]. Lastly, C-terminal truncated HBx has been reported to directly regulate miRNA transcription and promote hepatocellular proliferation [40].

3. Natural history

HBV carriers often are asymptomatic without significant liver injury because HBV replication in itself is not directly cytotoxic to hepatocytes [21, 41]. Hepatocellular injury occurs largely from host immune responses, both through major-histocompatibility-complex (MHC) class II-restricted, CD4+ helper T cells and MHC class I-restricted, CD8+ cytotoxic T lymphocytes [21, 42]. Four distinct phases comprise the natural history of HBV infection.

3.1. Acute "immune tolerant" phase

In the acute phase of infection with HBV, the "immune tolerant" phase is HBeAg (+) with high viral loads, normal serum alanine aminotransferase (ALT), and near normal liver histology [43]. When HBV is acquired in adulthood, this phase is very short [44]; however, perinatal and early childhood infection lead to a long "immune-tolerant" phase [45, 46]. The risk of progression to chronic carrier state differs greatly between those infected perinatally (90%) and as an adult (<1%) [44, 47, 48]. At the current time, antiviral treatment is not recommended

http://dx.doi.org/10.5772/65424

during the immune-tolerant phase but rather for the immune clearance phase. Interestingly, some recent reports have shown evidence of immune reactivity during the immune-tolerant stage [49–51]. As was presented by Zoulim and Mason, there is an argument to consider earlier treatment of CHB in order to prevent HCC [52].

3.2. "Immune clearance" phase

The "immune clearance" phase, developing during adolescence, is characterized by high viral load, HBeAg (+), and elevated ALT. Antiviral therapy is usually recommended during this phase. The salient feature of this phase is elevated ALT levels, which is a result of T-cell immune-mediated lysis of hepatocytes [53, 54]. The frequency of flares and duration of this phase are correlated with the risk of cirrhosis and HCC [55, 56]. High ALT level is a marker of vigorous host immune response, which is correlated with spontaneous HBeAg seroconversion. HBeAg seroconversion to anti-HBe is a pertinent outcome of this phase [57, 58].

3.3. "Inactive carrier" phase

Following HBeAg seroconversion, an "inactive HBsAg carrier" phase begins. It is marked by HBeAg (−), anti-HBe (+), normal ALT, and low or undetectable viral load [59]. Liver biopsy at this time would show mild hepatitis, minimal fibrosis, but cirrhosis may also be seen in patients who have experienced severe liver injury in the previous "immune clearance" phase [60]. Antiviral therapy is not indicated in this phase, but patients do need regular screening for HCC given the persistent risk while remaining positive for HBsAg and anti-HBc (IgG). Spontaneous seroclearance of HBsAg at a yearly incidence of 0.7–2.4% may happen after patients become HBeAg (−) [57, 61]. This phase may persist indefinitely.

3.4. "Reactivation/HBeAg-negative chronic hepatitis" phase

The last phase in the natural history of HBV infection is more recently recognized. The "reactivation of HBV replication/HBeAg-negative chronic hepatitis B" stage, also known as "e-CHB", is marked by HBeAg (−), anti-HBe (+), detectable viral load, elevated ALT, and continued necroinflammation on histology [62]. Patients may enter the "e-CHB" phase after some years in the "inactive carrier" phase or directly progress from HBeAg (+) chronic hepatitis to HBeAg (−) chronic hepatitis [63]. Many mutations in the viral core promoter and pre-core regions inhibit the synthesis of HBeAg without affecting HBV replication. Nucleotide 1896 is one of the most studied mutations associated with e-CHB in the pre-core region [64].

4. Prevention of HCC

4.1. Results of vaccination

Taiwan, a country with a high prevalence of chronic HBV, instituted a nationwide HBV vaccination program in 1984 for all citizens ranging from neonates to adults. A landmark paper published in the *New England Journal of Medicine* in 1997 reports the effect of vaccination on childhood HCC in Taiwan [65]. In 1984, the prevalence of seropositivity of HBsAg was 10.6% in six-year olds. Ten years after launching the vaccination campaign, this prevalence was reduced to <1% in six-year olds by 1994. The incidence of HCC in children ages 6–9 significantly declined from 0.52 per 100,000 for those born between 1974 and 1984 to 0.13 for those born between 1984 and 1986.

Given the availability of national health records, Taiwan is a country with tremendous potential for public health and epidemiological investigations. A newer study from the same group published recently re-examines the effect of HBV vaccination by comparing the rate of HCC in different time periods [66]. Between 1983 and 2011, 1509 patients were diagnosed with HCC. 1343 were born before and 166 were born after the HBV vaccination program began. The relative risk for HCC in patients 6–9 years old, 10–14 years old, 15–19 years old, and 20–26 years old who were vaccinated vs. unvaccinated were 0.26, 0.34, 0.37, and 0.42, respectively. Out of the 166 cases of HCC that occurred after HBV vaccination began in Taiwan, the two strongest risk factors were transmission of HBV from highly infectious mothers and incomplete immunization.

At this point, 180 countries have introduced infant HBV vaccination, and the global HBV vaccination coverage rate for the third dose is about 78% [67]. HBV vaccines are usually administered in three doses, with the second dose given one month after the first dose and the third dose given six months after the first dose. The dose recommended for adults is 10–20 μg and for infants and children 5–10 μg. With regard to the immunogenicity of HBV vaccines, over 90% of infants, children, and adolescents have protective serum anti-HBs antibody concentrations (>10 mIU/mL) after the vaccine series has been completed. However, host factors such as age older than 30, obesity, immunosuppression, and smoking have been linked to inadequate immunogenicity to the HBV vaccine.

Vaccination is most important for infants, particularly those born to HBsAg (+) mothers. In addition, the WHO recommends high-risk groups should also be vaccinated as well, including [1] people who frequently require blood transfusions, such as dialysis patients and recipients of solid organ transplantations [2]; people interned in prisons [3]; IV drug users [4]; household and sexual contacts of people with chronic HBV infection [5]; people with multiple sexual partners, health-care workers, and others who are exposed to blood or blood products through work [6]; and travelers who have not completed their HBV vaccine series. Although post-vaccination testing for immunity is not generally recommended, it has been the practice at our institution to conduct post-vaccination test to confirm the presence of anti-HBs at the protective level (>10 IU). For those who fail to produce antibody, it is important to rule out the occult HBV infection not uncommonly seen among the family members of HBV patients.

4.2. Surveillance for HCC

It is generally recommended to perform HCC surveillance in those with CHB and especially if the patient has cirrhosis. CHB is an independent risk factor for the development of HCC, which can occur even without cirrhosis. The surveillance method includes imaging, whether triple-phase CT or MRI with contrast, should occur every 6 months. The evidence for serological testing for alpha fetal protein (AFP) in surveillance for HCC is unclear; however, at our institution it is obtained at 6-month intervals with imaging.

A recent study shows the importance of HCC surveillance even in those with seroclearance of HBsAg [68]. In a retrospective analysis of 829 patients (mean age: 52.3 years; 575 males; 98 with cirrhosis) after HBsAg seroclearance, the estimated annual incidence of HCC was 2.85% and 0.29% in patients with and without cirrhosis, respectively. In non-cirrhotic patients, the annual rate of HCC was higher in males than females (0.40% vs. 0%, respectively). The study concludes that HCC surveillance should be considered for cirrhotic patients and non-cirrhotic male patients over age 50, even after HBsAg seroclearance, especially those infected with HBV genotype C.

4.3. Prevention of recurrent HCC post-resection, transplantation, and local tumor ablation

Antiviral therapy after tumor resection aims to improve prognosis by suppressing viral replication. Recent evidence indicates high serum HBV DNA levels, either preoperatively or postoperatively, is associated with a higher risk of HCC recurrence [69]. Furthermore, the incidence of HCC recurrence was significantly higher in patients who experienced acute postoperative exacerbations of hepatitis with high-serum concentrations of HBV DNA and sustained HBsAg expression postoperatively [70]. Antiviral therapy has been shown to induce the remission of active hepatitis, maintain liver function, and increase the likelihood of successful treatment for HCC recurrence even if recurrence developed after curative resection [71]. In addition, high levels of HBV DNA are significantly associated with shorter survival times, with the cause of death being HCC recurrence [71]. A recent meta-analysis shows that antiviral therapy with nucleos(t)ide analogs (NAs) reduces HCC-related mortality and HCC recurrence postoperatively, and improves overall survival in patients with HBV-related HCC [72].

There is a lack of evidence to guide the management of HBV after liver transplantation for HBV-related HCC; however, lifelong antivirals are used in most centers. In the case of transplantation for HBV cirrhosis, recurrent HBV may lead to graft loss and poor post-transplant survival. There is a direct relationship between the HBV VL at time of transplantation and the rate of HBV recurrence [73]. Since the study by Samuel et al. [74], hepatitis B immune globulin (HBIG) has been use as prophylaxis against HBV recurrence after liver transplantation for HBV cirrhosis.

We have reported favorable effects of antiviral therapy on the survival of HCC patients following local tumor ablation through interventional radiology [75]. We included 25 patients, who met criteria with a single HCC ≤ 7 cm and underwent tumor ablation with curative intent. Sixteen patients (diagnosed 1999 and after) received antiviral therapy and nine patients (diagnosed before 1999) did not. While there was no difference in their median tumor size and AFP, the survival was significantly different ($p < 0.001$). The median survival of the untreated was 16 months while that of the treated was 80 months. Fourteen of 16 treated patients are alive to date with two longest survivors alive for ≥151 months. Overall, there is evidence for lifelong antiviral therapy for patients with HCC treated with resection, transplantation, or local regional therapy.

5. Current treatment of hepatitis B

Since the advent of antiviral drugs, survival of patients with HBV has been remarkably improved. Current treatments for hepatitis B include nucleos(t)ide analogs (lamivudine, adefovir, entecavir, telbivudine, and tenofovir) and an interferon [pegylated-interferon alpha-2a (peg-IFN α-2a)] (**Table 1**) [4, 76]. The ultimate goal in the treatment of chronic hepatitis B is to prevent the development of HCC.

Name	Trade name	Strengths	Weaknesses	Approved
Pegylated interferon-2a	Pegasys	Finite duration of treatment Durable response post-treatment No known resistance	Needle injection High cost 65–70% fail to respond Significant side effects	1991 2005
Lamivudine	Epivir	Oral Safe with negligible side effects Effective and safe in pregnancy Least expensive	Long-term treatment is necessary High incidence of resistance	1998
Adefovir dipivoxil	Hepsera	Oral Low resistance	Long-term treatment is necessary Long-term treatment for renal toxicity Less potent than other treatments	2002
Entecavir	Baraclude	Oral Potent viral suppression Safe with negligible side effects Low resistance	Long-term treatment is necessary High cost	2005
Telbivudine	Tyzeka	Oral Potent viral suppression Effective and safe in pregnancy	Long-term treatment is necessary High incidence of resistance	2006
Tenofovir	Viread	Oral Potent viral suppression Safe with negligible side effects No known resistance so far Effective and safe in pregnancy	Long-term treatment is necessary	2008

Adapted from Halegoua-De Marzio and Hann [4].

Table 1. Current approved drugs for treatment of HBV.

5.1. Pegylated-interferon alpha-2a

Pegylated-interferon alpha-2a (peg-IFN α-2a) has replaced interferon alpha-2b due to better pharmacokinetic properties, weekly injection schedule, and similar efficacy. Its major mechanism of action is in immune modulation with a weak antiviral effect [77]. Peg-IFN α-2a has the highest rate of sustained response after 1 year of therapy, with a 27% rate of HBeAg seroconversion and 25% rate of loss of HBV DNA after 48 weeks of treatment [78, 79]. After 18 months of follow up, 4–6% of patients showed serum positivity for anti-HBs and had loss of HBsAg [78, 79]. Even after the end of treatment, 12–65% of patients had seroclearance of HBsAg within 5 years of losing HBeAg [80, 81]. A study of 542 patients, who received the medication for 48 weeks, shows patients with the best response include genotype A with HBV DNA <9 $\log_{10}$ copies/mL or ALT ≥ 2×ULN, or genotype B and C with ALT ≥ 2×ULN and low HBV DNA (<9 $\log_{10}$ copies/mL) [84]. Remission long after discontinuing therapy was associated with an early virological response, defined as suppressing levels to below 10^5 copies/mL within the first 2 weeks of therapy or >2 $\log_{10}$ decrease in serum HBV DNA [82, 83].

Peg-IFN α-2a only makes up about 10% of all hepatitis B prescriptions in the United States due to its substantial side effect profile and need for administration by injection [85].

5.2. Lamivudine

Approved by the Food and Drug Administration (FDA), lamivudine is a nucleoside analog reverse transcriptase inhibitor. Due to availability of other oral antivirals that have higher genetic barriers to resistance, lamivudine is not commonly used today. The most common reasons for its use currently are during pregnancy in HBsAg (+) women to perinatal transmission and during chemotherapy and immunosuppression to prevent reactivation of HBV in HBsAg (+) patients.

With 12 months of treatment, lamivudine is associated with 16–18% rate of HBeAg seroconversion [86]. In HBeAg (+) patients, the rate of HBeAg seroconversion increases with the duration of treatment, from 17% at 1 year to 27% at 2 years to 47% at 4 years [87]. Therapy for 1 year also results in 60–70% HBV DNA suppression in HBeAg (−) patients with chronic hepatitis B [88].

Lamivudine has been shown to decrease the rate of fibrosis and the incidence of HCC [89]. A study of 651 Asian patients with advanced fibrosis was stopped prematurely at 32 months because a significantly lower proportion of the lamivudine-treated group reached the primary endpoint of development of hepatic decompensation, HCC, or death from liver disease compared to placebo (7.8% vs. 17.7%) [89]. Lamivudine-treated patients have been observed to have a significant reduction in the incidence of HCC [90]. Reversal of fibrosis was significantly more likely to be seen on histology after 52 weeks of treatment with lamivudine than placebo [87].

Despite these positive attributes, there is a decrease in lamivudine usage due to its resistance profile. A large-scale safety study showed resistance rates of 23% at one year and 67% at five years of therapy in HBeAg (+) patients [91]. In a small study at our institution, lower resistance rate of 3% at one year and 10% at two years was found when 150 mg dose of lamivudine was used [92]. Pretreatment HBV DNA level is the most important factor for lamivudine resistance. Tenofovir has been shown to have stronger antiviral effect than adefovir against lamivudine-resistant HBV [93]. Furthermore, tenofovir monotherapy has been shown to be superior to adefovir and lamivudine combination therapy in lamivudine-resistant HBV [94].

5.3. Adefovir dipivoxil

Approved in 2002 by the FDA, adefovir dipivoxil is a nucleotide analog reverse transcriptase inhibitor. Treatment with adefovir for one year in HBeAg (+) patients leads to a 12% HBeAg seroconversion and 53% histological improvement [89, 95, 96]. Furthermore, HBeAg seroconversion is sustained in 91% of patients [97]. Development of resistance is associated with persistent viremia after 48 weeks of therapy. Rates of adefovir resistance at 1, 2, 4, and 5 years of therapy have been reported at 0%, 3%, 18%, and 29%, respectively [98]. Nevertheless, adefovir use is declining with the arrival of newer medications.

5.4. Entecavir

Approved by the FDA in 2005 for the treatment of CHB, entecavir is a nucleoside analog that inhibits HBV polymerase. It is administered as an oral dose of 0.5 mg/day, resulting in superior reduction of HBV DNA levels compared to lamivudine (6.98 $\log_{10}$ copies/mL vs. 5.4 $\log_{10}$ copies/mL) [99]. In a phase three clinical trial entecavir to lamivudine, those who received 52 weeks of entecavir achieved better virological response with HBV DNA < 400 copies/mL (67% entecavir vs. 36% lamivudine), normalization of ALT (78% vs. 70%), and histological improvement (72% vs. 62%) [99]. While entecavir is superior to lamivudine in HBeAg (−) patients, it does require indefinite treatment to maintain viral suppression and prevent relapse [100, 101]. After 6 years of therapy, 96% of HBeAg (+) CHB patients had histological improvement and 88% showed improved fibrosis scores even in cirrhosis [102]. Continuous entecavir treatment for up to 5 years in HBeAg (+) patients has been able to maintain HBV DNA suppression <300 copies/mL in 94% of patients [103].

In comparison to adefovir, entecavir has been shown to achieve viral suppression more rapidly within 14 days of initiating therapy [98]. Entecavir also has a higher rate of HBV clearance (58% vs. 19%) and ALT normalization (76% vs. 63%) when compared with adefovir after 48 weeks of treatment. No significant difference was observed in the rate of HBeAg loss or HBeAg seroconversion [104].

The incidence of HCC has been shown to decrease in entecavir-treated patients compared to non-treated. The five-year cumulative HCC incidence was 3.7% and 13.7% for entecavir-treated and control groups, respectively [105]. HBsAg loss has been associated with entecavir treatment [106, 107]. Compared to lamivudine treatment in HBeAg (+) patients, 96 weeks of entecavir treatment resulted in HBsAg loss in 5% of patients and 3% of lamivudine-treated patients [108]. Unlike HBeAg (+) patients, HBeAg (−) patients show no significant HBsAg loss on entecavir [109].

The biggest advantage of entecavir is its high genetic barrier and low resistance profile. The cumulative incidence of resistance after 6 years of entecavir in nucleoside-naïve patients is low at 1.2%. However, in lamivudine-refractory patients, the rate of resistance to entecavir is 57% at 6 years [110].

5.5. Telbivudine

Telbivudine is an L-nucleoside that is structurally related to lamivudine; it was approved by the FDA in 2006. It specifically inhibits HBV viral DNA synthesis, and it has been shown to be superior to lamivudine in both HBeAg (+) and HBeAg (−) patients with CHB. The seroconversion of HBeAg with telbivudine was found to be 22% and 30% at 1 and 2 years, respectively, in patients who are HBeAg (+) [111, 112]. In these patients, suppression of HBV DNA < 300 copies/mL was 60% and 56% at 1 and 2 years, respectively [105, 106]. Furthermore, recent evidence shows telbivudine has renoprotective effects, both in preventing adefovir-induced nephrotoxicity and improving renal function in liver transplant patients [113–116].

However, resistance to telbivudine has been reported at 21.6% and 8.6% after 2 years of therapy in HBeAg (+) and HBeAg (−) patients [117]. Predictive factors for response to telbivudine include ALT > 2×ULN at baseline or HBV DNA < 9 $\log_{10}$ copies/mL in HBeAg (+) patients [118, 119]. Telbivudine treatment has good therapeutic result in patients with low baseline HBV DNA and negative HBV DNA at week 24 [118].

Telbivudine is a pregnancy category B medication. A study of 186 pregnant Asian women with HBV DNA > 6,000,000 copies/mL, half received telbivudine from second trimester of pregnancy until 4 weeks postpartum and all infants received hepatitis B immune globulin (HBIG) within 24 h of birth, telbivudine treatment showed better outcomes compared with the control group with more women achieving undetectable HBV DNA (30% vs. 0%) [120]. Importantly, no infants born to women in the treatment group were HBsAg (+) compared to 8.7% in the control group.

5.6. Tenofovir

Tenofovir is the most recent nucleotide analog to be approved by the FDA in 2008. It is similar in structure to adefovir but more potent. Compared with adefovir in HBeAg (+) patients, 48 weeks of tenofovir led to more normalization of ALT (68% vs. 54%), stronger viral suppression defined as < 400 copies/mL (76% vs. 13%), histological improvement (67% vs. 12%), and HBsAg loss (3.2% vs. 0%) [121]. After 7 years of therapy, 99.3% of patients maintained viral suppression, 80% of patients achieved normalization of ALT, and no resistance was detected. In patients who are HBeAg (+), 54.5% achieved HBeAg (−) and 11.8% HBsAg (−). In HBeAg (−) patients, only 0.3% achieved HBsAg loss. There were 10 patients (1.7%) who had elevated serum creatinine ≥ 0.5 mg/dL above baseline while on tenofovir, and no significant changes in bone density was observed. HCC incidence has been recently reported to be decreased in tenofovir-treated HBV patients [122].

5.7. Hepatitis B during pregnancy

Newborns to mothers with CHB should receive hepatitis B immune globulin and the first dose of hepatitis B vaccine within 12 h of birth to prevent vertical transmission of HBV. Two subsequent doses of hepatitis B vaccine are administered within 6–12 months of age. Nevertheless, 7–32% of infants born to carrier mothers with high viral loads still become HBsAg (+) despite passive-active immunoprophylaxis [123, 124]. A Chinese study shows vertical transmission despite immunoprophylaxis failures occurred in HBeAg (+) mothers with HBV DNA levels >6 $\log_{10}$ copies/mL (>200,000 IU/mL) [125]. Therefore, it is very important to consider antiviral therapy in pregnant women with high levels of viremia, especially for mothers with infants who had previously failed immunoprophylaxis.

Both lamivudine and telbivudine have been used during the latter stages of pregnancy. They have comparable efficacy and safety in mothers and their newborns during 12 month post-partum observations, where the rate of vertical transmission was seen to be reduced when HBeAg (+) mothers with high viral loads received either lamivudine or telbivudine during the third trimester of pregnancy [121, 123, 126]. Currently, the use of oral antiviral agents during the first and second trimesters of pregnancy is not recommended.

Maternal HBV reactivation during pregnancy is uncommon but if encountered, antiviral therapy should be considered, especially if the reactivation is severe [126, 127]. Breastfeeding is not contraindicated for mothers who are on antiviral treatment as these medications are minimally excreted in breast milk and unlikely to cause significant toxicity [128].

5.8. Hepatitis B reactivation during chemotherapy or immunosuppressive therapy

With immunosuppressive therapy such as rituximab, chemotherapy, or corticosteroids, HBV reactivation can occur in HBsAg (+) carriers. Immunosuppression allows HBV replication and infection of hepatocytes, and reactivation usually occurs after discontinuation or withdrawal of immunosuppression as the immune system is reconstituted [129]. Reactivation leads to acute hepatitis, characterized by high levels of ALT and serum HBV DNA.

Lamivudine has been shown to be effective for prophylaxis of HBV reactivation during chemotherapy in a meta-analysis of 14 clinical trials [129]. It has been most effective when used for patients with low (<2000 IU/mL, < 10^4 copies/ml) or undetectable HBV DNA level and/or receiving a short course of immunosuppression for less than 6 months. Furthermore, for patients who are compliant with the medication, low resistance has been observed with a dose of 150 mg daily [92]. On the other hand, if the patient is undergoing a long course of chemotherapy or has a high viral load, nucleos(t)ide analogs such as tenofovir or entecavir are recommended due to their lower rate of resistance.

Asian patients should be screened for HBsAg prior to the initiation of chemotherapy or immunosuppressive therapy due to the high prevalence of CHB in Asia. These patients may be silent HBsAg (+) carriers who are unaware of their HBV status [130]. Patients who are HBsAg (−) but anti-HBc (+) should be tested for serum HBV DNA [80]. All HBsAg (+) patients who require immunosuppression or undergo bone marrow transplantation should be treated with antiviral prophylaxis [131]. Furthermore, any anti-HBc (+) patients, whether anti-HBs (+) or anti-HBs (−), who require such therapies should be considered as candidates for antiviral treatment [132]. Guidelines proposed by different societies for preventing HBV reactivation during immunosuppression were reviewed and summarized (**Table 2**) [132–136].

Society	Population (HBV DNA)	Prophylaxis	Prophylaxis type
AASLD [132]	Baseline HBV DNA <2000 IU/ml	Antiviral prophylaxis recommended	LAM or telbivudine (if IS < 12 months) or ETV > adefovir (if IS > 12 months)
	Baseline HBV DNA >2000 IU/ml	Antiviral prophylaxis recommended	LAM or telbivudine (if IS < 12 months) or ETV > adefovir (if IS > 12 months)
EASL [133]	Baseline HBV DNA <2000 IU/ml	Antiviral prophylaxis recommended	LAM
	Baseline HBV DNA >2000 IU/ml	Antiviral prophylaxis recommended	Antiviral w/ high barrier to resistance
AGA [134]	High risk (>10% HBVr incidence)	Antiviral prophylaxis recommended	Antiviral w/ high barrier to resistance
	Moderate risk (1–10% HBVr incidence)	Antiviral prophylaxis suggested or monitor	Antiviral w/ high barrier to resistance
	Low risk (<1% HBVr incidence)	None	N/A
APASL [135]	All HBsAg (+) patients	Antiviral prophylaxis recommended	ETV/TDF > LAM

AASLD, American Association for the Study of Liver Diseases; EASL, European Association for the Study of the Liver; AGA, American Gastroenterological Association; APASL, the Asian Pacific Association for the Study of the Liver; LAM, lamivudine; ETV, entecavir; TDF, tenofovir. Adapted from Wu and Hann [136].

Table 2. HBsAg (+) antiviral prophylactic guidelines for immunosuppression (IS) by society.

6. Seeking a cure for HBV

Firstly, defining the concept of HBV cure is important. The ultimate goal is eradication of cccDNA, also known as complete cure. However, functional cure (clearance of HBsAg, cessation of liver disease, even with persistent liver cccDNA) is achievable with current antivirals. Nonetheless, without eradication of HBV cccDNA, there remains a risk for HCC development even after years of successful antiviral treatment, especially in those with cirrhosis. Recent development of novel *in vitro* models has enriched the study of HBV pathogenesis and new antiviral strategies including immunotherapies.

Many new agents are in the pipeline. These include direct-acting antivirals (DAAs) and host-targeting agents (HTAs), which focus on targeting cccDNA in a number of different ways [28]. DAAs against HBV currently in development include novel polymerase inhibitors, capsid inhibitors, rcDNA-cccDNA conversion inhibitors, DNA cleavage enzymes, and small interfering RNA (siRNA)-based agents (**Table 3**) [137]. In addition, HTAs target sodium taurocholate co-transporting polypeptide (NTCP), host involvement in HBV secretion and budding, and immune responses (innate and adaptive) [28]. Novel agents to eradicate HBV would be a very important cancer cure given the role of hepatitis B virus in carcinogenesis.

Family/drug name	Mechanism	Status	Company
Nucleoside/nucleotide analogs			
Clevudine	Inhibits viral DNA polymerase	Approved in S. Korea and Philippines	Bukwang/Eisai
MIV-210 (lagociclovirvalactate)	Inhibits viral DNA polymerase	Phase II	Medivir/Daewoong
Besifovir (LB80380)	Inhibits viral DNA polymerase	Phase IIb	LG Life Sciences
Tenofovir alafenamide (GS-7340)	Inhibits viral DNA polymerase	Phase Ib	Gilead
CMX157	Inhibits viral DNA polymerase	Phase I	Chimerix
AGX-1009	Inhibits viral DNA polymerase	Phase I, China	Agenix
Non-nucleoside antivirals			
Myrcludex-B	Entry inhibitor	Phase Ia, Germany	Myr-GmbH
Bay 41-4109	Inhibits viral nucleocapsid	Phase I, Germany	AiCuris
GLS 4	Inhibits viral nucleocapsid	Phase I, China	Sunshine Lake
Phenylpropenamides	Inhibits viral encapsidation	Preclinical	
REP 9 AC	HBsAg release inhibitor	Phase Ib	REPLICor, Inc.
Nitazoxanide (alinia)	Small molecule	Preclinical	Romark Labs
dd-RNAi compound	Gene silencing	Preclinical	Benitec/Biomics
ARC-520	RNAi gene silencer	Phase I	Arrowhead Research
Immune-based			
Zadaxin (thymosin-alpha 1)	Immunomodulator	Orphan drug approval in United States for liver cancer	SciClone
NOV-205 (BAM 205)	Immunomodulator	Approved in Russia	Novelos
GS-9620	TLR7-agonist	Phase I	Gilead
GI-13020	HBV antigen	Preclinical	Global Immune
DV-601	Therapeutic HBV vaccine	Phase Ib	Dynavax

Adapted from Wang and Chen [137].

Table 3. Emerging drugs against HBV.

Conflict of interest

BN declares no conflict of interest, and HWH receives clinical research grants from Bristol-Myers Squibb and Gilead Sciences.

Author details

Bolin Niu[1] and Hie-Won Hann[1,2*]

*Address all correspondence to: hie-won.hann@jefferson.edu

1 Division of Gastroenterology and Hepatology, Department of Medicine, Thomas Jefferson University Hospital, Philadelphia, PA, USA

2 Liver Disease Prevention Center, Department of Medicine, Thomas Jefferson University Hospital, Philadelphia, PA, USA

References

[1] Gerlich WH. Medical virology of hepatitis B: how it began and where we are now. Virol. J. 2013;10:239.

[2] Blumberg BS, Alter HJ, Visnich S. A "new" antigen in leukemia sera. JAMA. 1965;191:541–546.

[3] Blumberg BS. Australia antigen and the biology of hepatitis B. Science. 1977;197:17–25.

[4] Halegoua-De Marzio D, Hann HW. Then and now: the progress in hepatitis B treatment over the past 20 years. World J. Gastroenterol. 2014;20:401–413.

[5] Dane DS, Cameron CH, Briggs M. Virus-like particles in serum of patients with Australia-antigen-associated hepatitis. Lancet Lond. Engl. 1970;1:695–698.

[6] Millman I, Loeb LA, Bayer ME, Blumberg BS. Australia antigen (a hepatitis-associated antigen): purification and physical properties. J. Exp. Med. 1970;131:1190–1199.

[7] Galibert F, Mandart E, Fitoussi F, Tiollais P, Charnay P. Nucleotide sequence of the hepatitis B virus genome (subtype ayw) cloned in *E. coli*. Nature. 1979;281:646–650.

[8] Szmuness W, Stevens CE, Harley EJ, Zang EA, Oleszko WR, William DC, et al. Hepatitis B vaccine: demonstration of efficacy in a controlled clinical trial in a high-risk population in the United States. N. Engl. J. Med. 1980;303:833–841.

[9] Beasley RP, Hwang LY, Lin CC, Chien CS. Hepatocellular carcinoma and hepatitis B virus. A prospective study of 22 707 men in Taiwan. Lancet Lond. Engl. 1981;2:1129–1133.

[10] Schweitzer A, Horn J, Mikolajczyk RT, Krause G, Ott JJ. Estimations of worldwide prevalence of chronic hepatitis B virus infection: a systematic review of data published between 1965 and 2013. Lancet Lond. Engl. 2015;386:1546–1555.

[11] Huang V, Li W, Tsai J, Begier E. Cancer mortality among Asians and Pacific Islanders in New York City, 2001–2010. J. Cancer Epidemiol. 2013;2013:986408.

[12] Pollack HJ, Kwon SC, Wang SH, Wyatt LC, Trinh-Shevrin C, AAHBP Coalition. Chronic hepatitis B and liver cancer risks among Asian immigrants in New York City: Results from a large, community-based screening, evaluation, and treatment program. Cancer Epidemiol. Biomark. Prev. Publ. Am. Assoc. Cancer Res. Cosponsored Am. Soc. Prev. Oncol. 2014;23:2229–2239.

[13] Benvegnù L, Gios M, Boccato S, Alberti A. Natural history of compensated viral cirrhosis: a prospective study on the incidence and hierarchy of major complications. Gut. 2004;53:744–749.

[14] Yu MW, Chang HC, Liaw YF, Lin SM, Lee SD, Liu CJ, et al. Familial risk of hepatocellular carcinoma among chronic hepatitis B carriers and their relatives. J. Natl. Cancer Inst. 2000;92:1159–1164.

[15] Ohnishi K, Iida S, Iwama S, Goto N, Nomura F, Takashi M, et al. The effect of chronic habitual alcohol intake on the development of liver cirrhosis and hepatocellular carcinoma: relation to hepatitis B surface antigen carriage. Cancer. 1982;49:672–677.

[16] Tsubota A, Arase Y, Ren F, Tanaka H, Ikeda K, Kumada H. Genotype may correlate with liver carcinogenesis and tumor characteristics in cirrhotic patients infected with hepatitis B virus subtype adw. J. Med. Virol. 2001;65:257–265.

[17] Yu M-W, Yeh S-H, Chen P-J, Liaw Y-F, Lin C-L, Liu C-J, et al. Hepatitis B virus genotype and DNA level and hepatocellular carcinoma: a prospective study in men. J. Natl. Cancer Inst. 2005;97:265–272.

[18] Baptista M, Kramvis A, Kew MC. High prevalence of 1762(T) 1764(A) mutations in the basic core promoter of hepatitis B virus isolated from black Africans with hepatocellular carcinoma compared with asymptomatic carriers. Hepatol. Baltim. Md. 1999;29:946–953.

[19] Kao J-H, Chen P-J, Lai M-Y, Chen D-S. Basal core promoter mutations of hepatitis B virus increase the risk of hepatocellular carcinoma in hepatitis B carriers. Gastroenterology. 2003;124:327–334.

[20] Borgia G, Carleo MA, Gaeta GB, Gentile I. Hepatitis B in pregnancy. World J. Gastroenterol. 2012;18:4677–4683.

[21] Ganem D, Prince AM. Hepatitis B virus infection—natural history and clinical consequences. N. Engl. J. Med. 2004;350:1118–1129.

[22] Franceschi S, Montella M, Polesel J, La Vecchia C, Crispo A, Dal Maso L, et al. Hepatitis viruses, alcohol, and tobacco in the etiology of hepatocellular carcinoma in Italy. Cancer Epidemiol. Biomark. Prev. Publ. Am. Assoc. Cancer Res. Cosponsored Am. Soc. Prev. Oncol. 2006;15:683–689.

[23] Fattovich G, Stroffolini T, Zagni I, Donato F. Hepatocellular carcinoma in cirrhosis: incidence and risk factors. Gastroenterology. 2004;127:S35–S50.

[24] Yang JD, Kim WR, Coelho R, Mettler TA, Benson JT, Sanderson SO, et al. Cirrhosis is present in most patients with hepatitis B and hepatocellular carcinoma. Clin. Gastroenterol. Hepatol. Off. Clin. Pract. J. Am. Gastroenterol. Assoc. 2011;9:64–70.

[25] Yang H-I, Lu S-N, Liaw Y-F, You S-L, Sun C-A, Wang L-Y, et al. Hepatitis B e antigen and the risk of hepatocellular carcinoma. N. Engl. J. Med. 2002;347:168–174.

[26] Chen C-J, Yang H-I, Iloeje UH, REVEAL-HBV Study Group. Hepatitis B virus DNA levels and outcomes in chronic hepatitis B. Hepatol. Baltim. Md. 2009;49:S72–S84.

[27] Chen J-D, Yang H-I, Iloeje UH, You S-L, Lu S-N, Wang L-Y, et al. Carriers of inactive hepatitis B virus are still at risk for hepatocellular carcinoma and liver-related death. Gastroenterology. 2010;138:1747–1754.

[28] Zeisel MB, Lucifora J, Mason WS, Sureau C, Beck J, Levrero M, et al. Towards an HBV cure: state-of-the-art and unresolved questions—report of the ANRS workshop on HBV cure. Gut. 2015;64:1314–1326.

[29] Schulze A, Gripon P, Urban S. Hepatitis B virus infection initiates with a large surface protein-dependent binding to heparan sulfate proteoglycans. Hepatol. Baltim. Md. 2007;46:1759–1768.

[30] Yan H, Zhong G, Xu G, He W, Jing Z, Gao Z, et al. Sodium taurocholate cotransporting polypeptide is a functional receptor for human hepatitis B and D virus. eLife. 2012;1:e00049.

[31] Summers J, Mason WS. Replication of the genome of a hepatitis B-like virus by reverse transcription of an RNA intermediate. Cell. 1982;29:403–415.

[32] Das K, Xiong X, Yang H, Westland CE, Gibbs CS, Sarafianos SG, et al. Molecular modeling and biochemical characterization reveal the mechanism of hepatitis B virus polymerase resistance to lamivudine (3TC) and emtricitabine (FTC). J. Virol. 2001;75:4771–4779.

[33] Kuo C-Y, Wang J-C, Wu C-C, Hsu S-L, Hwang G-Y. Effects of hepatitis B virus X protein (HBx) on cell-growth inhibition in a CCL13-HBx stable cell line. Intervirology. 2008;51:26–32.

[34] Hsieh A, Kim H-S, Lim S-O, Yu D-Y, Jung G. Hepatitis B viral X protein interacts with tumor suppressor adenomatous polyposis coli to activate Wnt/β-catenin signaling. Cancer Lett. 2011;300:162–172.

[35] Yamashita T, Ji J, Budhu A, Forgues M, Yang W, Wang H-Y, et al. EpCAM-positive hepatocellular carcinoma cells are tumor-initiating cells with stem/progenitor cell features. Gastroenterology. 2009;136:1012–1024.

[36] Kuo T-C, Chao CC-K. Hepatitis B virus X protein prevents apoptosis of hepatocellular carcinoma cells by upregulating SATB1 and HURP expression. Biochem. Pharmacol. 2010;80:1093–1102.

[37] Toh ST, Jin Y, Liu L, Wang J, Babrzadeh F, Gharizadeh B, et al. Deep sequencing of the hepatitis B virus in hepatocellular carcinoma patients reveals enriched integration events, structural alterations and sequence variations. Carcinogenesis. 2013;34:787–798.

[38] Jung S-Y, Kim Y-J. C-terminal region of HBx is crucial for mitochondrial DNA damage. Cancer Lett. 2013;331:76–83.

[39] Sze KMF, Chu GKY, Lee JMF, Ng IOL. C-terminal truncated hepatitis B virus x protein is associated with metastasis and enhances invasiveness by C-Jun/matrix metalloproteinase protein 10 activation in hepatocellular carcinoma. Hepatol. Baltim. Md. 2013;57:131–139.

[40] Yip W-K, Cheng AS-L, Zhu R, Lung RW-M, Tsang DP-F, Lau SS-K, et al. Carboxyl-terminal truncated HBx regulates a distinct microRNA transcription program in hepatocellular carcinoma development. PLoS One. 2011;6:e22888.

[41] de Franchis R, Meucci G, Vecchi M, Tatarella M, Colombo M, Del Ninno E, et al. The natural history of asymptomatic hepatitis B surface antigen carriers. Ann. Intern. Med. 1993;118:191–194.

[42] Chisari FV, Ferrari C. Hepatitis B virus immunopathogenesis. Annu. Rev. Immunol. 1995;13:29–60.

[43] Chu CM, Karayiannis P, Fowler MJ, Monjardino J, Liaw YF, Thomas HC. Natural history of chronic hepatitis B virus infection in Taiwan: studies of hepatitis B virus DNA in serum. Hepatol. Baltim. Md. 1985;5:431–434.

[44] Tassopoulos NC, Papaevangelou GJ, Sjogren MH, Roumeliotou-Karayannis A, Gerin JL, Purcell RH. Natural history of acute hepatitis B surface antigen-positive hepatitis in Greek adults. Gastroenterology. 1987;92:1844–1850.

[45] Fattovich G, Bortolotti F, Donato F. Natural history of chronic hepatitis B: special emphasis on disease progression and prognostic factors. J. Hepatol. 2008;48:335–352.

[46] Villa E, Fattovich G, Mauro A, Pasino M. Natural history of chronic HBV infection: special emphasis on the prognostic implications of the inactive carrier state versus chronic hepatitis. Dig. Liver Dis. Off. J. Ital. Soc. Gastroenterol. Ital. Assoc. Study Liver. 2011;43 Suppl 1:S8–S14.

[47] Beasley RP, Hwang LY, Lin CC, Leu ML, Stevens CE, Szmuness W, et al. Incidence of hepatitis B virus infections in preschool children in Taiwan. J. Infect. Dis. 1982;146:198–204.

[48] Beasley RP, Trepo C, Stevens CE, Szmuness W. The e antigen and vertical transmission of hepatitis B surface antigen. Am. J. Epidemiol. 1977;105:94–98.

[49] Bertoletti A, Kennedy PT. The immune tolerant phase of chronic HBV infection new perspectives on an old concept. Cell Mol. Immunol. 2015; 12:258–63.

[50] Kennedy PT, Sandalova E, Jo J, et al. Preserved T-cell function in children and young adults with immune-tolerant chronic hepatitis B. Gastroenterology 2012;143:637–645.

[51] Levy O. Innate immunity of the newborn: basic mechanisms and clinical correlates. Nat. Rev. Immunol. 2007;7,379–390.

[52] Zoulim F, Mason WS. Reasons to consider earlier treatment of chronic HBV infections. Gut. 2012;61,333–336 doi:10.1136/gutjnl-2011-300937.

[53] Tsai SL, Chen PJ, Lai MY, Yang PM, Sung JL, Huang JH, et al. Acute exacerbations of chronic type B hepatitis are accompanied by increased T cell responses to hepatitis B core and e antigens. Implications for hepatitis B e antigen seroconversion. J. Clin. Invest. 1992;89:87–96.

[54] Chu CM, Liaw YF. Intrahepatic distribution of hepatitis B surface and core antigens in chronic hepatitis B virus infection. Hepatocyte with cytoplasmic/membranous hepatitis B core antigen as a possible target for immune hepatocytolysis. Gastroenterology. 1987;92:220–225.

[55] Liaw YF, Tai DI, Chu CM, Chen TJ. The development of cirrhosis in patients with chronic type B hepatitis: a prospective study. Hepatol. Baltim. Md. 1988;8:493–496.

[56] McMahon BJ, Holck P, Bulkow L, Snowball M. Serologic and clinical outcomes of 1536 Alaska Natives chronically infected with hepatitis B virus. Ann. Intern. Med. 2001;135:759–768.

[57] Liaw Y-F. Hepatitis flares and hepatitis B e antigen seroconversion: implication in anti-hepatitis B virus therapy. J. Gastroenterol. Hepatol. 2003;18:246–252.

[58] Yuen M-F, Yuan H-J, Hui C-K, Wong DK-H, Wong W-M, Chan AO-O, et al. A large population study of spontaneous HBeAg seroconversion and acute exacerbation of chronic hepatitis B infection: implications for antiviral therapy. Gut. 2003;52:416–419.

[59] Chu C-M, Liaw Y-F. Genotype C hepatitis B virus infection is associated with a higher risk of reactivation of hepatitis B and progression to cirrhosis than genotype B: a longitudinal study of hepatitis B e antigen-positive patients with normal aminotransferase levels at baseline. J. Hepatol. 2005;43:411–417.

[60] Yim HJ, Lok AS-F. Natural history of chronic hepatitis B virus infection: what we knew in 1981 and what we know in 2005. Hepatol. Baltim. Md. 2006;43:S173–S181.

[61] Zacharakis GH, Koskinas J, Kotsiou S, Papoutselis M, Tzara F, Vafeiadis N, et al. Natural history of chronic HBV infection: a cohort study with up to 12 years follow-up in North Greece (part of the Interreg I-II/EC-project). J. Med. Virol. 2005;77:173–179.

[62] Hadziyannis SJ, Vassilopoulos D. Hepatitis B e antigen-negative chronic hepatitis B. Hepatol. Baltim. Md. 2001;34:617–624.

[63] Hsu Y-S, Chien R-N, Yeh C-T, Sheen I-S, Chiou H-Y, Chu C-M, et al. Long-term outcome after spontaneous HBeAg seroconversion in patients with chronic hepatitis B. Hepatol. Baltim. Md. 2002;35:1522–1527.

[64] Carman WF, Jacyna MR, Hadziyannis S, Karayiannis P, McGarvey MJ, Makris A, et al. Mutation preventing formation of hepatitis B e antigen in patients with chronic hepatitis B infection. Lancet Lond. Engl. 1989;2:588–591.

[65] Chang MH, Chen CJ, Lai MS, Hsu HM, Wu TC, Kong MS, et al. Universal hepatitis B vaccination in Taiwan and the incidence of hepatocellular carcinoma in children. Taiwan Childhood Hepatoma Study Group. N. Engl. J. Med. 1997;336:1855–1859.

[66] Chang M-H, You S-L, Chen C-J, Liu C-J, Lai M-W, Wu T-C, et al. Long-Term Effects of Hepatitis B Immunization of Infants in Preventing Liver Cancer. Gastroenterology. 2016;151:472–480.

[67] Kao J-H. Hepatitis B vaccination and prevention of hepatocellular carcinoma. Best Pract. Res. Clin. Gastroenterol. 2015;29:907–917.

[68] Kim G-A, Lee HC, Kim M-J, Ha Y, Park EJ, An J, et al. Incidence of hepatocellular carcinoma after HBsAg seroclearance in chronic hepatitis B patients: a need for surveillance. J. Hepatol. 2015;62:1092–1099.

[69] Urata Y, Kubo S, Takemura S, Uenishi T, Kodai S, Shinkawa H, et al. Effects of antiviral therapy on long-term outcome after liver resection for hepatitis B virus-related hepatocellular carcinoma. J. Hepato-Biliary-Pancreat. Sci. 2012;19:685–696.

[70] Kubo S, Hirohashi K, Tanaka H, Tsukamoto T, Shuto T, Higaki I, et al. Virologic and biochemical changes and prognosis after liver resection for hepatitis B virus-related hepatocellular carcinoma. Dig. Surg. 2001;18:26–33.

[71] Qu L-S, Jin F, Huang X-W, Shen X-Z. High hepatitis B viral load predicts recurrence of small hepatocellular carcinoma after curative resection. J. Gastrointest. Surg. Off. J. Soc. Surg. Aliment. Tract. 2010;14:1111–1120.

[72] Wong JS-W, Wong GL-H, Tsoi KK-F, Wong VW-S, Cheung SY-S, Chong C-N, et al. Meta-analysis: the efficacy of anti-viral therapy in prevention of recurrence after curative treatment of chronic hepatitis B-related hepatocellular carcinoma. Aliment. Pharmacol. Ther. 2011;33:1104–1112.

[73] Degertekin B, Han S-HB, Keeffe EB, Schiff ER, Luketic VA, Brown RS, et al. Impact of virologic breakthrough and HBIG regimen on hepatitis B recurrence after liver transplantation. Am. J. Transplant. Off. J. Am. Soc. Transplant. Am. Soc. Transpl. Surg. 2010;10:1823–1833.

[74] Samuel D, Muller R, Alexander G, Fassati L, Ducot B, Benhamou JP, et al. Liver transplantation in European patients with the hepatitis B surface antigen. N. Engl. J. Med. 1993;329:1842–1847.

[75] Hann HW, Coben R, Brown D, Needleman L, Rosato E, Min A, et al. A long-term study of the effects of antiviral therapy on survival of patients with HBV-associated hepatocellular carcinoma (HCC) following local tumor ablation. Cancer Med. 2014;3:390–396.

[76] Ayoub WS, Keeffe EB. Review article: current antiviral therapy of chronic hepatitis B. Aliment. Pharmacol. Ther. 2011;34:1145–1158.

[77] Dianzani F. Biological basis for the clinical use of interferon. Gut. 1993;34:S74–S76.

[78] Lau GKK, Piratvisuth T, Luo KX, Marcellin P, Thongsawat S, Cooksley G, et al. Peginterferon Alfa-2a, lamivudine, and the combination for HBeAg-positive chronic hepatitis B. N. Engl. J. Med. 2005;352:2682–2695.

[79] Janssen HLA, van Zonneveld M, Senturk H, Zeuzem S, Akarca US, Cakaloglu Y, et al. Pegylated interferon alfa-2b alone or in combination with lamivudine for HBeAg-positive chronic hepatitis B: a randomised trial. Lancet Lond. Engl. 2005;365:123–129.

[80] Tong MJ, Pan CQ, Hann HW, Kowdley KV, Han SH, Min AD, Leduc TS. The management of chronic hepatitis B in Asian Americans. Dig. Dis. Sci. 2011;56:3143–316281.

[81] Lau DT, Everhart J, Kleiner DE, Park Y, Vergalla J, Schmid P, et al. Long-term follow-up of patients with chronic hepatitis B treated with interferon alfa. Gastroenterology. 1997;113:1660–1667.

[82] Fried MW, Piratvisuth T, Lau GKK, Marcellin P, Chow W-C, Cooksley G, et al. HBeAg and hepatitis B virus DNA as outcome predictors during therapy with peginterferon alfa-2a for HBeAg-positive chronic hepatitis B. Hepatol. Baltim. Md. 2008;47:428–434.

[83] Hansen BE, Buster EHCJ, Steyerberg EW, Lesaffre E, Janssen HLA. Prediction of the response to peg-interferon-alfa in patients with HBeAg positive chronic hepatitis B using decline of HBV DNA during treatment. J. Med. Virol. 2010;82:1135–1142.

[84] Buster EHCJ, Hansen BE, Lau GKK, Piratvisuth T, Zeuzem S, Steyerberg EW, et al. Factors that predict response of patients with hepatitis B e antigen-positive chronic hepatitis B to peginterferon-alfa. Gastroenterology. 2009;137:2002–2009.

[85] Zoulim F, Perrillo R. Hepatitis B: reflections on the current approach to antiviral therapy. J. Hepatol. 2008;48 Suppl 1:S2–S19.

[86] Dienstag JL, Schiff ER, Wright TL, Perrillo RP, Hann HW, Goodman Z, et al. Lamivudine as initial treatment for chronic hepatitis B in the United States. N. Engl. J. Med. 1999;341:1256–1263.

[87] Chang T-T, Lai C-L, Chien R-N, Guan R, Lim S-G, Lee C-M, et al. Four years of lamivudine treatment in Chinese patients with chronic hepatitis B. J. Gastroenterol. Hepatol. 2004;19:1276–1282.

[88] Liaw Y-F, Leung N, Kao J-H, Piratvisuth T, Gane E, Han K-H, et al. Asian-Pacific consensus statement on the management of chronic hepatitis B: a 2008 update. Hepatol. Int. 2008;2:263–283.

[89] Liaw Y-F, Sung JJY, Chow WC, Farrell G, Lee C-Z, Yuen H, et al. Lamivudine for patients with chronic hepatitis B and advanced liver disease. N. Engl. J. Med. 2004;351:1521–1531.

[90] Eun JR, Lee HJ, Kim TN, Lee KS. Risk assessment for the development of hepatocellular carcinoma: according to on-treatment viral response during long-term lamivudine therapy in hepatitis B virus-related liver disease. J. Hepatol. 2010; 53,118–125

[91] Lok ASF, Lai C-L, Leung N, Yao G-B, Cui Z-Y, Schiff ER, et al. Long-term safety of lamivudine treatment in patients with chronic hepatitis B. Gastroenterology. 2003;125:1714–1722.

[92] Chae HB, Hann H-W. Baseline HBV DNA level is the most important factor associated with virologic breakthrough in chronic hepatitis B treated with lamivudine. World J. Gastroenterol. 2007;13:4085–4090.

[93] Hann HW, Chae HB, Dunn SR. Tenofovir (TDF) has stronger antiviral effect than adefovir (ADV) against lamivudine (LAM)-resistant hepatitis B virus (HBV). Hepatol. Int. 2008;2:244–249.

[94] Yang D-H, Xie Y-J, Zhao N-F, Pan H-Y, Li M-W, Huang H-J. Tenofovir disoproxil fumarate is superior to lamivudine plus adefovir in lamivudine-resistant chronic hepatitis B patients. World J. Gastroenterol. 2015;21:2746–2753.

[95] Marcellin P, Chang T-T, Lim SG, Tong MJ, Sievert W, Shiffman ML, et al. Adefovir dipivoxil for the treatment of hepatitis B e antigen-positive chronic hepatitis B. N. Engl. J. Med. 2003;348:808–816.

[96] Hadziyannis SJ, Tassopoulos NC, Heathcote EJ, Chang T-T, Kitis G, Rizzetto M, et al. Adefovir dipivoxil for the treatment of hepatitis B e antigen-negative chronic hepatitis B. N. Engl. J. Med. 2003;348:800–807.

[97] Schiff ER, Lai C-L, Hadziyannis S, Neuhaus P, Terrault N, Colombo M, et al. Adefovir dipivoxil therapy for lamivudine-resistant hepatitis B in pre- and post-liver transplantation patients. Hepatol. Baltim. Md. 2003;38:1419–1427.

[98] Hadziyannis SJ, Tassopoulos NC, Heathcote EJ, Chang T-T, Kitis G, Rizzetto M, et al. Long-term therapy with adefovir dipivoxil for HBeAg-negative chronic hepatitis B for up to 5 years. Gastroenterology. 2006;131:1743–1751.

[99] Chang T-T, Gish RG, de Man R, Gadano A, Sollano J, Chao Y-C, et al. A comparison of entecavir and lamivudine for HBeAg-positive chronic hepatitis B. N. Engl. J. Med. 2006;354:1001–1010.

[100] Shouval D, Lai C-L, Chang T-T, Cheinquer H, Martin P, Carosi G, et al. Relapse of hepatitis B in HBeAg-negative chronic hepatitis B patients who discontinued successful entecavir treatment: the case for continuous antiviral therapy. J. Hepatol. 2009;50:289–295.

[101] Lai C-L, Shouval D, Lok AS, Chang T-T, Cheinquer H, Goodman Z, et al. Entecavir versus lamivudine for patients with HBeAg-negative chronic hepatitis B. N. Engl. J. Med. 2006;354:1011–1020.

[102] Chang T-T, Liaw Y-F, Wu S-S, Schiff E, Han K-H, Lai C-L, et al. Long-term entecavir therapy results in the reversal of fibrosis/cirrhosis and continued histological improvement in patients with chronic hepatitis B. Hepatol. Baltim. Md. 2010;52:886–893.

[103] Chang T-T, Lai C-L, Kew Yoon S, Lee SS, Coelho HSM, Carrilho FJ, et al. Entecavir treatment for up to 5 years in patients with hepatitis B e antigen-positive chronic hepatitis B. Hepatol. Baltim. Md. 2010;51:422–430.

[104] Leung N, Peng C-Y, Hann H-W, Sollano J, Lao-Tan J, Hsu C-W, et al. Early hepatitis B virus DNA reduction in hepatitis B e antigen-positive patients with chronic hepatitis B: a randomized international study of entecavir versus adefovir. Hepatol. Baltim. Md. 2009;49:72–79.

[105] Hosaka T, Suzuki F, Kobayashi M, Seko Y, Kawamura Y, Sezaki H, et al. Long-term entecavir treatment reduces hepatocellular carcinoma incidence in patients with hepatitis B virus infection. Hepatol. Baltim. Md. 2013;58:98–107.

[106] Chen Y-C, Sheen I-S, Chu C-M, Liaw Y-F. Prognosis following spontaneous HBsAg seroclearance in chronic hepatitis B patients with or without concurrent infection. Gastroenterology. 2002;123:1084–1089.

[107] Chu C-M, Liaw Y-F. Hepatitis B surface antigen seroclearance during chronic HBV infection. Antivir. Ther. 2010;15:133–143.

[108] Gish RG, Chang T-T, Lai C-L, de Man R, Gadano A, Poordad F, et al. Loss of HBsAg antigen during treatment with entecavir or lamivudine in nucleoside-naïve HBeAg-positive patients with chronic hepatitis B. J. Viral Hepat. 2010;17:16–22.

[109] Reijnders JGP, Deterding K, Petersen J, Zoulim F, Santantonio T, Buti M, et al. Antiviral effect of entecavir in chronic hepatitis B: influence of prior exposure to nucleos(t)ide analogues. J. Hepatol. 2010;52:493–500.

[110] Tenney DJ, Rose RE, Baldick CJ, Pokornowski KA, Eggers BJ, Fang J, et al. Long-term monitoring shows hepatitis B virus resistance to entecavir in nucleoside-naïve patients is rare through 5 years of therapy. Hepatol. Baltim. Md. 2009;49:1503–1514.

[111] Liaw Y-F, Gane E, Leung N, Zeuzem S, Wang Y, Lai CL, et al. 2-Year GLOBE trial results: telbivudine Is superior to lamivudine in patients with chronic hepatitis B. Gastroenterology. 2009;136:486–495.

[112] Lai C-L, Gane E, Liaw Y-F, Hsu C-W, Thongsawat S, Wang Y, et al. Telbivudine versus lamivudine in patients with chronic hepatitis B. N. Engl. J. Med. 2007;357:2576–2588.

[113] Gane EJ, Deray G, Liaw Y-F, Lim SG, Lai C-L, Rasenack J, et al. Telbivudine improves renal function in patients with chronic hepatitis B. Gastroenterology. 2014;146:138–146.

[114] Lee M, Oh S, Lee HJ, Yeum T, Lee J, Yu SJ, et al. Telbivudine protects renal function in patients with chronic hepatitis B infection in conjunction with adefovir-based combination therapy. J. Viral Hepat. 2014;21:873–881.

[115] Li W, Zhang D. Influence of monotherapy with telbivudine or entecavir on renal function in patients with chronic hepatitis B. Zhonghua Gan Zang Bing Za Zhi Zhonghua Ganzangbing Zazhi Chin. J. Hepatol. 2015;23:407–411.

[116] Perrella A, Lanza A, Pisaniello D, DiCostanzo G, Calise F, Cuomo O. Telbivudine prophylaxis for hepatitis B virus recurrence after liver transplantation improves renal function. Transplant Proc. 2014;46:2319–21.

[117] Sonneveld MJ, Janssen HLA. Chronic hepatitis B: peginterferon or nucleos(t)ide analogues? Liver Int. Off. J. Int. Assoc. Study Liver. 2011;31 Suppl 1:78–84.

[118] Zeuzem S, Gane E, Liaw Y-F, Lim SG, DiBisceglie A, Buti M, et al. Baseline characteristics and early on-treatment response predict the outcomes of 2 years of telbivudine treatment of chronic hepatitis B. J. Hepatol. 2009;51:11–20.

[119] Hann HW. Telbivudine for the treatment of hepatitis B. Expert Opin. Pharmacother. 2010; 11:2243–2249.

[120] Han G-R, Cao M-K, Zhao W, Jiang H-X, Wang C-M, Bai S-F, et al. A prospective and open-label study for the efficacy and safety of telbivudine in pregnancy for the prevention of perinatal transmission of hepatitis B virus infection. J. Hepatol. 2011;55:1215–1221.

[121] Marcellin P, Heathcote EJ, Buti M, Gane E, de Man RA, Krastev Z, et al. Tenofovir disoproxil fumarate versus adefovir dipivoxil for chronic hepatitis B. N. Engl. J. Med. 2008;359:2442–2455.

[122] Kim WR, Loomba R, Berg T, Schall REA, Yee LJ, Dinh PV, et al. Impact of long-term tenofovirdisoproxilfumarate on incidence of hepatocellular carcinoma in patients with chronic hepatitis B. Cancer 2015; 121, 3631–3638.

[123] Xu W-M, Cui Y-T, Wang L, Yang H, Liang Z-Q, Li X-M, et al. Lamivudine in late pregnancy to prevent perinatal transmission of hepatitis B virus infection: a multicentre, randomized, double-blind, placebo-controlled study. J. Viral Hepat. 2009;16:94–103.

[124] Wiseman E, Fraser MA, Holden S, Glass A, Kidson BL, Heron LG, et al. Perinatal transmission of hepatitis B virus: an Australian experience. Med. J. Aust. 2009;190:489–492.

[125] Zou H, Chen Y, Duan Z, Zhang H, Pan C. Virologic factors associated with failure to passive-active immunoprophylaxis in infants born to HBsAg-positive mothers. J. Viral Hepat. 2012;19:e18–e25.

[126] Zhang H, Pan CQ, Pang Q, Tian R, Yan M, Liu X. Telbivudine or lamivudine use in late pregnancy safely reduces perinatal transmission of hepatitis B virus in real-life practice. Hepatol. Baltim. Md. 2014;60:468–476.

[127] Hung J-H, Chu C-J, Sung P-L, Chen C-Y, Chao K-C, Yang M-J, et al. Lamivudine therapy in the treatment of chronic hepatitis B with acute exacerbation during pregnancy. J. Chin. Med. Assoc. JCMA. 2008;71:155–158.

[128] Shapiro RL, Holland DT, Capparelli E, Lockman S, Thior I, Wester C, et al. Antiretroviral concentrations in breast-feeding infants of women in Botswana receiving antiretroviral treatment. J. Infect. Dis. 2005;192:720–727.

[129] Loomba R, Rowley A, Wesley R, Liang TJ, Hoofnagle JH, Pucino F, et al. Systematic review: the effect of preventive lamivudine on hepatitis B reactivation during chemotherapy. Ann. Intern. Med. 2008;148:519–528.

[130] Weinbaum C, Williams I, Mast E, Wang S, Finelli L, Wasley A, et al. Recommendations for identification and public health management of persons with chronic hepatitis B virus infection. MMWR. 2008;57:1–20.

[131] Civan J, Hann HW. Giving rituximab in patients with occult or resolved hepatitis B virus infection: are the current guidelines good enough? Expert Opin. Drug Saf. 2015;14:865–875.

[132] Lok ASF, McMahon BJ. Chronic hepatitis B: update 2009. Hepatol. Baltim. Md. 2009;50:661–662.

[133] European Association for the Study of the Liver. EASL clinical practice guidelines: management of chronic hepatitis B virus infection. J. Hepatol. 2012;57:167–185.

[134] Reddy KR, Beavers KL, Hammond SP, Lim JK, Falck-Ytter YT, American Gastroenterological Association Institute. American Gastroenterological Association Institute guideline on the prevention and treatment of hepatitis B virus reactivation during immunosuppressive drug therapy. Gastroenterology. 2015;148:215–219.

[135] Liaw Y-F, Kao J-H, Piratvisuth T, Chan HLY, Chien R-N, Liu C-J, et al. Asian-Pacific consensus statement on the management of chronic hepatitis B: a 2012 update. Hepatol. Int. 2012;6:531–561.

[136] Wu RM, Hann HW. Hepatitis B virus (HBV) reactivation following immunosuppression in HBsAg (+) carriers. North Am. J. Med. Sci. Oct. 2015;8:191.

[137] Wang X-Y, Chen H-S. Emerging antivirals for the treatment of hepatitis B. World J. Gastroenterol. 2014;20:7707–7717.

Chapter 6

Diagnosis of Hepatocellular Carcinoma

Ayse Kefeli, Sebahat Basyigit and
Abdullah Ozgur Yeniova

Additional information is available at the end of the chapter

http://dx.doi.org/10.5772/64992

Abstract

Hepatocellular carcinoma (HCC) is one of the commonest cancers worldwide, particularly in the developing countries HCC occurs predominantly in patients with underlying chronic liver disease and cirrhosis, especially due to chronic hepatitis C virus (HCV) and hepatitis B virus (HBV) infection. Tumors progress with local expansion, intrahepatic spread, and distant metastases, and the life expectancy of patients with HCC is poor, with a mean survival of 6–20 months. Thus, developing effective and efficient care for patients with HCC must become a significant subject. Removal of HCC by surgical, transplantation or resection of the tumors, means offers the best chance for possible cure. Criteria for such intervention have been refined over the last decade to optimize long-term survival in selected patients with Milan criteria. Not many patients are candidate given the advanced stage of their cancer at diagnosis or degree of liver disease. The other main limiting factor is inadequate organ storage. Unfortunately, many patients die when they are waiting a donor organ. Local ablative therapies may be effective for time saving as a bridge therapy, and may provide palliation, in these patients. Diagnostic tools commonly used include radiographic imaging, and rarely serum markers and liver biopsy. A suspicious lesion on the ultrasound generally requires additional imaging studies to confirm the diagnosis of the tumor. Histologic confirmation is not required in a patient at increased risk for hepatocellular carcinoma whose lesion(s) fulfill criteria for hepatocellular carcinoma which are presence of typical features, including hypervascularity during arterial phase followed by decreased enhancement (washout) during portal venous phases on computerized tomography or has increased T2 signal intensity on magnetic resonance imaging.

Keywords: hepatocellular carcinoma, alpha fetoprotein, computerized tomography, magnetic resonance imaging

1. Introduction

Hepatocellular carcinoma (HCC) is the most common primary tumor of the liver that usually develops in the setting of chronic liver disease. It is the fifth most common cancer in men and the eighth most common in women and is the second leading cause of cancer-related death in the world [1]. Moreover, incidence of HCC is increasing despite limited number of cancer registries, underdiagnosis of HCC, particularly in developing countries. Therefore, the ability to make a diagnosis of HCC at an early time has a critical role to providing effective treatment, including curative treatment such as surgical resection, liver transplantation. Hereby, surveillance program has been developed to provide early treatment and updated guidelines recommend that groups were specified for which surveillance who has chronic liver disease, was likely to be cost-effective because the HCC incidence was high enough [2–6]. Eventually, surveillance programs with the purpose of early detection of HCC, primarily through serum markers as alpha-fetoprotein (AFP) assessment and hepatic imaging, have led to archive to early diagnosis and curative treatment in patients with HCC [7]. When hepatic lesion is identified by surveillance program, the diagnosis of HCC can be made by the use of dynamic imaging series, tumor markers, and rarely liver biopsy. Imaging modalities have primary role to establishing the diagnosis of HCC but serum tumor markers and liver biopsy continue to have important role, particularly in the setting of small or atypical hepatic lesion. On the other hand, unfortunately, no universal guidelines for diagnosis exist, which may be because of the differences in the diagnostic approach between Eastern and Western institutions. The aim of this chapter is to provide an extensive review of the current modalities employed for the diagnosis of HCC, including serum markers, radiological techniques and histological evaluation, and comparison international guidelines for the diagnostic approach to HCC.

2. Diagnosis of Hepatocellular Carcinoma

The diagnostic approach to the solid liver lesion is commonly determined by the size of the lesion. The diagnostic approach differs according to whether lesion is lesser or larger than 1 cm. The American Association for the Study of Liver Diseases (ASLD) and Korean Liver Cancer study Group-National Cancer Centre Korea (KLCSG-NCC) guidelines recommend follow-up ultrasound (US) every three-six months if the lesions are lesser than 1 cm and require definitive contrast-enhanced imaging with either 4-phase computed tomography (CT) or magnetic resonance imaging (MRI) (**Figure 1**) if the lesions are larger than 1 cm; otherwise European Association for the Study of the Liver (EASL) guidelines have different algorithm which had three ways; first one is which nodules are lesser than 1 cm, second one is in diameter 1–2 cm, and third one is larger than 2 cm. On the other hand, Asian Pacific Association for the Study of the Liver the Asian Pacific Association for the Study of the Liver (APASL) guideline ignores the size of the liver lesion. Recent guidelines have some diversity, and thus, all algorithms of guidelines were presented in figures (**Figures 1–4**) [2–6].

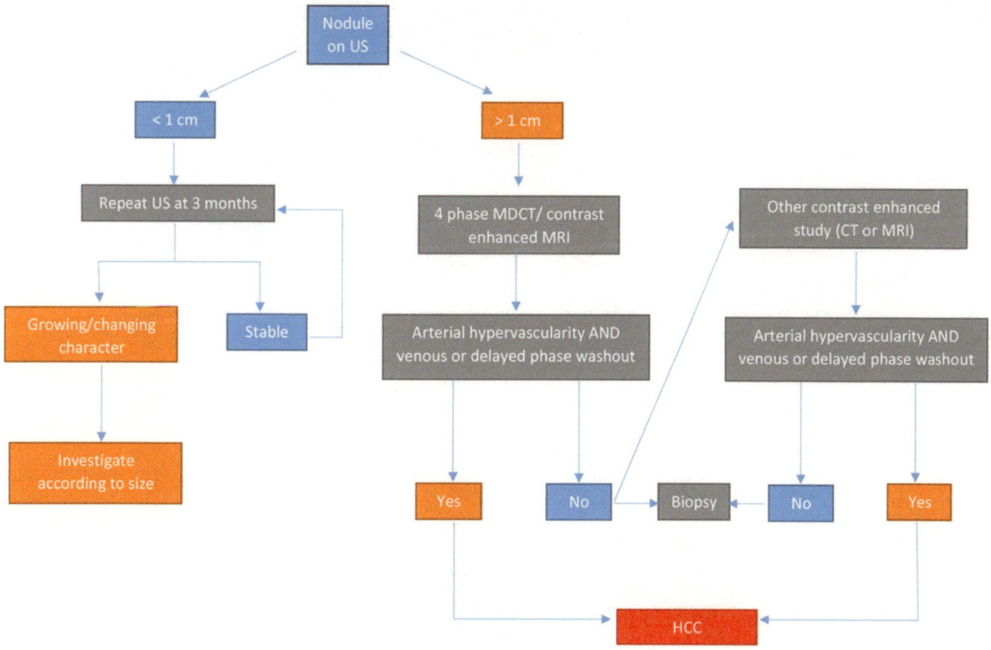

Figure 1. Diagnostic algorithm of AASLD guideline for nodule by detected US in patients at risk of HCC.

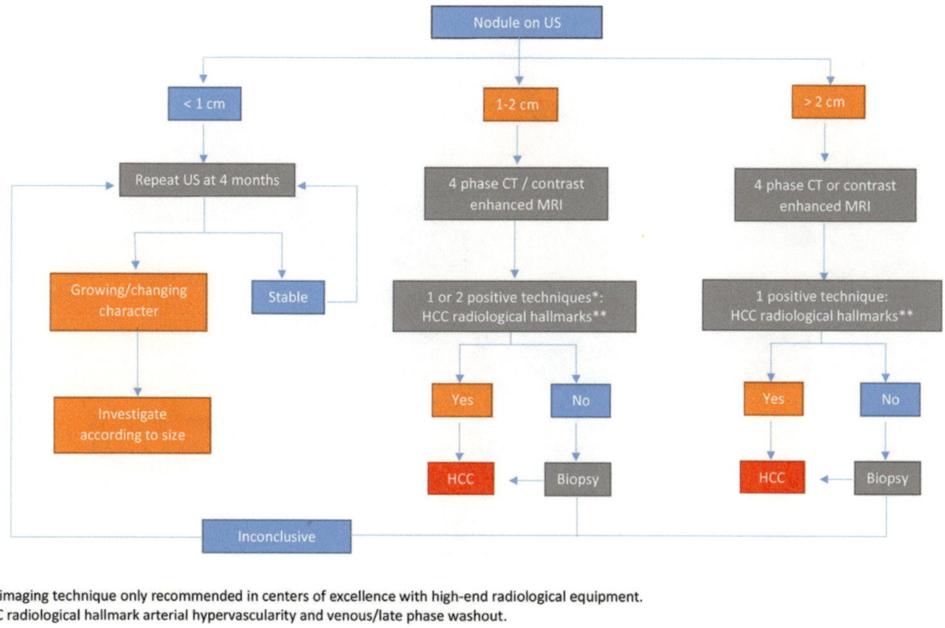

Figure 2. Diagnostic algorithm of EASL guideline for nodule by detected US in patients at risk of HCC.

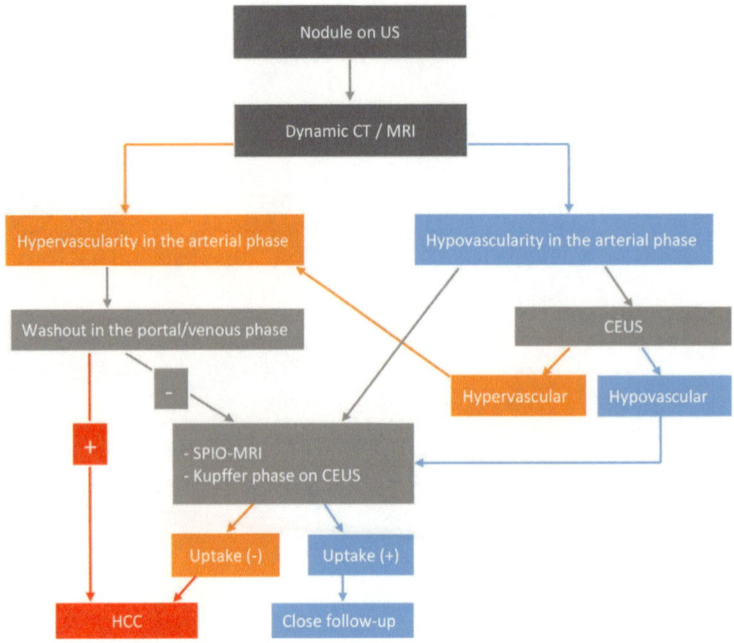

Figure 3. Diagnostic algorithm of APASL guideline for nodule by detected US in patients at risk of HCC.

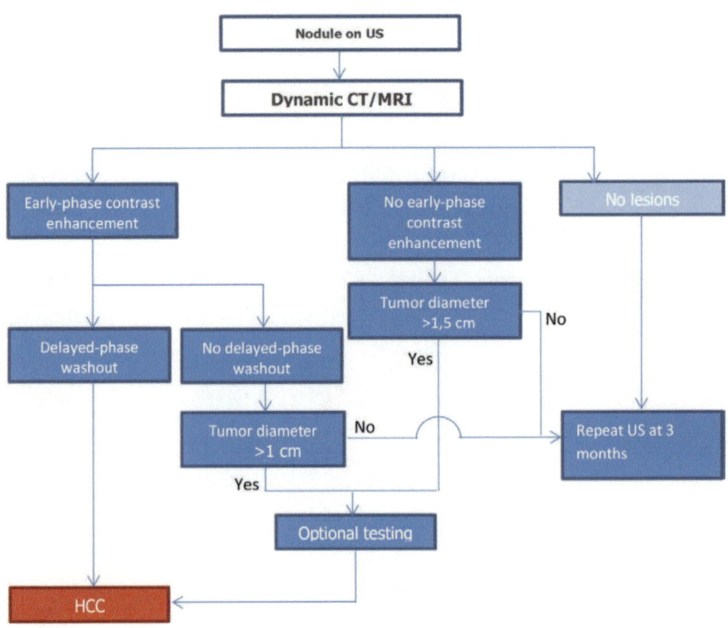

Figure 4. Diagnostic algorithm of JAPAN for nodule guideline by detected US in patients at risk of HCC.

Histologic confirmation is not required in a patient at increased risk of hepatocellular carcinoma whose lesion(s) fulfill criteria for hepatocellular carcinoma which are the presence of typical features on 4-phase CT or MRI, including hypervascularity during arterial phase followed by decreased enhancement (washout) during portal venous phases on CT or has increased T2 signal intensity on MRI. However, if the diagnosis remains unclear, the lesions did not have these specific features, and the results will affect the patient's management, and a biopsy of the lesions is indicated. Biopsy is rarely needed due to valuable contribution of serum markers on diagnosis of HCC. Although elevated serum AFP levels had been evaluated in guidelines previously, almost all of recent guidelines no longer include measurement of serum AFP in the diagnostic algorithm for hepatic nodules found on surveillance program [2, 3].

With the Asian, American, and European guidelines, Liver Imaging Reporting and Data System (LI-RADS) has been developed to address the limitations of prior imaging-based criteria including the lack of established consensus regarding the exact definitions of imaging features, binary categorization (either definite or not definite HCC), and failure to consider non-HCC malignancies [8].

Comparison of the EASL, AASLD, APASL, and LI-RADS guidelines are summarized in **Table 1**.

	EASL	AASLD	APASL	JAPAN	LI-RADS
Target population	Cirrhosis	Hep B carriers, cirrhosis	Cirrhosis only with Hep B or Hep C	All patients at high risk of HCC	All patients at high risk of HCC
Targeted lesion	Detected nodule by US	Detected nodule by US	Detected nodule by US and elevated AFP	Detected nodule by US and elevated AFP, AFP-L3, DCP	All nodules
Imaging modality	4-phase MDCT, CE-MRI	4-phase MDCT, CE-MRI	CT, CEUS, SPIO-MRI	CT, CEUS, Gd-EOB-DTPA-enhanced MRI, CT angiography	CT, MRI with extracellular and hepatobiliary agent
Diagnostic criteria	Larger than 1 cm	Larger than 1 cm	Washout on PVP, DP or	AP enhancement	AP enhancement
	AP enhancement	AP enhancement	High SPIO-MR signal or	Washout on DP	Washout on PVP, DP
	Washout on PVP, DP	Washout on PVP, DP	Defect in KP on CEUS	Larger than1 or 1.5 cm	Capsule appearance
			*Regardless of the size		
Number of requiredexam	≥2 cm: one exam 1–2 cm: two exams	One exam	One exam	One exam	One exam
Serum marker	N/A	N/A	Only for small nodules (<1 cm)	Yes	N/A
Category of diagnosis	HCC	HCC	HCC	HCC	LR-1 definitely benign
	Not HCC	Not HCC	Not HCC	Not HCC	LR-2 probably benign
	Indeterminate	Indeterminate	Indeterminate	Indeterminate	LR-3 indeterminate

	EASL	AASLD	APASL	JAPAN	LI-RADS
					LR-4 probably HCC
					LR-5 definitely HCC
					LR-5V definitely tumor invading vein
					LR-M probably malignancy but not specific for HCC
Diagnosis of subcentimetre HCC without biopsy	No	No	Yes (tumor marker + imaging)	No	Yes (probably HCC)
Biopsy required	Yes	Yes	No	Yes	Yes (LR-4, LR-M)

AASLD: Association for the Study of Liver Diseases; AFP: alpha-fetoprotein; AP: arterial phase; CHB: chronic hepatitis B; CHC: chronic hepatitis C; DP: delayed phase; EASL: European Association for the Study of the Liver; 4-phase MDCT: +phase multidetector computerized tomography; CE-MRI: contrast-enhanced magnetic resonance imaging; HCC: hepatocellular carcinoma; KLCSG-NCC: Korean Liver Cancer Study Group-National Cancer Center; LC: liver cirrhosis; LI-RADS: Liver Imaging Reporting and Data System; N/A: not applicable; PVP: portal venous phase; TP: transitional phase; US: ultrasonography; KP: Kupfer.

Table 1. Comparison of EASL, AASLD, APASL guidelines, and LI-RADS.

2.1. Serum markers

Ideal biomarkers should provide or contribute to diagnose and to monitor a disease, with a sufficient sensibility and specificity, to define its stage as well as to allow an easy and reproducible screening in the target population, with a low cost.

Serum AFP concentration is the most commonly used marker for HCC. Although several other serologic markers [such as des-gamma-carboxyprothrombin (DCP), glypican 3] may signify the presence of HCC, they are just used in combination with the serum AFP which may improve the diagnostic accuracy. These markers are not common used in alone in routine clinical practice.

2.1.1. Alpha-fetoprotein

However, serum levels of AFP do not correlate always with other clinical features of HCC such as size, stage, or prognosis, and AFP is the most common used marker for HCC. Because of AFP is normally produced during gestation by the fetal liver and yolk sac, the serum concentration of AFP can be increased during pregnancy with tumors of gonadal origin (both germ cell and non-germ cell) and in a variety of other malignancies [9]. Elevated serum AFP can also be seen in patients with chronic liver disease without HCC such as acute or chronic viral hepatitis, particularly in hepatitis C [10].

However, the accuracy of AFP has been critically challenged, and there is growing debate about its continued use in HCC surveillance programs, and AFP appears to be beneficial in clinical practice. In addition, many guidelines including EASL and ASLD no longer recommend measuring AFP level for surveillance of HCC. Only Asian Guideline recommends US and AFP every 6 months. However, a rise in serum AFP in a patient with cirrhosis or hepatitis B alerts the physician on possible HCC development.

In practice, it is generally accepted that serum levels greater than 500 mcg/L (normal in most laboratories is between 10 and 20 mcg/L) in a high-risk patient are diagnostic of HCC [11]. On the other hand, HCC is often diagnosed at a lower AFP level in patients undergoing screening [9] because all tumors do not secrete AFP, and serum concentrations are normal in up to 40% of small HCCs [12]. Elevated serum levels of AFP are commonly associated with HCC causing on advanced-stage fibrosis. Persistently elevated AFP values in a patient with cirrhosis have an increased risk of developing HCC compared with those who have fluctuating or normal levels (29% vs 13 and 2.4%, respectively, in one report) [13].

The sensitivity, specificity, and predictive value for the serum AFP in the diagnosis of HCC is still controversial issue. There is no strict cutoff value. Commonly accepted value is >20 mcg/L and a review which have five studies showed that sensitivity was 41–65% and specificity was 80–94% based upon a cutoff value of >20 mcg/L [14].

An increase in AFP level may be has a greater diagnostic accuracy than one time measurement of AFP whether higher than cutoff value. Using longitudinal AFP measurements could have identified an increase in AFP. Requiring an increase in AFP level of ≥2 from its nadir in the prior year maintained high sensitivity of surveillance while increasing specificity. This finding confirms prior studies [15].

Although ASLD and EASL guidelines recommend using US alone to achieve this goal given concerns about the suboptimal sensitivity and specificity of AFP [2, 3], and when AFP used in combination with US, its sensitivity reaches up to 63% for early-stage HCC [16].

Despite the poor reliability and low sensitivity of serum AFP for the diagnosis of HCC, it has emerged as an important prognostic marker, especially in patients undergoing resection and those being considered for liver transplantation. In addition, an increase in AFP is associated with increased tumor size and stage, extrahepatic metastasis, portal vein thrombosis, and decreased survey. Patients with AFP levels >1000 mcg/L have an extremely high risk of recurrent disease following transplantation, irrespective of the tumor size [17, 18].

2.1.2. AFP-L3

AFP-L3 is molecular variant of AFP, in which different isoforms of AFP, which can be identified through electrophoretic techniques relied on specific lectins, have long been reported in the biomedical literature [19]. Because of the limitations of serum AFP measurements, several other molecular variants of AFP, such as AFP-L3, have been evaluated for diagnosis or estimating prognosis in patients with HCC. Lens culinaris agglutinin-reactive AFP (AFP-L3) is a newly developed assay, highly sensitive fraction of AFP (hs-AFP-L3) that has been used as a diagnostic and prognostic marker of HCC. In patients with AFP < 20 ng/mL, measurements of AFP-L3% by the highly sensitive method before treatment was more useful for diagnosis and prognosis of HCC than by the conventional method [20].

Furthermore, since hs-AFP-L3% increases before HCC is detectable by various advanced imaging modalities, this assay may help identify benign liver disease patients with a higher risk of HCC [21].

2.1.3. MicroRNAs

Recently, miRNAs have been widely reported as a new class of clinical biomarkers and potential therapeutic targets for cancers. Because miRNAs act as key factors in several biological processes, such as growth, cell proliferation, differentiation, apoptosis, and carcinogenesis. HBV- or HCV-related HCC development and progression are associated with a significant and important deregulation of serum/plasma and liver tissues' profiles of miRNAs, as it has been widely reported by several studies. Thus, this evidence makes miRNAs potential and useful biomarkers for diagnosis, staging, progression, prognosis, and response to treatment. Therefore, in the last years, a large series of studies has been performed to investigate the correlation between specific miRNAs levels and/or profiles in body fluids and HCC [22, 23].

miRNAs have some usefulness characteristics, including the possibility to detect these molecules in serum/plasma samples, that may be easily collected, and their high stability, even in conditions that are generally known to induce RNAs degradation, such as fluctuations in temperature and pH levels as well as long-term storage [24, 25]. Although some studies showed that miRNA panels can be used to discriminate HCC patients from cancer-free controls, and could be a blood-based early detection biomarker for HCC screening, and demonstrated as important regulators in HCC pathogenesis, definitive conclusions about relationship between the majority of miRNAs and HCC remain to be explored [26–28].

2.1.4. Des-gamma-carboxyprothrombin

DCP, also known as the protein induced by vitamin K absence or antagonist II (PIVKA-II), is an abnormal form of the coagulation protein, prothrombin. The vitamin K-dependent carboxylase responsible for the carboxylation is absent in many HCC cells, and an abnormal prothrombin with all or some of unconverted glutamic acid is secreted. Therefore, this non-carboxylated form (DCP) has been used as an HCC biomarker [29, 30].

The sensitivities for AFP, AFP-L3%, and DCP were 68, 62, and 73%, respectively. When the three markers were combined, the sensitivity was increased to 86%. In another study, DCP levels were shown to correlate with tumor size and metastatic HCC. Several studies that are compared to AFP and DCP had the highest sensitivity (67–63% vs 73–87% for DCP), specificity was the highest in DCP in comparison with AFP (91% vs 78% respectively), and the highest positive predictive value (87%) in patients with HCC [31, 32]. APASL guideline recommends simultaneous measurement of AFP and DCP [4]. In addition, elevated serum DCP is significantly related to portal vein invasion and/or intrahepatic metastasis. It recommends simultaneous measurements of serum alpha-fetoprotein and protein induced by vitamin K absence for detecting hepatocellular carcinoma [31, 32].

DCP can be elevated in other conditions besides HCC. Conditions such as obstructive jaundice, intrahepatic cholestasis causing chronic decrease in vitamin K, and ingestion of drugs such as warfarin or wide-spectrum antibiotics can result in high concentrations of DCP. In addition, 25–50% of patients with HCC will have a DCP value within the reference range. Because of this, a normal DCP value does not rule out HCC.

Simultaneous determinations of AFP and DCP are useful for monitoring recurrence in patients with HCC after treatment, but the decrease to normal levels of a single marker does not always indicate the absence of tumor recurrence [33].

2.1.5. Glypican-3

Glypican (GPC) is a family of heparan sulfate proteoglycans that are bound to the cell surface by a lipid anchor. Six members (GPC1~6) of this family have been identified. New finding of recent research is that GPC-3 expression is closely associated with hepatocyte malignant transformation [34] and is a specific oncofetal biomarker for HCC diagnosis [35].

A number of studies showed that a very high specificity (90–100%) associated with serum GPC-3 in patients with HCC, but the sensitivity of serum GPC-3 remained relatively low; however, if GPC-3 measured combined with AFP, sensitivity appears to improve [36, 37].

2.1.6. Proteomic profiling

The fields of proteomic-based biomarker discovery have applied advanced tools to identify early changes in protein and metabolite expression in HCC. Although, with robust validation, it is anticipated that from these candidates will rise a high-performance noninvasive test able to diagnose early HCC and related condition, a meta-analysis which is reviewed 22 studies, showed only six assessed the diagnostic performance of the biomarker candidates proposed [38]. Therefore, these biomarkers have not been currently recommended for surveillance or diagnosis.

2.1.7. Other serum markers

Other serum markers of HCC that have been studied include the following:

- Tumor-associated isoenzymes of gamma-glutamyl transpeptidase: Isoenzymes were present in 42% of hepatocellular carcinoma patients with a normal serum alpha-fetoprotein concentration and in 50% of those with a non-diagnostic value [39].
- Urinary transforming growth factor beta-1: Transforming Growht Factor (TGF)-beta1 showed a high specificity (99%), but the sensitivity was 53.1%. The determination of both markers TGF-beta1 and AFP in parallel significantly increased the diagnostic accuracy (90.1%) and sensitivity (84%), with a high specificity (98%) and positive likelihood ratio [40].
- Serum alpha-L-fucosidase activity [41].
- Human carboxylesterase 1 [42].
- Acetylcarnitine [43].

2.2. Imaging studies

Imaging studies have main role to make a diagnosis of HCC. While Japan, and KLCSG-NCC guidelines' recommendations are based on serum biomarkers and imaging studies, APASL,

EASL guideline and ASLD guidelines' recommendations are just based on imaging findings for diagnosis of HCC. US, CT, MRI, and angiography are the imaging tests which are most commonly used for the diagnosis of HCC. Basically, a unique dynamic radiological behavior (contrast uptake in the arterial phase and early washout on portal phase or delayed phase by CT, MRI, angiography, or contrast-enhanced US) represented the backbone of radiological diagnosis of early HCC [2–6].

HCC can have a variety of size and appearances on imaging studies; such as small hypo-hyper vascular nodules or massive mass, which may have necrosis, fat and/or calcification, nodular multiple masses of variable attenuation which may also have central necrosis, and infiltrative diffuse lesion [44].

2.2.1. Ultrasound

US is the preferred modality for surveillance of HCC in patients with chronic liver disease, and if a lesion is found on US, the lesion/lesions is/are evaluated by advance imaging tests [2–6].

While US has many advantages including low-cost, noninvasive, high availability, and high specificity, it has several disadvantages such as low sensitivity and depending on the operator. Thus, US should be used as a screening test, not as a diagnostic test for HCC. Otherwise, contrast-enhanced ultrasound (CEUS) can be used as a diagnostic test because it is as sensitive as dynamic CT or MRI in the diagnosis of HCC [4].

HCC can be appeared variable imaging structure; mostly small focal HCC appears hypoechoic compared with normal liver, larger lesions which are heterogeneous due to fibrosis, fatty change, necrosis, and calcification [45]. A peripheral halo of hypoechogenicity may be seen with focal fatty sparing, diffuse lesion which may be difficult to identify or distinguish from background cirrhosis [46].

2.2.2. Computerized tomography

Accurate technical performance of 4-phase CT scanning with imaging in the hepatic arterial and venous–portal venous, as well as delayed contrast images, is extremely important to characterize the lesions in detecting HCC because there are sequential changes in the supplying vessels and hemodynamic state during hepatocarcinogenesis [47]. If early vascular imaging is not performed, some lesions can be missed. It is important to use high injection rates and appropriate bolus timing. Sensitivity of good-quality 4-phase CT scanning for the detection of patients with tumors is 60–94.4%, in tumor larger than 1 cm, and its sensitivity reduced by 33–45% for detecting tumors smaller than 1 cm [48]. The hallmark of HCC during CT scan is the presence of arterial enhancement followed by washout meaning becoming indistinct or hypoattenuating of the tumor in the portal-venous and/or delayed. The presence of arterial enhancement followed by washout has a sensitivity and specificity of 90 and 95%, respectively [49–52].

Small, arterially enhancing nodules are common in the cirrhotic liver, and majority of these nodules are benign [53, 54]. Thus, every attempt, including imaging follow-up or biopsy, should be made to characterize these nodules [55].

In patients with HCC, unenhanced CT typically shows an isohypodense mass. If the mass is large, central areas of necrosis may be seen that are typically hypodense during this imaging phase.

In the hepatic arterial phase, HCCs typically are hyperdense (relative to hepatic parenchyma) and arterioportal shunt can occur as they are hypervascular tumors. Therefore, wedge-shaped perfusion abnormality due to arterioportal shunts can be seen and can result in a focal fatty change in the normal liver or focal fatty sparing in the diffusely fatty liver [56]. A halo of focal fatty sparing may also be seen around an HCC in an otherwise fatty liver [57].

The portal venous phase coincides with peak parenchymal enhancement is characterized by enhancement of hepatic veins as well as portal veins. In this phase, small lesions may be isodense or hypodense and distinguish from the parenchyma is difficult, as the remainder of the liver increases in attenuation. Larger lesions with necrotic regions remain hypodense [58].

The portal venous and delayed phases can also evaluate nodule diameter, depicting hypovascular nodules including low- or high-grade dysplastic nodules, early HCCs, and well-differentiated HCC. Portal blood flow may be maintained in some cases of dysplastic nodules and early HCC but reduced in other nodules, although the pathology remains because of early HCC, in which arterial blood flow has not yet increased. In addition, these phases can also identify complication of HCC, such as portal venous or hepatic invasion and vascular thrombosis [59]. Moreover, CT can be assessed to establish for other complications such as bleeding and hemoperitoneum.

A vascular mass or a large necrotic mass strongly suggests HCC; however, other hepatic lesions, benign or malignant, can mimic HCC on CT. On the other hand, false-negative CT imaging also can occur. In case of a cirrhotic liver with elevated AFP, and if the diagnosis is not absolute, MRI or other imaging modalities can assist in this differentiation.

2.2.3. Magnetic resonance imaging

MRI is the best test for evaluating HCC in patients with liver lesion detected by abnormal US. HCC appearance varies on MRI depending on multiple factors, such as hemorrhage, degree of fibrosis, histologic pattern, degree of necrosis, and the amount of fatty change.

HCC on T1-weighted images may be isointense, hypointense, or hyperintense relative to the liver. On T2-weighted images, HCC is usually hyperintense. Precontrast and postcontrast MRI has a 70–85% chance of detecting a solitary mass of HCC [60]. However, MRI sensitivity is the lowest when evaluating tumors <2 cm in diameter [51].

MRI can help differentiate cirrhotic nodules from HCC: (1) If the mass is bright on T2-weighted images, it is HCC until proven otherwise; (2) if the mass is dark on T1- and T2-weighted images, it is a siderotic regenerative nodule or siderotic dysplastic nodule; (3) if the mass is bright on T1-weighted images and dark or isointense on T2-weighted images, it is a dysplastic nodule or low-grade HCC [61].

Hepatocyte-specific contrast-enhanced MRI including such as gadolinium-enhanced MRI typically demonstrates an increasing number of subcentimetre cirrhotic nodules and that are often confirmed as HCCs or high-grade dysplastic nodules by these techniques [62]. The diagnosis can be confirmed as HCC nodules if these subcentimetre hypervascular nodules show arterial phase enhancement and "washout", diffusion restriction or hyperintensity on T2-weighted imaging and hypointensity on the hepatobiliary phase.

However, dysplastic nodules and, less likely, regenerative nodules can show similar enhancement. The degree of enhancement varies, particularly with the degree of necrosis in larger tumors. In addition, a "flash filling" haemangioma can have rapid arterial enhancement but could be differentiated by lack of washout on delayed images. Besides, keep in mind that gadolinium-based contrast agents have been linked to the development of nephrogenic systemic fibrosis or nephrogenic fibrosing dermopathy [63].

Recent studies showed that contrast agents other than gadolinium-based contrast media might demonstrate HCC. Super paramagnetic iron oxide (SPIO) particles used alone or in conjunction with gadolinium-based contrast agents [64] have been shown to be highly sensitive for the detection of HCC, particularly for small tumors. Double-contrast MR imaging (SPIO and gadolinium) is highly sensitive (92%) in the diagnosis of hepatocellular carcinomas of 10 mm or larger, but success in the definition of tumors smaller than 10 mm is still problematic [64, 65]. When uptake by Kupffer cells is reduced in the Kupffer phase of SPIO-enhanced MRI, malignancy should be highly suspected [64, 66].

A recent study showed that dynamic gadobenate dimeglumine (which is hepatocyte selective agent and shows extracellular distribution)-enhanced MRI has a sensitivity of 80–85% and a positive predictive value of 65–66% in the detection of HCC. The technique, however, is of limited value for detecting and characterizing lesions smaller than 1 cm in diameter [67].

The only hepatocyte-selective contrast agent that has been approved for clinical use is mangafodipir trisodium can evaluate questionable lesions in the liver. Mangafodipir trisodium is taken up by normal hepatocytes and masses that contain hepatocytes, causing increased signal intensity on T1-weighted images. This agent may help differentiate a tumor of hepatocellular origin, such as HCC, from secondary hepatic masses [68].

Although MRI is the most useful test to make a diagnosis, the nodules sometimes might not distinguish. In case the nodules have not specific features of HCC and the diagnosis is still unclear, advance imaging modalities or histological examination is needed.

2.2.4. Other imaging modalities

The less invasive imaging studies including dynamic CT, MRI, and CEUS have replaced conventional angiography for the diagnosis of HCC [69]. The role of positron emission tomography (PET) in the diagnostic and staging evaluation of HCC still remains uncertain. Several studies have suggested a role for [18F] fluorodeoxyglucose (FDG)-PET scanning for the detection of primary HCCs, tumor staging, assessing response to therapy, and for predicting prognosis as an adjunct to CT [70, 71]. The sensitivity of PET in diagnosis of HCC was 55% compared with 90% for CT scanning, although only PET detected some tumors (including distant metastases). Well-differentiated and low-grade tumors had lower activity on PET and correspondingly lower PET scores [71, 72]. However, FDG-PET might be a useful imaging modality for identifying extrahepatic metastases, although sensitivity is limited for lesions 1 cm or smaller [73].

2.3. Pathology

Pathological diagnosis of HCC is recommended for all nodules occurring in non-cirrhotic livers, and for those patients with inconclusive or atypical imaging appearance in cirrhotic livers. While taking a biopsy in lesions 1–2 cm and in lesions >2 cm with atypical vascularization on dynamic imaging was recommended by EASL, ASLD, and Japan guideline, APASL and KLCSG-NCC guidelines recommend either biopsy or follow-up could be used for indeterminate nodules on imaging workup [2–7].

Sensitivity of liver biopsy depends upon location, size, and expertise and might range between 70 and 90% for all tumor sizes. However, there is no recommendation on prioritizing strategy for indeterminate nodules. The issue is also related to the need of risk stratification of atypical nodules in cirrhosis using ancillary findings. Importantly, "threshold growth" is included as a main diagnostic criterion in LI-RADS and the Organ Procurement and Transplantation Network (OPTN) system introduced by the United Network for Organ Sharing (UNOS). OPTN-UNOS guidelines allow the diagnosis of arterial-phase hyperenhancing HCCs using threshold growth, defined as growth >50% in ≤6 months [74].

Pathological diagnosis is particularly complex for small nodules because minute biopsy specimens may not contain intratumoral portal tracts, thus precluding the detection of stromal invasion. Therefore, core biopsy is commonly used to diagnosis for these small nodules. Core liver biopsy is definitely superior to fine-needle aspiration, because the increased amount of tissue obtained is appropriate for the valuation of both architectural and cytologic features. Furthermore, the tissue block obtained obtains materials for marker studies. Fine-needle aspiration is usually used for the evaluation of large lesions that are likely to be moderately to poorly differentiate [75].

The histologic appearance of HCC can range from well differentiated (with individual hepatocytes appearing nearly identical to normal hepatocytes) to poorly differentiated lesions consisting of large multinucleate anaplastic tumor giant cells. Central necrosis of large tumors is common. Bile globules and acidophilic (hyaline) inclusions are occasionally present.

In some cases, dysplasia rather than carcinoma is diagnosed. There is an ongoing debate about the usefulness of various grades of dysplasia in predicting the ultimate development of HCC in dysplastic nodules.

In case of, the diagnosis is not clearly HCC, and sample should be stained with CD34, CK7, glypican 3, HSP-70, and glutamine synthetase to improve diagnostic accuracy [3]. Additional staining can be considered to detect progenitor cell features (K19 and EpCAM) or assess neovascularization (CD34) [2].

3. Summary

Early diagnosis of HCC is too important because early diagnosis of HCC provides curative treatment of HCC. The risk population for HCC should be determined and these patients should be entered into a surveillance program. When a nodule/nodules detected, convenient test should be used to identify the nodule. Recent guidelines are practical and recommend noninvasive criteria in terms of implementing diagnostic criteria using four-phase CT or contrast-enhanced MRI, and establishing criteria for subcentimetre-sized HCCs. Although there are several remaining issues including diagnostic criteria of non-hypervascular hypointense nodules, almost all suspicious lesion of liver can be defined by serum markers, imaging series, and contribution of biopsy because the characteristics of HCC are sufficiently clear.

Conflict of interest

No conflict of interest was declared by the authors.

Financial disclosure

The authors declared that this study has received no financial support.

Author details

Ayse Kefeli[1*], Sebahat Basyigit[2] and Abdullah Ozgur Yeniova[1]

*Address all correspondence to: aysekefeli@hotmail.com

1 Gastroenterology Department, Gaziosmanpasa University, Tokat, Turkey

2 Gastroenterology Department, Artvin State Hospital, Artvin, Turkey

References

[1] Jemal A, Bray F, Center MM, Ferlay J, Ward E, Forman CA. Global cancer statistics. Cancer J Clin. 2011;61(2):69.

[2] European Association for the Study of the Liver, European Organisation for Research and Treatment of Cancer. EASL-EORTC clinical practice guidelines: management of hepatocellular carcinoma. J Hepatol. 2012;56:908–943.

[3] Bruix J, Sherman M. American Association for the Study of Liver Diseases. Management of hepatocellular carcinoma: an update. Hepatology. 2011;53:1020–1022.

[4] Omata M, Lesmana L, Tateishi R, Chen P,Lin S et al. Asian Pacific Association for the Study of the Liver consensus recommendations on hepatocellular carcinoma. Hepatol Int. 2010;4:439–474

[5] Kudo M, Matsui O, Izumi N, Iijima H, Kadoya M, Imai Y, et al. JSH consensus-based clinical practice guidelines for the management of hepatocellular carcinoma: 2014 update by the Liver Cancer Study Group of Japan. Liver Cancer. 2014;3:458–468.

[6] Korean Liver Cancer Study Group (KLCSG); National Cancer Center, Korea (NCC) 2014 Korean Liver Cancer Study Group-National Cancer Center Korea practice guideline for the management of hepatocellular carcinoma. Korean J Radiol. 2015;16:465–522.

[7] Sangiovanni A, Del Ninno E, Fasani P, De Fazio C, Ronchi G, et al. Increased survival of cirrhotic patients with a hepatocellular carcinoma detected during surveillance. Gastroenterology. 2004;126(4):1005–1014.

[8] American College of Radiology. Liver imaging reporting and data system (LI-RADS). American College of Radiology. [Accessed August 1, 2015]. Web site. http://www.acr.org/Quality-Safety/Resources/LIRADS Published May 25, 2014.

[9] El-Bahrawy M. Alpha-fetoprotein-producing non-germ cell tumours of the female genital tract. Eur J Cancer. 2010;46:1317.

[10] Collier J, Sherman M. Screening for hepatocellular carcinoma. Hepatology. 1998;27:273.

[11] Wu JT. Serum alpha-fetoprotein and its lectin reactivity in liver diseases: a review. Ann Clin Lab Sci. 1990;20:98.

[12] Chen DS, Sung JL, Sheu JC, Lai MY, How SW, et al. Serum alpha-fetoprotein in the early stage of human hepatocellular carcinoma. Gastroenterology. 1984;86:1404.

[13] Colombo M, de Franchis R, Del Ninno E, Sangiovanni A, De Fazio C et al. Hepatocellular carcinoma in Italian patients with cirrhosis. N Engl J Med. 1991;325:675.

[14] Gupta S, Bent S, Kohlwes J. Test characteristics of alpha-fetoprotein for detecting hepatocellular carcinoma in patients with hepatitis C. A systematic review and critical analysis. Ann Intern Med. 2003;139:46.

[15] Lee E1, Edward S, Singal AG, Lavieri MS, Volk M. Improving screening for hepatocellular carcinoma by incorporating data on levels of α-fetoprotein, over time. Clin Gastroenterol Hepatol. 2013;11:437–440.

[16] Mehta A, Singal AG. Hepatocellular carcinoma surveillance: does alpha-fetoprotein have a role? Gastroenterology. 2015;149(3):816–8817.

[17] Ioannou GN, Perkins JD, Carithers RL Jr. Liver transplantation for hepatocellular carcinoma: impact of the MELD allocation system and predictors of survival. Gastroenterology. 2008;134:1342.

[18] Pomfret EA, Washburn K, Wald C, Nalesnik MA, Douglas D et al. Report of a national conference on liver allocation in patients with hepatocellular carcinoma in the United States. Liver Transpl. 2010;16:262.

[19] Mizejewski GJ. Alpha-fetoprotein structure and function: relevance to isoforms, epitopes, and conformational variants. Exp Biol Med. 2001;226(5):377–408.

[20] Toyoda H, Kumada T, Tada T, Kaneoka Y, Maeda A, et al. Clinical utility of highly sensitive Lens culinaris agglutinin-reactive alpha-fetoprotein in hepatocellular carcinoma patients with alpha-fetoprotein <20 ng/mL. Cancer Sci. 2011;102(5):1025–1031.

[21] Oda K, Ido A, Tamai T, Matsushita M, Kumagai K, et al. Highly sensitive lens culinaris agglutinin-reactive α-fetoprotein is useful for early detection of hepatocellular carcinoma in patients with chronic liver disease. Oncol Rep. 2011;26(5):1227–1233.

[22] Chen X, Ba Y, Ma L, Cai X, Yin Y, et al. Characterization of microRNAs in serum: a novel class of biomarkers for diagnosis of cancer and other diseases. Cell Res. 2008;18(10): 997–1006.

[23] Yu L, Gong X, Sun L, Zhou Q, Lu B, Zhu L. The circular RNA Cdr1as act as an oncogene in hepatocellular carcinoma through targeting miR-7 expression. PLoS One. 2016;11(7):e0158347.

[24] Arroyo JD, Chevillet JR, Kroh EM, Ruf IK, Pritchard CC, et al. Argonaute2 complexes carry a population of circulating microRNAs independent of vesicles in human plasma. Proc Natl Acad Sci USA. 2011;108:5003–5008.

[25] Boeri M, Verri C, Conte D, Roz L, Modena P, et al. MicroRNA signatures in tissues and plasma predict development and prognosis of computed tomography detected lung cancer. Proc Natl Acad Sci USA. 2011;108:3713–3718.

[26] Cho WC. MicroRNAs: potential biomarkers for cancer diagnosis, prognosis and targets for therapy. Int J Biochem Cell Biol. 2010;42:1273–1281.

[27] Wen Y, Han J, Chen J, Dong J, Xia Y, et al. Plasma miRNAs as early biomarkers for detecting hepatocellular carcinoma. Int J Cancer. 2015;137(7):1679–1690. doi:10.1002/ijc.29544.

[28] Khoury S, Tran N. Circulating microRNAs: potential biomarkers for common malignancies. Biomarkers Med. 2015;9:131–151.

[29] Carr B, Kanke F, Wise M, Satomura S. Clinical evaluation of Lens culinaris agglutinin-reactive alpha-fetoprotein and des-gamma-carboxyprothrombin in histologically proven hepatocellular carcinoma in the United States. Dig Dis Sci. 2007;52:776–778.

[30] Ishii M, Gama H, Chida N, Ueno Y, Shinzawa H, et al. South Tohoku District Study Group. Am J Gastroenterol? 2000;95(4):1036–1040.

[31] Bertino G, Ardiri AM, Calvagno GS, Bertino N, Boemi PM. Prognostic and diagnostic value of des-gamma-carboxyprothrombin in liver cancer. Drug News Perspect. 2010;23(8):498–508.

[32] Durazo FA, Blatt LM, Corey WG, Lin JH, Han S, et al. Des-gamma-carboxyprothrombin, alpha-fetoprotein and AFP-L3 in patients with chronic hepatitis, cirrhosis and hepatocellular carcinoma. J Gastroenterol Hepatol. 2008;23:1541–1548.

[33] Aoyagi Y, Oguro M, Yanagi M, Mita Y, Suda T, et al. Clinical significance of simultaneous determinations of alpha-fetoprotein and des-gamma-carboxyprothrombin in monitoring recurrence in patients with hepatocellular carcinoma. Cancer. 1996;77(9): 1781.

[34] Yao M, Yao DF, Bian YZ, Zhang CG, Qiu LW, et al. Oncofetal antigen glypican-3 as a promising early diagnostic marker for hepatocellular carcinoma. Hepatobiliary Pancreat Dis Int. 2011;10:289–294.

[35] Li B, Liu H, Shang HW, Li P, Li N, Ding HG. Diagnostic value of glypican-3 in alpha fetoprotein negative hepatocellular carcinoma patients. Afr Health Sci. 2013;13:703–709.

[36] Hippo Y, Watanabe K, Watanabe A, Midorikawa Y, Yamamoto S, et al. Identification of soluble NH2-terminal fragment of glypican-3 as a serological marker for early-stage hepatocellular carcinoma. Cancer Res. 2004;64(7):2418–2423.

[37] Hui Liu, Peng Li, Yun Zhai, Chun-FengQu, Li-Jie Zhang, et al. Diagnostic value of glypican-3 in serum and liver for primary hepatocellular carcinoma. World J Gastroenterol. 2010;16(35):4410–4415.

[38] Kimhofer T, Fye H, Taylor-Robinson S, Thursz M, and Holmes E. Proteomic and metabonomic biomarkers for hepatocellular carcinoma: a comprehensive review. Br J Cancer. 2015;112(7):1141–1156.

[39] Kew MC, Wolf P, Whittaker D, Rowe P. Tumour-associated isoenzymes of gamma-glutamyl transferase in the serum of patients with hepatocellular carcinoma. Br J Cancer. 1984;50(4):451.

[40] Tsai JF, Jeng JE, Chuang LY, Yang ML, Ho MS, et al. Clinical evaluation of urinary transforming growth factor-beta1 and serum alpha-fetoprotein as tumour markers of hepatocellular carcinoma. Br J Cancer. 1997;75(10):1460.

[41] Takahashi H, Saibara T, Iwamura S, Tomita A, Maeda T, et al. Serum alpha-L-fucosidase activity and tumor size in hepatocellular carcinoma. Hepatology. 1994;19(6):1414.

[42] Na K, Jeong SK, Lee MJ, Cho SY, Kim SA, et al. Human liver carboxylesterase 1 outperforms alpha-fetoprotein as biomarker to discriminate hepatocellular carcinoma from other liver diseases in Korean patients. Int J Cancer. 2013;133(2):408–415.

[43] Lu Y, Li N, Gao L, Xu YJ, Huang C, et al. Acetylcarnitine is a candidate diagnostic and prognostic biomarker of hepatocellular carcinoma. Canc Res. 2016;76(10):2912–2920.

[44] Reynolds AR, Furlan A, Fetzer DT, asatomi E, Borhani AA, et-al. Infiltrative hepatocellular carcinoma: what radiologists need to know. Radiographics. 2015;35(2):371–386.

[45] Lau WY. Hepatocellular Carcinoma. World Scientific Pub Pte Ltd Co Inc., Singapore 596224; 2008. ISBN: 9812707999. P. 193–199

[46] Malhi H, Grant EG, Duddalwar V. Contrast-enhanced ultrasound of the liver and kidney. Radiol. Clin. North Am. 2014;52(6):1177–1190.

[47] Kim TK, Jang HJ, Wilson SR. Imaging diagnosis of hepato-cellular carcinoma with differentiation from other pathology. Clin Liver Dis. 2005;9:253–279.

[48] Ma Y, Zhang XL, Li XY, Zhang L, Su HH, Zhan CY. Value of computed tomography and magnetic resonance imaging in diagnosis and differential diagnosis of small hepatocellular carcinoma. Nan Fang Yi Ke Da XueXueBao. 2008;28(12):2235–2238.

[49] Marrero JA, Hussain HK, Nghiem HV, Umar R, Fontana RJ, Lok AS. Improving the prediction of hepatocellular carcinoma in cirrhotic patients with an arterially-enhancing liver mass. Liver Transpl. 2005;11:281–289.

[50] Kim SH, Choi BI, Lee JY, Kim SJ, So YH, Eun HW. Diagnostic accuracy of multi-/single-detector CT and contrast- enhanced MRI in the detection of hepatocellular carcinomas meeting the Milan criteria before liver transplantation. Intervirology. 2008;51(Suppl 1): 52–60.

[51] Krinsky GA, Lee VS, Theise ND, Weinreb JC, Rofsky NM, et al. Hepatocellular carcinoma and dysplastic nodules in patients with cirrhosis: prospective diagnosis with MR imaging and explantation correlation. Radiology. 2001;219:445–454.

[52] Ebara M, Ohto M, Watanabe Y, Kimura K, Saisho H, et al. Diagnosis of small hepatocellular carcinoma: correlation of MR imaging and tumor histologic studies. Radiology. 1986;159:371–377.

[53] Holland AE, Hecht EM, Hahn WY, Kim DC, Babb JS, et al. Importance of small (B20-mm) enhancing lesions seen only during the hepatic arterial phase at MR imaging of the cirrhotic liver: evaluation and comparison with whole explanted liver. Radiology. 2005;237:938–944.

[54] Baron RL, Peterson MS. From the RSNA refresher courses: screening the cirrhotic liver for hepatocellular carcinoma with CT and MR imaging: opportunities and pitfalls. Radiographics. 2001;21:117–132.

[55] Willatt JM, Hussain HK, Adusumilli S, Marrero JA. MR Imaging of hepatocellular carcinoma in the cirrhotic liver: challenges and controversies. Radiology. 2008;247:311–330.

[56] Choi BI, Lee KH, Han JK, Lee JM. Hepatic arterioportal shunts: dynamic CT and MR features. Korean J Radiol. 2002;3(1):1–15.

[57] Kim KW, Kim MJ, Lee SS, Kim HJ, Shin YM, et-al. Sparing of fatty infiltration around focal hepatic lesions in patients with hepatic steatosis: sonographic appearance with CT and MRI correlation. AJR Am J Roentgenol. 2008;190(4):1018–1027.

[58] Hong HS, Kim HS, Kim MJ, De Becker J, Mitchell DG, Kanematsu M. Single breath-hold multiarterial dynamic MRI of the liver at 3T using a 3D fat-suppressed keyhole technique. J Magn Reson Imaging. 2008;28(2):396–402.

[59] Takayasu K, Furukawa H, Wakao F, Muramatsu Y, Abe H et al. CT diagnosis of early hepatocellular carcinoma: sensitivity, findings, and CT-pathologic correlation. AJR Am J Roentgenol. 1995;164(4):885–890.

[60] Bialecki ES, Di Bisceglie AM. Diagnosis of hepatocellular carcinoma. HPB (Oxford). 2005;7(1):26–34.

[61] Hanna RF, Aguirre DA, Kased N, Emery SC, Peterson MR, Sirlin CB. Cirrhosis-associated hepatocellular nodules: correlation of histopathologic and MR imaging features. RadioGraphics. 2008;28(3):747–769.

[62] Golfieri R, Grazioli L, Orlando E, Dormi A, Lucidi V, et al. Which is the best MRI marker of malignancy for atypical cirrhotic nodules: hypointensity in hepatobiliary phase alone or combined with other features? Classification after Gd-EOB-DTPA administration. J Magn Reson Imaging. 2012;36:648–657.

[63] Marckmann P, Skov L, Rossen K, Dupont A, Damholt MB, et al. Nephrogenic systemic fibrosis: suspected causative role of gadodiamide used for contrast-enhanced magnetic resonance imaging. J Am SocNephrol. 2006;17(9):2359–2362.

[64] Bhartia B, Ward J, Guthrie JA, Robinson PJ. Hepatocellular carcinoma in cirrhotic livers: double-contrast thin-section MR imaging with pathologic correlation of explanted tissue. AJR Am J Roentgenol. 2003;180:577–584.

[65] Ward J, Guthrie JA, Scott DJ, Atchley J, Wilson D, et al. Hepatocellular carcinoma in the cirrhotic liver: double- contrast MR imaging for diagnosis. Radiology. 2000;216:154–162.

[66] Imai Y, Murakami T, Yoshida S, Nishikawa M, Ohsawa M, et al. Super paramagnetic iron oxide-enhanced magnetic resonance images of hepatocellular carcinoma: correlation with histological grading. Hepatology. 2000;32:205–212.

[67] Choi SH, Lee JM, Yu NC, Suh KS, Jang JJ, et al. Hepatocellular carcinoma in liver transplantation candidates: detection with gadobenate dimeglumine-enhanced MRI. AJR Am J Roentgenol. 2008;191:529–536.

[68] Semelka RC, Helmberger TK. Contrast agents for MR imaging of the liver. Radiology. 2001;218:27–38.

[69] Kanematsu M, Hoshi H, Imaeda T, Murakami T, Inaba Y, et al. Detection and characterization of hepatic tumors: value of combined helical CT hepatic arteriography and CT during arterial portography. AJR Am J Roentgenol. 1997;168:1193–1198.

[70] Yang SH, Suh KS, Lee HW, Cho EH, Cho JY, et al. The role of (18)F-FDG-PET imaging for the selection of liver transplantation candidates among hepatocellular carcinoma patients. Liver Transpl. 2006;12:1655–1660.

[71] Khan MA, Combs CS, Brunt EM, Lowe VJ, Wolverson MK, et al. Positron emission tomography scanning in the evaluation of hepatocellular carcinoma. J Hepatol. 2000;32:792–797.

[72] Trojan J, Schroeder O, Raedle J, Baum RP, Herrmann G, et al. Fluorine-18 FDG positron emission tomography for imaging of hepatocellular carcinoma. Am J Gastroenterol. 1999;94:3314–3319.

[73] Sugiyama M, Sakahara H, Torizuka T, Kanno T, Nakamura F, et al. 18F-FDG PET in the detection of extra- hepatic metastases from hepatocellular carcinoma. J Gastroenterol. 2004;39:961–968.

[74] Wald C, Russo MW, Heimbach JK, Hussain HK, Pomfret EA, Bruix J. New OPTN/UNOS policy for liver transplant allocation: standardization of liver imaging, diagnosis, classification, and reporting of hepatocellular carcinoma. Radiology. 2013;266:376–382.

[75] International Consensus Group for Hepatocellular Neoplasia. Pathologic diagnosis of early hepatocellular carcinoma: a report of the international consensus group for hepatocellular neoplasia. Hepatol. 2009;49:658–664.

Chapter 7

Onco-Surgical Management of Liver Metastases from Colorectal Cancer

Irinel Popescu and Sorin Tiberiu Alexandrescu

Additional information is available at the end of the chapter

http://dx.doi.org/10.5772/65223

Abstract

Metastatic disease is the main cause of death in patients with colorectal cancer and the most frequent location of metastases is in the liver. The treatment of liver metastases of colorectal origin is multimodal and should be based on a multidisciplinary team decision. A systematic review of the literature revealed that the number of liver metastases, their maximum size, CEA level, advanced age of the patients, and presence of extrahepatic disease are no longer contraindications to liver resection. The resectability rate of colorectal liver metastases increased from 10 to almost 40%, enabling 5-year overall survival rates higher than 30%. Short-term and long-term results achieved by simultaneous resection (SR) are similar to those achieved by staged resections in patients with synchronous colorectal liver metastases. Whenever possible, major hepatectomies should be replaced by ultrasound-guided limited liver resections, and primary tumor should be approached in a minimally invasive manner. Even initially unresectable colorectal liver metastases could be rendered resectable by an aggressive multimodal approach ("two-stage" hepatectomies, hepatectomy after portal vein embolization/ligation, resection after conversion chemotherapy, and hepatectomy associated with ablation). The presence of extrahepatic metastases is no longer a contraindication to liver resection, when extrahepatic disease is resectable. Repeat hepatectomy improves survival in patients with recurrent liver metastases.

Keywords: colorectal liver metastases, liver resection, survival, liver re-resection, unresectable liver metastases

1. Introduction

Colorectal cancer is the third cause of cancer-related death among adult patients [1]. Most of the patients with colorectal carcinoma decease due to the metastatic disease, and only a small percentage of these patients die due to the complications of the primary tumor or other comorbidities. Thus, in order to increase the life expectancy of patients with colorectal cancer, it is mandatory to improve the therapeutic strategies addressed to the metastatic colorectal cancer (mCRC). Because more than two thirds of the patients with colorectal cancer will develop liver metastases during their lifetime, it is obvious that the improvements in the treatment of liver metastases will translate into higher survival rates for these patients [2].

In this chapter, the current therapeutic strategies and the potential future trends in the onco-surgical treatment of colorectal liver metastases (CLMs) are presented.

2. Treatment of liver metastases from colorectal cancer

Nowadays, the treatment of colorectal liver metastases is multimodal, including liver resection, ablative therapies, chemotherapy, targeted therapies, and interventional radiology (radioembolization, chemoembolization, and portal vein embolization).

The most recent studies revealed that the highest survival rates have been achieved by complete resection of CLMs. Thus, an international database including more than 25,000 patients treated for CLMs (collected from 313 centers all over the world) revealed that the 5-year overall survival (OS) rate achieved by liver resection was 42%, while the 5-year overall survival rate achieved by ablative therapies was 26% (p value < 0.001). Moreover, the 5-year overall survival rate achieved by nonsurgical therapies was only 6% (p value < 0.001) [3].

2.1. Pretherapeutic evaluation

The main objectives of pretherapeutic evaluation are as follows: (1) confirmation of the presence of liver metastases, (2) assessment of extrahepatic metastases, and (3) evaluation of liver metastases resectability.

2.1.1. Confirmation of liver metastases

The presence of metastatic disease should be determined in all the patients diagnosed with colorectal cancer, at the time of their primary tumor diagnosis. The metastases identified at that time are considered as synchronous metastases, as well as the metastases detected during the operation addressed to the primary tumor (even when they were not revealed by preoperative evaluation). However, patients without synchronous metastases who underwent a curative-intent resection of the colorectal primary tumor should be periodically followed-up because up to 50% of them will develop metastases of colorectal origin [4]. These metastases are considered as metachronous colorectal metastases.

The evaluation performed to diagnose metastases from colorectal cancer is based on the CT scan of the thorax, abdomen, and pelvis. Sometimes, when the CT scan cannot rule out the presence of liver metastases, magnetic resonance imaging (MRI) could be useful because its specificity is higher than that of CT scan.

http://dx.doi.org/10.5772/65223

2.1.2. *Assessment of extrahepatic metastases*

When the presence of extrahepatic disease is suspected, PET/CT should be performed in order to achieve a correct pretherapeutic evaluation. Moreover, in the past few years, the NCCN and ESMO guidelines suggested a routine performance of PET/CT scan in patients with resectable CLMs, to assess the extension of the disease [5].

Whenever the patient shows signs or symptoms suggestive for brain metastases, a head CT scan should be performed; similarly, when bone metastases are suspected, a bone scintigraphy is mandatory.

2.1.3. *Evaluation of liver metastases resectability*

The paradigm regarding the CLMs resectability has changed over the past two decades. Thus, in the early 1990s, the following situations were considered as contraindications for liver metastases resection: (a) the presence of more than four CLMs, (b) the size of liver metastases exceeding 5 cm of maximum diameter, (c) the presence of extrahepatic metastases, and (d) the advanced age of the patient (usually older than 70 years). During the past few years, one by one, each of these contraindications has been challenged by the results reported by different authors, based on smaller or larger cohorts of patients undergoing liver resection for CLMs exceeding these criteria.

At present, the largest database including patients with CLMs who underwent surgery with the intention of curative resection is LiverMetSurvey—an international registry of patients operated in 313 centers from 70 countries [3]. According to the report released by the managers of this database in December 2015, important observations regarding the usefulness of liver resection in different groups of patients were presented.

a. Although the survival rates achieved in patients with up to 3 CLMs were statistically significant, higher than those reported in patients with 4 or more CLMs, even in patients with more than 7 CLMs, the 5-year overall survival (OS) rate (achieved by curative-intent hepatectomy) was 26% [3]. These results suggested that the number of CLMs should not represent a contraindication to liver resection.

b. Regarding the size of CLMs, although the highest survival rates were achieved in the group of patients with liver metastases lower than 3 cm, the 5-year OS rates were higher than 35% also in patients with CLMs larger than 5 cm [3].

c. In patients with synchronous hepatic and extrahepatic metastases who underwent curative-intent surgery for both liver metastases and extrahepatic metastases, the 5-year OS rate was 22%, significantly lower than those achieved in patients with liver-only metastases (5-year OS rate—44%). However, the 22% survival rate in 5 years is obviously higher than the survival rates achieved by palliative treatment in patients with mCRC (6% rate in 5 years according to the same database) [3]. Thus, the presence of concomitant extrahepatic disease is no longer considered as a contraindication to surgery, when the entire metastatic burden could be resected.

d. Because the life expectancy increased significantly in most countries, more and more elderly patients, with a good clinical status, were diagnosed with CLMs. The results presented by the LiverMetSurvey database revealed that in patients older than 70 years, the 5-year OS rate was 38% [3]. Thus, curative-intent hepatectomy is a worthwhile operation even in elderly patients and the age should not be considered as a contraindication for liver resection if the patient's performance status is good.

Because almost all the traditional contraindications to liver resection are no longer valid nowadays, the definition of the CLMs resectability should be based on a technical/practical point of view, taking into account what remains after liver resection.

At present, technical criteria of resectability include the anticipated ability to [6]

1. perform a margin-negative resection (R0);
2. preserve at least two contiguous liver segments with adequate vascular inflow, outflow, and biliary drainage;
3. preserve adequate future liver remnant (FLR) volume (at least 20–30% of functional liver volume in patients with normal liver and 30–35% of functional liver volume in patients pretreated with chemotherapy).

Moreover, in patients with a marginal FLR volume and/or underlying liver disease, the ability of FLR to function effectively should be assessed (frequently based on the appropriate regenerative response after portal vein embolization – PVE) [6].

Based on these criteria, the indications of liver resection for CLMs broadened over the past two decades, providing increased resectability rates in patients with CLMs. Thus, at present, it is considered that among the patients newly diagnosed with CLMs, almost 25% are initially resectable, whereas 75% are initially unresectable metastases.

Regarding the potentiality to resect CLMs, ESMO classified the patients with liver metastases in four groups [7]:

Group 0: Primarily, technically R0-resectable liver metastases and no "biological" relative contraindications (e.g., progressive disease during neo-adjuvant treatment, etc.).

Group 1: Potentially resectable metastatic disease with curative intention.

Group 2: Disseminated disease, technically "never"/unlikely resectable.

Group 3: Never-resectable metastatic disease.

2.2. Initially resectable CLMs: Group 0

Regarding the onco-surgical approach to CLMs, there are some differences between patients presenting synchronous CLMs (SCLMs) and patients who develop metachronous CLMs (MCLMs). These different strategies should mainly take into account the concomitant presence of the primary tumor and liver metastases in patients with SCLMs and the need to remove both tumor locations.

2.2.1. Synchronous colorectal liver metastases

The first approach used in patients with SCLMs is consisted of two stages. During the first stage, the resection of the primary tumor is performed; and subsequently, usually 2–3 months later, the resection of liver metastases is performed. This strategy is called ***delayed liver resection (DR)*** and theoretically presents a few advantages as presented below.

Due to the progress made in liver surgery and anesthesiology, in the late 1990s some centers started to perform, in selected patients, simultaneous resection of the primary tumor and liver metastases. The advantages postulated by the promoters of this ***simultaneous resection approach (SR)*** include the comfort of the patient (who avoids two surgical procedures under general anesthesia), the avoidance of progression to unresectability of CLMs (which is possible in the DR approach, during the interval between the two operations), and it is cost-effective [8–10].

However, the partisans of the DR approach advocate that this strategy is based on two theoretical assumptions: (a) DR avoids the association of two resections, thus reduces the risks of postoperative complications and mortality, and increases the safety of the procedure; (b) the biological behavior of the tumor could be assessed during the observation period between the two operations, thus allowing a better selection of the patients and improving the oncologic outcome [11, 12].

2.2.1.1. Safety of the procedure

Although the SR was looked upon with caution during the first few years after its launch, the results reported over the past two decades revealed that in patients with colon tumors and liver metastases requiring minor hepatectomies, the morbidity and mortality rates achieved by SR were similar to those observed in patients undergoing DR [13–16].

However, if the primary tumor is complicated with perforation or obstruction, due to the poor clinical condition of the patient, it is advisable to avoid the simultaneous resection and this situation is considered a common reason for DR.

In patients with rectal tumors and/or requiring major hepatectomies, the SR is still controversial because some authors reported significantly higher morbidity and mortality rates after SR in such instances than those shown by DR [16]. By these reasons, a consensus conference on CLMs management suggested caution in performing SR in such patients and recommended a staged approach (either delayed liver resection or liver-first approach) [17].

The ***liver-first approach*** is a new surgical strategy that consists of initial resection of liver metastases and subsequent resection of the primary tumor [18]. This approach is recommended especially in patients with border-line resectable CLMs (**Figure 1**) and/or rectal cancers. The advantages of this new approach over the classical delayed liver resection are as follows:

- When CLMs are border-line resectable at the time of the diagnosis, if a DR is scheduled, there is a major risk of metastases progression after the primary tumor resection, making the metastases unresectable and missing the chance of a potentially curative resection. This scenario could be avoided by the initial removal of CLMs. Because, in such situations, the complete resection of metastases usually requires a major hepatectomy (**Figure 2**), it is recommended to avoid the performance of a simultaneous resection in order to decrease the postoperative morbidity and mortality rates. Thus, the resection of the primary tumor could usually be postponed for few weeks, with a low risk of developing primary tumor complications.

- Moreover, if the primary tumor involves the rectum, in order to decrease the risk of local recurrence, it is advisable to perform preoperative radiotherapy. Because during radiotherapy the patient does not receive Oxaliplatin or Irinotecan and the interval between the start of radiotherapy and the time of rectal resection is usually longer than 3 months, the risk of CLMs progression to unresectability is high. Thus, the initial resection of CLMs avoids their progression to unresectability and allows the optimal treatment of the primary tumor, offering the highest chance of survival to these patients (**Figure 3**).

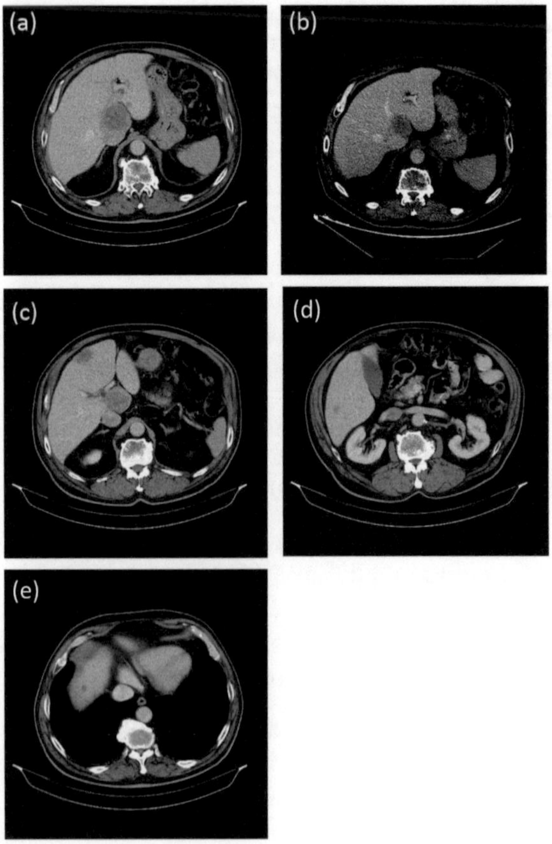

Figure 1. Abdominal CT scan of a 73-year-old patient with middle rectal adenocarcinoma and synchronous multiple liver metastases [5]: (a) segments 3 and 1 (caudate lobe) liver metastases; (b) the caudate lobe metastasis is adjacent to the inferior vena cava (IVC) and encases the middle hepatic vein; (c) segment 4 metastasis; (d) segment 6 metastasis; (e) segment 8 metastasis.

http://dx.doi.org/10.5772/65223

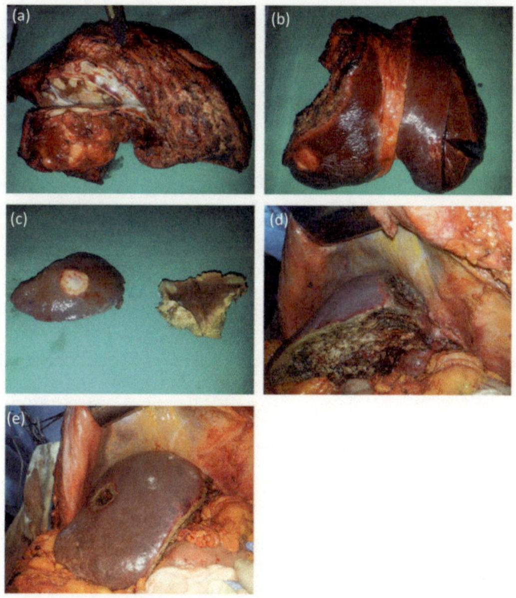

Figure 2. Liver-first approach (left hepatectomy extended to segment 1 and metastasectomies for the segment 6 and 8 CLMs): (a) specimen of left hepatectomy extended to segment 1, depicting the segment 1 metastasis with encasement of the middle hepatic vein; (b) the same specimen with segment 3 and 4 metastases; (c) specimens of metastasectomies for segment 6 and 8 CLMs; (d and e) intraoperative images of the remnant liver after complete resection of CLMs.

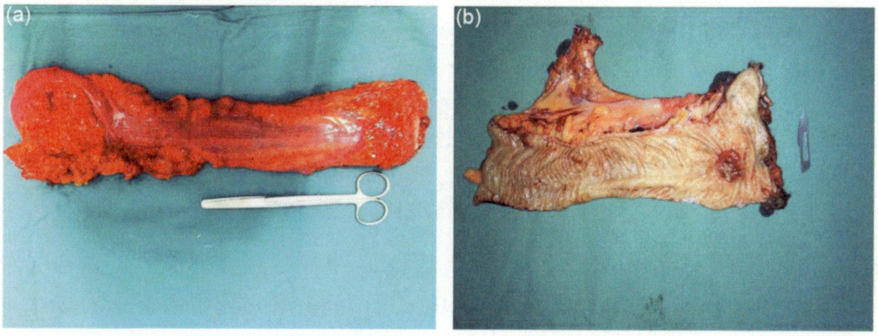

Figure 3. Specimen of low anterior rectal resection performed after short-course radiotherapy (the patient underwent radiotherapy after liver-first resection): (a) the specimen of low anterior rectal resection with total mesorectal excision; (b) the same specimen, transected (at least 2 cm distal resection margin).

2.2.1.2. Oncologic outcome

Regarding the postulated advantages offered by the "observation period," most of the series published until now revealed that the overall survival rates achieved by SR were similar to those achieved by staged resections [8, 13, 19]. Thus, the speculated advantage of "better selection of patients by DR" does not seem to be supported by the practice. This could be explained by the fact that most patients underwent chemotherapy between the two operations, and in the era of modern chemotherapy the progression-free survival rates are longer than 6 months [20]. Thus, the information provided by the "test of time" between the two operations is mitigated by the chemotherapy.

Moreover, a recent retrospective study, based on the results observed in patients enrolled in LiverMetSurvey, revealed that in patients with synchronous CLMs, the preoperative chemotherapy did not improve overall survival [21].

In conclusion, at present, most authors recommend the following approaches:

- Simultaneous resection (SR) in patients with uncomplicated colon tumors and synchronous CLMs requiring minor hepatectomies.
- Delayed resection (DR) in patients with obstruction or perforation of the primary tumor and synchronous CLMs.
- Liver-first approach in patients with border-line resectable CLMs (requiring major hepatectomies) and/or rectal carcinoma

2.2.2. Metachronous colorectal liver metastases

In patients with initially resectable metachronous CLMs, the up-front surgery could be recommended.

Preoperative chemotherapy may be useful especially in patients with a high clinical risk score (CRS). The clinical risk score is calculated by assigning one point to each of the following factors: multiple CLMs, metastases diameter larger than 5 cm, CEA level higher than 200 U/ml, node-positive status of primary tumor (pathological), and disease-free interval less than 12 months [22]. A recent study revealed that neo-adjuvant chemotherapy significantly improved the survival rate in patients with a high clinical risk score (CRS 3–5), whereas in patients with a low risk profile (CRS 0–2) neo-adjuvant chemotherapy might not be beneficial [23].

However, the postoperative (adjuvant) chemotherapy is universally recommended at present, being considered almost mandatory after resection of CLMs, irrespective of the time of their appearance (synchronous or metachronous). The goals of postoperative chemotherapy are to increase both the disease-free survival (DFS) and overall survival (OS) rates [5].

2.3. Potentially resectable CLMs: Group 1

In this group, those patients who cannot undergo a complete resection of CLMs at the time of diagnosis, but are resectable by applying several onco-surgical strategies are included.

Thus, the goal of the treatment in this group should be conversion to resectability.

The following strategies will be able to render resectable the initially unresectable CLMs:

2.3.1. *Liver resection following portal vein embolization or ligation*

When the complete resection of CLMs would leave in place at least two adjacent liver segments, but the FLR volume is not large enough to avoid the risk of postoperative liver failure, it might be possible to enlarge the volume of the FLR by performing portal vein ligation (PVL) or embolization (PVE) [24–26].

This strategy is especially useful in patients presenting CLMs confined to the right hemiliver and segment 4. In such instances, frequently the volume of segments 2 and 3 is lower than 25–30% of functional liver volume (FLV). The right portal branch ligation or embolization could induce the hypertrophy of segments 2–3 (FLR), thus ensuring a volume of the FLR higher than 25–30% of FLV in 2–8 weeks after the procedure [24, 27]. The same therapeutic approach could be applied in patients with CLMs confined to the right hemiliver and presenting a small left hemiliver (the volume of segments 2–4 is lower than 25–30% of the FLV).

The occlusion of the right portal branch will induce the atrophy of the right hemiliver and compensatory hypertrophy of the left hemiliver [28]. Thus, the ratio of FLR hypertrophy regularly ranges between 20 and 50% and the volume of segments 2 and 3 (or of the left hemiliver) will often exceed 25–30% of the FLV [24, 27, 29, 30]. Consequently, a right trisectionectomy or right hepatectomy could be safely performed in more than 60% of the patients undergoing PVE/PVL, achieving the 5-year overall survival rates higher than 30% [24, 27, 30, 31].

The evaluation of FLR and FLV is usually based on software-assisted image postprocessing programs that provide volume measurements taking into account the actual anatomy of a specific patient (identified by CT scan), where FLV = volume of the entire liver – volume of the tumor. FLR represents the volume of the segments that are planned to be left in place after the scheduled curative liver resection.

Unfortunately, in almost one third of these patients, the complete resection of the metastatic disease could not be achieved, either due to the insufficient hypertrophy of the FLR or due to the development of new metastases in the FLR during the interval between PVL/PVE and the scheduled hepatectomy [24, 27, 32].

In order to overcome these drawbacks of portal vein occlusion, recently, a new strategy has been launched, aiming to increase the resectability rates in such patients.

2.3.2. *ALPPS (associating liver partition and portal vein ligation for staged hepatectomy)*

This surgical approach consists of association of the right portal branch ligation with transection of liver parenchyma during the same operative procedure. It was observed that this strategy enables a more rapid and greater hypertrophy of the FLR [33–35]. Thus, 7–10 days after this operation, the percentage of FLR volume hypertrophy ranges between 40 and 80% [33, 35], allowing the subsequent performance of R0 resection in almost 90–100% of the patients subjected to this new approach [36, 37].

Moreover, it was proved that in patients who failed to achieve adequate FLR hypertrophy after PVE, the performance of ALPPS was effective, inducing a FLR gain that allowed subsequent R0 resection [37, 38].

Because the hypertrophy of the FLR produced by ALPPS is 11-fold faster than those induced by PVL/PVE [34], this new strategy allows the complete resection of the tumor in a shorter period of time (7–14 days after the first stage), providing additional advantages, such as: (1) decreases the risk of disease progression between the two stages of the operation [36, 39]; (2) allows a more rapid recovery of the patient, decreasing the length of hospital stay [36]; and (3) the adjuvant chemotherapy could be started sooner than in patients undergoing PVL/PVE [36].

The main disadvantage of ALPPS is the high rate of major postoperative complications (27–41%) and mortality (8–12.5%) [34, 35, 37, 40, 41]. To decrease the morbidity and mortality rates, some authors recommended avoiding the performance of ALPPS in patients older than 60 years and to circumvent the ligation of the right bile duct during the first operation [34, 40–42]. Other factors associated with a dismal outcome are obesity, poststage one biliary fistula, and infected/bilious peritoneal fluid at the time of the second-stage operation [37].

However, a thorough selection of patients and a meticulous surgical technique could overcome these drawbacks, allowing the complete resection of initially unresectable CLMs in most patients scheduled for this approach.

2.3.3. Two-stage liver resection

This strategy is mainly recommended in patients presenting multiple bilobar CLMs, whose resection is not feasible during a single operative procedure because the volume of the remnant liver would be too small to avoid the postoperative liver failure [28, 43, 44]. Thus, the goal of complete resection of CLMs could be achieved by combining two liver resections. During the first operation, the liver metastases from the FLR (usually left hemiliver or segments 2–3) are resected by metastasectomies, sparing as much as possible of the remnant functional liver. Consequently, the second-stage operation aims at the complete removal of CLMs, frequently by a right hepatectomy or a right trisectionectomy [28, 43, 44].

Because the volume of the FLR is commonly insufficient (due to the liver resections already performed during the first operation), PVL could be carried out in the first stage. If the PVL was not performed during the first operation and the CT scan evaluation made before the second stage would reveal an insufficient volume of the FLR, a PVE could be underwent before the second surgery. Therefore, the hypertrophy of the FLR achieved by portal vein occlusion will allow the safe performance of the second operation, avoiding the risk of postoperative liver failure.

In the series reported until now, the resectability rates achieved by this approach ranged between 60 and 80%, and the 3-year overall survival (OS) rates were higher than 35% [28, 43–45].

2.3.4. *Liver resection after downsizing chemotherapy*

This onco-surgical approach is usually performed in patients with few large metastases, whose initial resection would not preserve an adequate volume of the remnant liver parenchyma [28, 46, 47]. The goal of the treatment is to achieve the shrinkage of the tumors to such an extent that makes possible their resection.

In such patients with potentially resectable CLMs (Group 1), it is recommended to start an intense chemotherapy regimen, usually consisting of three chemotherapic drugs (5-FU, Oxaliplatin, and Irinotecan—FOLFOXIRI) and a monoclonal antibody [5]. In patients with RAS-wild-type tumors the use of an anti-EGFR (epidermal growth factor receptor) monoclonal antibody (Cetuximab or Panitumumab) is recommended, whereas in patients with RAS-mutant tumors the use of anti-VEGF (vascular endothelial growth factor) agent (Bevacizumab) is advocated.

The response to the treatment should be assessed every 2 months after the therapy commences (by CT scan or MRI) and the patient should be referred to the surgery as soon as the metastases became resectable. The continuation of the oncologic therapy beyond this time point could expose the patient to three dangerous scenarios:

- After the initial response to the oncologic therapy, the metastases could regrow, closing the "window of opportunity" for liver resection. Thus, the patient misses the chance of a potentially curative liver resection due to the useless continuation of chemotherapy [28].

- Due to the hepatic toxicity of both Oxaliplatin and Irinotecan, there is a high risk of an impaired liver function secondary to the long-course chemotherapy (usually more than six cycles) [48–50]. Oxaliplatin induces vascular disorders causing the appearance of the so-called "blue-liver," whereas Irinotecan induces steatohepatitis (NASH—nonalcoholic steatohepatitis) that generates the so-called "yellow-liver" [48–50]. When liver resection is performed in such patients, the morbidity and mortality rates increase dramatically, especially when major hepatectomies are needed [51–53]. Thus, to avoid the higher postoperative morbidity and mortality rates in patients whose CLMs were rendered to resectability after downsizing chemotherapy is mandatory to perform liver resection as soon as the metastases became resectable. Moreover, data derived from the LiverMetSurvey database revealed that the higher the number of chemotherapy cycles or lines, the lower the survival after liver resection [3].

- If the chemotherapy is prolonged too much, some liver metastases could become unidentifiable on CT scan or MRI. Unfortunately, this clinical/radiologic complete response is not equivalent to pathologic complete response, and it was well established that in more than 80% of cases the viable tumor cells are still present at the site of initial liver metastases (although they could not be found radiologically or intraoperatively) [54]. These lesions are called "vanishing metastases" and their initial sites should be resected in order to avoid their recurrence. However, this goal is difficult, especially when the metastases were originally located deep in the liver parenchyma. The metastases that could not be resected because they are not identified intraoperatively are called "missing metastases." In such instances, it is recommended to have a close follow-up of the patients in order to identify, as soon as possible, the "reappearance" of CLMs and perform their resection. In patients with "missing metastases," intra-arterial chemotherapy could also be offered which seems to decrease the recurrence rates [55].

By using 5-FU and Oxaliplatin, the Paul Brousse group reported a rate of conversion to resectability of 13% [49, 56], whereas more recent series reported even higher conversion rates (up to 28%) by using intense chemotherapy regimens associated with targeted therapies [57].

In patients who underwent curative-intent resection of initially unresectable CLMs downsized by chemotherapy, the disease-free survival (DFS) and overall survival (OS) rates were statistically significant lower than those achieved in patients undergoing R0 resection for initially resectable CLMs [28, 56]. However, the 5-year OS rates (higher than 25%) achieved by patients rendered to resectability after chemotherapy are statistically significant, higher than those reported in patients who received only palliative oncologic treatment (6% at 5 years) [3, 56]. These results justify the efforts to render the resectability of the initially unresectable CLMs by conversion chemotherapy [28].

Moreover, early tumor shrinkage (the decrease of CLMs size with more than 20%, according to RECIST criteria, after 8 weeks of treatment) induced by the combination of chemotherapy with anti-EGFR agents (Cetuximab or Panitumumab) correlates with a higher rate of conversion to resectability [58, 59]. Meanwhile, early tumor shrinkage is a strong predictor of favorable outcome, both in patients undergoing liver resection and in patients whose CLMs could not be rendered to resectability [59, 60]. In patients who experienced early tumor shrinkage and underwent curative-intent liver resection, the 5-year OS rates were statistically significant, higher than those reported in patients rendered to resectability but who did not experience early tumor shrinkage [59].

2.3.5. Liver resection associated with ablative treatment

This strategy aims at the complete clearance of the liver and is especially recommended in patients with multiple bilobar CLMs that cannot be completely resected.

The ablative therapies are represented by radiofrequency ablation (RFA), microwave ablation and cryosurgery. The most widely used ablative therapy is RFA and most studies revealed that the local recurrence rates after RFA of CLMs smaller than 3 cm are similar to those achieved by liver resection [61].

For this reason, in patients with multiple bilobar CLMs the resection of the bulk metastatic burden (usually by a major hepatectomy—right hepatectomy or right trisectionectomy) and RFA of the small liver metastases from the remnant liver could be performed.

This approach is also of particular interest in patients with multiple CLMs, one of which is ill-located (e.g., in the proximity of hepato-caval confluence or portal vein bifurcation). Usually, the resection of such ill-located metastasis requires the removal of a large volume of normal liver parenchyma, increasing the risk of postoperative liver failure. Performing RFA for that metastasis avoids a major hepatectomy, sparing a large volume of nontumoral liver parenchyma, without compromising the oncologic outcome. In such instances, all the liver metastases could be resected, except for the ill-located one, which can be treated by ablation.

This strategy (also called CARe—combined ablation and resection) has recently gained wide acceptance because current studies [62] revealed that the long-term outcomes achieved by CARe (5-year OS rates up to 37%) are similar to those achieved by the other strategies used to render the resectability of the initially unresectable CLMs. Thus, the DFS and OS rates achieved by this approach are similar to those achieved by "two-stage" hepatectomies in the setting of multiple bilobar CLMs [63]. Moreover, the morbidity and mortality rates after CARe tend to be lower than those reported after "two-stage" liver resections [63].

However, these favorable long-term outcomes cannot be achieved if the diameter of the metastasis that will be ablated is larger than 3 cm or if the tumor is not completely ablated.

2.4. Disseminated disease, technically "never"/unlikely resectable: Group 2

In this group of patients, the therapeutic intention is rather palliative [5] and, obviously, the medical oncologist should start the treatment. According to the ESMO guidelines, the preferred option for the first line therapy is a cytotoxic doublet in combination with a targeted agent [5]. For symptomatic patients with RAS-wild type tumors, the association of FOLFOX/FOLFIRI with an anti-EGFR agent (Cetuximab or Panitumumab) seems to be the preferred therapy, whereas in the other patients the association of a cytotoxic doublet with Bevacizumab should be proposed.

When imaging re-evaluation shows evidence of favorable response of CLMs to the first-line treatment, the therapy should be reconsidered based on a multidisciplinary team decision.

Thus, if liver metastases became resectable, the patient should be referred to surgery. Even when CLMs were not rendered to resectability, oligometastatic patients could benefit from ablative therapies. In this situation, the ablation of the metastases could be performed percutaneously by an interventional radiologist. Although the DFS rates are lower than those achieved by liver resection, this approach could offer a period of chemotherapy discontinuation until the disease progresses [5].

In patients who did not become eligible for surgery or ablation, the de-escalation of the initial combination should be considered [5], in order to achieve a prolonged progression-free interval with good symptom control and, eventually, a higher overall survival rate.

2.5. Never-resectable metastatic disease: Group 3

This group includes the patients with bulk metastatic burden (frequently hepatic and extra-hepatic) who cannot be rendered to resectability by anyone of the above-mentioned strategies.

The goal of the treatment should be the prevention of tumor progression as long as possible and the prolongation of life with minimal treatment load [5], without aiming maximal tumor shrinkage because conversion to resectability was ruled out *ab initio*. These goals might be achieved by either of the two approaches: (1) cytotoxic doublet (FOLFOX or FOLFIRI) usually associated with a monoclonal antibody, shifting to the other doublet on progression; (2) escalation strategy, starting with a fluoropyrimidine drug frequently associated with Bevacizumab, followed (on progression) by a cytotoxic doublet associated with a targeted agent [5].

At present, the interventional oncology techniques (e.g., selective internal radiation therapy, SIRT, and chemoembolization using drug-eluting beads Irinotecan, DEBIRI) are usually used in the second or the third-line therapy, but their efficacy is still under evaluation.

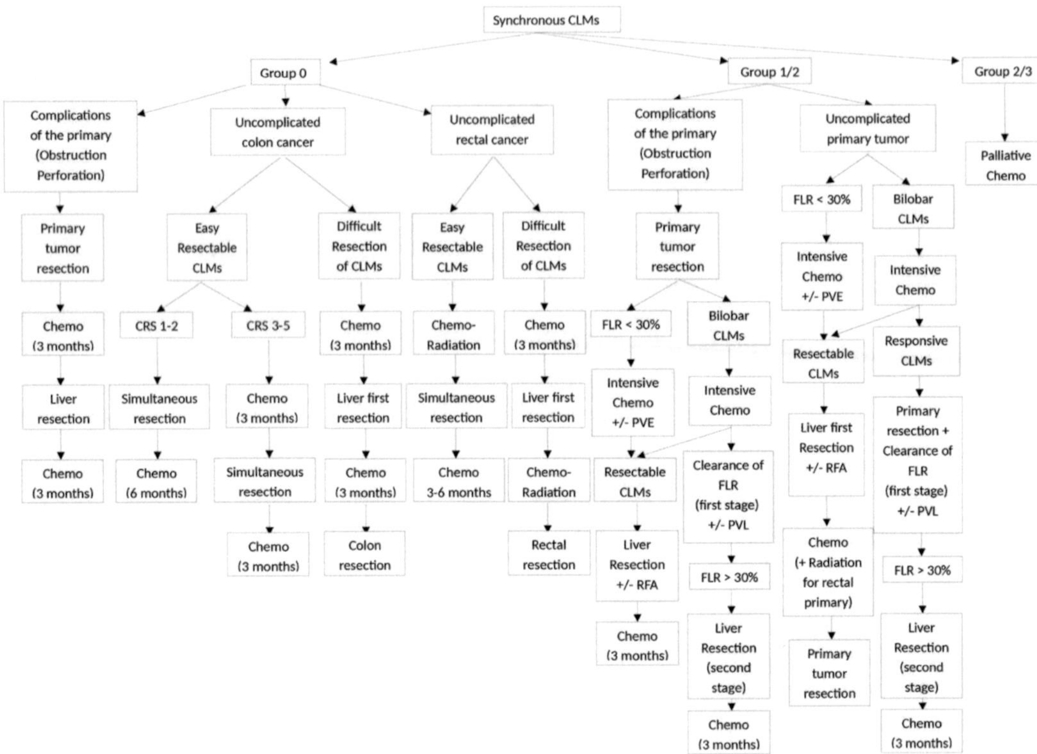

Table 1. Algorithm for onco-surgical management of patients with synchronous CLMs.

A meta-analysis revealed that DEBIRI achieved higher progression free survival (PFS) rates and better quality of life than standard oncologic therapy, when used in the second or the third-line treatment (after disease progression on previous lines of systemic chemotherapy) [64]. Moreover, a randomized controlled trial compared the results of FOLFOX+Bevacizumab versus FOLFOX+DEBIRI+Bevacizumab in the first-line treatment of patients with initially unresectable CLMs. It was observed that the combination of FOLFOX, DEBIRI, and Bevacizumab achieved higher response rates, higher resectability rates, and significantly higher PFS rates than the standard combination of FOLFOX with Bevacizumab [65].

Thus, it is possible that future studies will establish a more prominent role for these therapies in the treatment of patients with initially unresectable CLMs.

In conclusion, the algorithm for onco-surgical management of CLMs is presented in **Table 1** (synchronous CLMs) and **Table 2** (metachronous CLMs).

http://dx.doi.org/10.5772/65223

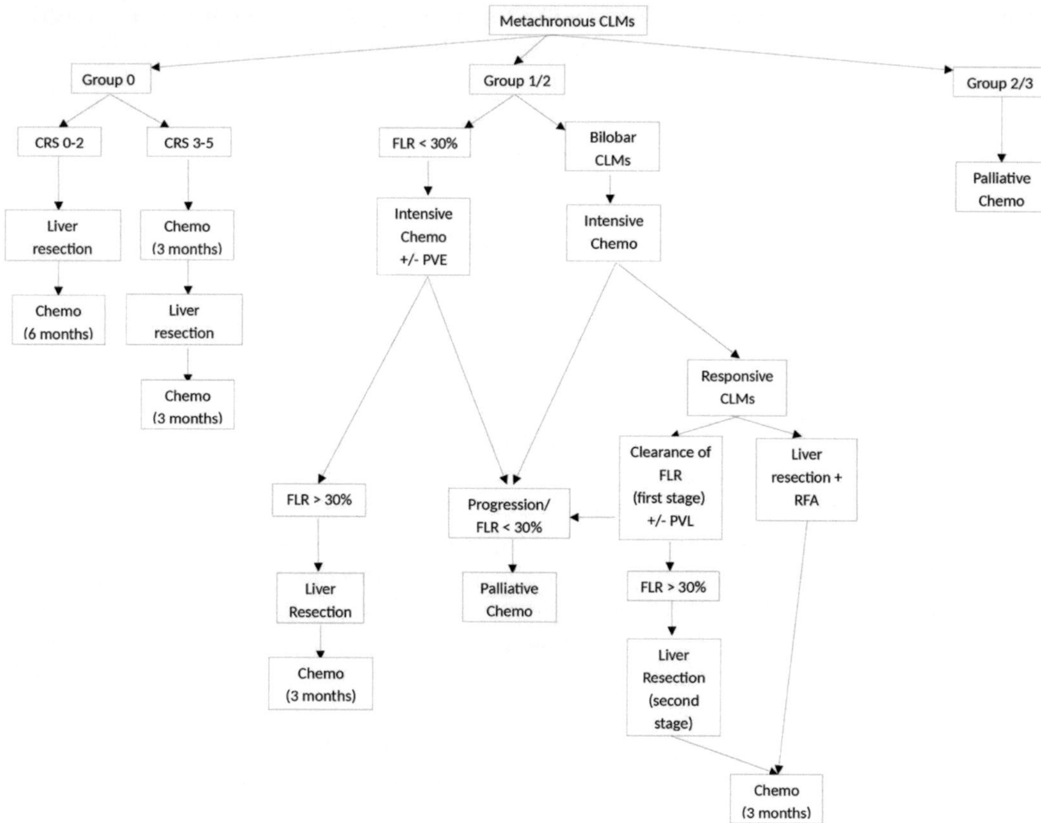

Table 2. Algorithm for onco-surgical management of patients with metachronous CLMs.

2.6. Technical issues in surgery of CLMs

During the past decade, the classical paradigms regarding the minimal resection margins that should be achieved, the adequate type of liver resection and the modality of surgical approach to liver metastases and primary tumor have been challenged by recent advances in surgery, anesthesiology, and medical oncology.

2.6.1. Resection margins

The classical paradigm regarding the width of resection margins postulated that a minimum margin of 10 mm is mandatory, to avoid the local recurrence. Later on, it was revealed that even narrower resection margins could be accepted if the metastasis is located in close proximity of bilio-vascular structures that should be preserved. Thus, Tanaka et al. reported a local recurrence rate of 2.8% in patients who underwent resection of CLMs with margins ranging between 2 and 4 mm and no local recurrence when resection margins were wider than 4 mm [66].

Therefore, at present, the resection of CLMs is recommended whenever a negative resection margin (R0) could be achieved [6].

Moreover, recent papers have revealed that in patients who primarily underwent R1 resection (CLMs located in contact with intrahepatic vascular structures that should be preserved) and subsequently modern postoperative chemotherapy, the overall survival rates were similar to those observed in patients who underwent R0 resections (p value > 0.05) [67, 68].

2.6.2. Types of liver resections

In the late 1990s, it was considered that anatomical liver resections offer superior long-term outcomes than nonanatomical hepatectomies because the rate of positive resection margins would be higher when nonanatomical resections were performed [69]. Later on, most authors revealed that the survival rates were similar irrespective of the type of liver resection, as long as complete resection (R0) of liver metastases could be achieved [22, 70].

Moreover, a considerable disadvantage of anatomical resections is related to the higher volume of nontumoral liver parenchyma that is removed, especially when major hepatectomies are performed. This issue has a negative impact on both the short-term and long-term outcomes. For example, a large retrospective study revealed that the number of liver segments resected and blood loss were the only predictors for both postoperative morbidity and mortality [71]. The authors concluded that reductions in the number of resected liver segments and blood loss are primarily responsible for the decrease in the perioperative mortality rate [71]. Moreover, because the recurrence rate of CLMs after an initial complete resection is up to 66% [72, 73] and the highest survival rates in patients with recurrent CLMs are achieved by liver re-resections [74–76], it is obvious that a parenchyma-sparing hepatectomy should be always performed, in order to increase the possibility of subsequent liver resections.

Consequently, whenever possible, major liver resections should be replaced by parenchyma-sparing hepatectomies in order to decrease the perioperative morbidity and mortality rates and to offer the chance of repeat hepatectomies in patients with recurrent CLMs, thus prolonging their survival. For these reasons, at present, most authors recommend the performance of (ultrasound-guided) limited liver resections in patients with CLMs instead of major anatomical hepatectomies [72, 77, 78].

2.6.3. Surgical approach

At present, laparoscopic colorectal resection offers similar morbidity, mortality, and survival rates as open resection of colorectal cancers [79]. Moreover, the laparoscopic approach decreases the blood loss, and ensures a more rapid postoperative recovery and shorter hospital stay [80]. By these reasons, in patients with synchronous CLMs, it is recommended to perform laparoscopic resection of the primary tumor and resection of liver metastases by an open approach, either during the same operative time (simultaneous resection) or as a staged procedure (delayed liver resection or liver-first resection). The simultaneous performance of colorectal resection by laparoscopy and liver resection by the open approach is particularly useful in patients presenting left colon or rectal tumor and liver metastases located in the right hemiliver [80].

Due to the technological progress made in the past few years, the rectal tumors have been approached more frequently by robotic surgery, and the morbidity, mortality, and survival rates are similar to those achieved by laparoscopic or open approach [81]. Because the anatomical structures of the pelvis are better visualized during robotic procedures, we recommend, in patients with rectal cancer and synchronous CLMs, the robotic resection of the primary tumor and resection of liver metastases by open surgery [82].

The progresses in laparoscopy also allowed the performance of liver resection by this approach. A meta-analysis revealed that laparoscopic liver resections enable lower blood loss and shorter hospital stay than open hepatectomies [83]. Moreover, a retrospective study reported a lower morbidity rate after laparoscopic hepatectomies than in patients undergoing liver resection by open approach [84]. Both of the above mentioned papers revealed that in patients undergoing laparoscopic liver resections for malignant diseases, the rates of complete resection (R0) were similar to those achieved in patients undergoing open hepatectomies [83, 84]. Regarding the long-term results achieved by laparoscopic resection of malignant liver tumors, the survival rates were similar to those achieved by open surgery [85–88]. Based on these outcomes, in the last period, in experienced centers, laparoscopic resection of CLMs is more frequently performed, even in patients scheduled for simultaneous resection of the primary tumor and liver metastases [82, 89, 90].

2.7. Recurrent CLMs

Almost two thirds of patients who underwent complete resection (R0) of CLMs will develop recurrent metastases, most of them during the first three years after the initial resection [72, 73]. The same therapeutic modalities are available to treat the recurrent CLMs and the highest survival rates are achieved by repeat liver resection [74–76, 91–93]. In the past few years, an increasing number of patients underwent a third, fourth, or even more liver resection and the available data suggest that the higher the number of repeated liver resections, the higher the survival rates [3, 75, 93]. Thus, the repeat liver resection is one of the most important therapeutic tools that contribute to a significant prolongation of overall survival in patients with CLMs.

Regarding the technical aspects, repeat liver resections presents some peculiar features, which could increase the risk of intraoperative and postoperative complications:

- Due to the previous liver resection, most patients develop perihepatic adhesions, thus increasing the risk of visceral (stomach, duodenum, and colon) or vascular (portal vein, inferior vena cava) injuries.

- The liver parenchyma is frailer as a consequence of the liver regeneration process (after the previous liver resection) and due to the hepatotoxicity induced by the prior chemotherapy. Thus, the amount of blood loss during the repeat liver resection could be higher than through the first hepatectomy, increasing the risk of postoperative complications.

- Because a part of the functional liver parenchyma has already been resected and previous chemotherapy could induce steatohepatitis or intrahepatic vascular injuries, the risk of postoperative liver failure after repeat hepatectomies is higher than after the first operation. To avoid this potentially fatal postoperative complication, it is advisable to perform parenchyma sparing hepatectomies both at the time of primary liver resection and during the subsequent hepatectomies.

However, recent studies revealed that the morbidity and mortality rates after liver re-resection are not statistically significant, higher than those induced by the first operation [91].

2.8. Surgery in patients with hepatic and extrahepatic colorectal metastases

Although the presence of extrahepatic metastases was considered a major contraindication to liver resection for CLMs, the data presented during the last decade revealed that liver resection might be beneficial even in the presence of extrahepatic disease, when the entire metastatic burden could be resected [94, 95]. However, the performance of FDG-PET is mandatory prior to surgery, to assess the complete extent of metastatic disease.

Obviously, the survival rates are lower than those achieved in patients presenting liver-only colorectal metastases, but the 5-year overall survival rates up to 22% achieved in patients with concomitant extrahepatic disease seem to justify the efforts to accomplish the complete resection of metastatic disease [59].

The resection of the entire metastatic burden could be achieved during a single operation (liver resection associated with resection of intra-abdominal metastases – e.g., hepatic pedicle lymph nodes metastases, ovarian metastases, peritoneal metastases, adrenal metastases, etc.) or by staged operations (e.g., initial resection of liver metastases, followed by resection of lung metastases in a second stage).

In patients presenting hepatic and peritoneal metastases, along with liver resection, cytoreductive surgery (CRS) associated with hyperthermic intraperitoneal chemotherapy (HIPEC) should be offered, in order to achieve the highest survival rates [96, 97].

The favorable prognostic factors seem to be up to five liver metastases, extrahepatic disease confined only to the lung, primary tumor located on the left colon, and the CEA level lower than 10 ng/ml [98].

Acknowledgements

This study was financially supported by EEA-JRP-RO-NO-2013-1-0363, contract no. 4SEE/30.06.2014.

Author details

Irinel Popescu and Sorin Tiberiu Alexandrescu*

*Address all correspondence to: stalexandrescu@yahoo.com

"Dan Setlacec" Center of General Surgery and Liver Transplantation, Fundeni Clinical Institute, Bucharest, Romania

References

[1] Jemal A, Murray T, Ward E, Samuels A, Tiwari RC, Ghafoor A, Feuer EJ, Thun MJ: Cancer statistics, 2005. CA Cancer J Clin 2005;55:10–30.

[2] McLoughlin JM, Jensen EH, Malafa M: Resection of colorectal liver metastases: current perspectives. Cancer Control 2006;13:32–41.

[3] LiverMet Survey: LiverMetSurvey Statistics December 2015. https://livermetsurvey manettis org:8443/SASStoredProcess/do.

[4] McMillan DC, McArdle CS: Epidemiology of colorectal liver metastases. SurgOncol 2007;16:3–5.

[5] Van CE, Cervantes A, Nordlinger B, Arnold D: Metastatic colorectal cancer: ESMO Clinical Practice Guidelines for diagnosis, treatment and follow-up. Ann Oncol 2014;25 Suppl 3:iii1–iii9.

[6] Adams RB, Aloia TA, Loyer E, Pawlik TM, Taouli B, Vauthey JN: Selection for hepatic resection of colorectal liver metastases: expert consensus statement. HPB (Oxford) 2013;15:91–103.

[7] Schmoll HJ, Van CE, Stein A, Valentini V, Glimelius B, Haustermans K, Nordlinger B, van de Velde CJ, Balmana J, Regula J, Nagtegaal ID, Beets-Tan RG, Arnold D, Ciardiello F, Hoff P, Kerr D, Kohne CH, Labianca R, Price T, Scheithauer W, Sobrero A, Tabernero J, Aderka D, Barroso S, Bodoky G, Douillard JY, El GH, Gallardo J, Garin A, Glynne-Jones R, Jordan K, Meshcheryakov A, Papamichail D, Pfeiffer P, Souglakos I, Turhal S, Cervantes A: ESMO Consensus Guidelines for management of patients with colon and rectal cancer. A personalized approach to clinical decision making. Ann Oncol 2012;23:2479–2516.

[8] Jaeck D, Bachellier P, Guiguet M, Boudjema K, Vaillant JC, Balladur P, Nordlinger B: Long-term survival following resection of colorectal hepatic metastases. Association Francaise de Chirurgie. Br J Surg 1997;84:977–980.

[9] Popescu I, Alexandrescu S: Hepatic metastasis of colorectal cancer—current therapeutic possibilities. Chirurgia (Bucur) 2010;105:155–169.

[10] Weber JC, Bachellier P, Oussoultzoglou E, Jaeck D: Simultaneous resection of colorectal primary tumour and synchronous liver metastases. Br J Surg 2003;90:956–962.

[11] Belghiti J: Métastases hépatiques synchroneset resecables des cancers colorectaux: y a-t il un délai minimum a respecter avant de faire la résectionhépatique. [Synchronous and resectable hepatic metastases of colorectal cancer: should there be a minimum delay before hepatic resection?] Ann Chir 1990;44:427–429.

[12] Nordlinger B, Guiguet M, Vaillant JC, Balladur P, Boudjema K, Bachellier P, Jaeck D: Surgical resection of colorectal carcinoma metastases to the liver. A prognostic scoring

system to improve case selection, based on 1568 patients. Association Francaise de Chirurgie. Cancer 1996;77:1254–1262.

[13] Alexandrescu S, Hrehoret D, Ionel Z, Croitoru A, Anghel R, Popescu I: Simultaneous resection of the primary colorectal tumor and liver metastases—a safe and effective operation. Chirurgia (Bucur) 2012;107:298–307.

[14] Jaeck D, Bachellier P, Weber JC, Boudjema K, Mustun A, Paris F, Schaal JC, Wolf P: Stratégie chirurgicale dans le traitement des métastases hépatiques synchrones des cancers colorectaux. Analysed'unesérie de 59 malades opérés. Chirurgie 1999 [Surgical strategy in the treatment of synchronous hepatic metastases of colorectal cancers. Analysis of a series of 59 operated on patients];124:258–263.

[15] Luo Y, Wang L, Chen C, Chen D, Huang M, Huang Y, Peng J, Lan P, Cui J, Cai S, Wang J: Simultaneous liver and colorectal resections are safe for synchronous colorectal liver metastases. J Gastrointest Surg 2010;14:1974–1980.

[16] Reddy SK, Pawlik TM, Zorzi D, Gleisner AL, Ribero D, Assumpcao L, Barbas AS, Abdalla EK, Choti MA, Vauthey JN, Ludwig KA, Mantyh CR, Morse MA, Clary BM: Simultaneous resections of colorectal cancer and synchronous liver metastases: a multi-institutional analysis. Ann Surg Oncol 2007;14:3481–3491.

[17] Adam R, De GA, Figueras J, Guthrie A, Kokudo N, Kunstlinger F, Loyer E, Poston G, Rougier P, Rubbia-Brandt L, Sobrero A, Tabernero J, Teh C, Van CE, Jean-Nicolas V: The oncosurgeryapproach to managing liver metastases from colorectal cancer: amultidisciplinary international consensus. Oncologist 2012;17(10):1225–39.

[18] Mentha G, Roth AD, Terraz S, Giostra E, Gervaz P, Andres A, Morel P, Rubbia-Brandt L, Majno PE: 'Liver first' approach in the treatment of colorectal cancer with synchronous liver metastases. Dig Surg 2008;25:430–435.

[19] Mayo SC, Pulitano C, Marques H, Lamelas J, Wolfgang CL, de SW, Choti MA, Gindrat I, Aldrighetti L, Barrosso E, Mentha G, Pawlik TM: Surgical management of patients with synchronous colorectal liver metastasis: a multicenter international analysis. J Am Coll Surg 2013;216:707–716.

[20] Reddy SK, Barbas AS, Clary BM: Synchronous colorectal liver metastases: is it time to reconsider traditional paradigms of management? Ann Surg Oncol 2009;16:2395–2410.

[21] Bonney GK, Coldham C, Adam R, Kaiser G, Barroso E, Capussotti L, Laurent C, Verhoef C, Nuzzo G, Elias D, Lapointe R, Hubert C, Lopez-Ben S, Krawczyk M, Mirza DF: Role of neoadjuvant chemotherapy in resectable synchronous colorectal liver metastasis; An international multi-center data analysis using LiverMetSurvey. J Surg Oncol 2015;111:716–724.

[22] Fong Y, Fortner J, Sun RL, Brennan MF, Blumgart LH: Clinical score for predicting recurrence after hepatic resection for metastatic colorectal cancer: analysis of 1001 consecutive cases. Ann Surg 1999;230:309–318.

[23] Ayez N, van der Stok EP, Grunhagen DJ, Rothbarth J, van ME, Eggermont AM, Verhoef C: The use of neo-adjuvant chemotherapy in patients with resectable colorectal liver metastases: clinical risk score as possible discriminator. Eur J Surg Oncol 2015;41:859–867.

[24] Azoulay D, Castaing D, Smail A, Adam R, Cailliez V, Laurent A, Lemoine A, Bismuth H: Resection of nonresectable liver metastases from colorectal cancer after percutaneous portal vein embolization. Ann Surg 2000;231:480–486.

[25] Makuuchi M, Thai BL, Takayasu K, Takayama T, Kosuge T, Gunven P, Yamazaki S, Hasegawa H, Ozaki H: Preoperative portal embolization to increase safety of major hepatectomy for hilar bile duct carcinoma: a preliminary report. Surgery 1990;107:521–527.

[26] Popescu I, David L, Brasoveanu V, Boros M, Hrehoret D: Two-stage hepatectomy: an analysis of a single center's experience. MagySeb 2006;59:184–189.

[27] Popescu I, Alexandrescu S, Croitoru A, Boros M: Strategies to convert to resectability the initially unresectable colorectal liver metastases. Hepatogastroenterology 2009;56:739–744.

[28] PopescuI, Alexandrescu ST: Surgical options for initially unresectable colorectal liver metastases. HPB Surg 2012;2012:454026.

[29] Farges O, Belghiti J, Kianmanesh R, Regimbeau JM, Santoro R, Vilgrain V, Denys A, Sauvanet A: Portal vein embolization before right hepatectomy: prospective clinical trial. Ann Surg 2003;237:208–217.

[30] Jaeck D, Bachellier P, Nakano H, Oussoultzoglou E, Weber JC, Wolf P, Greget M: One or two-stage hepatectomy combined with portal vein embolization for initially nonresectable colorectal liver metastases. Am J Surg 2003;185:221–229.

[31] Abdalla EK, Hicks ME, Vauthey JN: Portal vein embolization: rationale, technique and future prospects. Br J Surg 2001;88:165–175.

[32] Abulkhir A, Limongelli P, Healey AJ, Damrah O, Tait P, Jackson J, Habib N, Jiao LR: Preoperative portal vein embolization for major liver resection: a meta-analysis. Ann Surg 2008;247:49–57.

[33] de SE, Alvarez FA, Ardiles V: How to avoid postoperative liver failure: a novel method. World J Surg 2012;36:125–128.

[34] Schadde E, Ardiles V, Slankamenac K, Tschuor C, Sergeant G, Amacker N, Baumgart J, Croome K, Hernandez-Alejandro R, Lang H, de SE, Clavien PA: ALPPS offers a better chance of complete resection in patients with primarily unresectable liver tumors compared with conventional-staged hepatectomies: results of a multicenter analysis. World J Surg 2014;38:1510–1519.

[35] Schnitzbauer AA, Lang SA, Goessmann H, Nadalin S, Baumgart J, Farkas SA, Fichtner-Feigl S, Lorf T, Goralcyk A, Horbelt R, Kroemer A, Loss M, Rummele P, Scherer MN,

Padberg W, Konigsrainer A, Lang H, Obed A, Schlitt HJ: Right portal vein ligation combined with in situ splitting induces rapid left lateral liver lobe hypertrophy enabling 2-staged extended right hepatic resection in small-for-size settings. Ann Surg 2012;255:405–414.

[36] Tanaka K, Matsuo K, Murakami T, Kawaguchi D, Hiroshima Y, Koda K, Endo I, Ichikawa Y, Taguri M, Tanabe M: Associating liver partition and portal vein ligation for staged hepatectomy (ALPPS): short-term outcome, functional changes in the future liver remnant, and tumor growth activity. Eur J Surg Oncol 2015;41:506–512.

[37] Truant S, Scatton O, Dokmak S, Regimbeau JM, Lucidi V, Laurent A, Gauzolino R, Castro BC, Pequignot A, Donckier V, Lim C, Blanleuil ML, Brustia R, Le Treut YP, Soubrane O, Azoulay D, Farges O, Adam R, Pruvot FR: Associating liver partition and portal vein ligation for staged hepatectomy (ALPPS): impact of the inter-stages course on morbi-mortality and implications for management. Eur J Surg Oncol 2015;41:674–682.

[38] Tschuor C, Croome KP, Sergeant G, Cano V, Schadde E, Ardiles V, Slankamenac K, Claria RS, de SE, Hernandez-Alejandro R, Clavien PA: Salvage parenchymal liver transection for patients with insufficient volume increase after portal vein occlusion – an extension of the ALPPS approach. Eur J Surg Oncol 2013;39:1230–1235.

[39] de SE, Clavien PA: Playing Play-Doh to prevent postoperative liver failure: the "ALPPS" approach. Ann Surg 2012;255:415–417.

[40] Dokmak S, Belghiti J: Which limits to the "ALPPS" approach? Ann Surg 2012;256:e6–e7.

[41] Nadalin S, Capobianco I, Li J, Girotti P, Konigsrainer I, Konigsrainer A: Indications and limits for associating liver partition and portal vein ligation for staged hepatectomy (ALPPS). Lessons learned from 15 cases at a single centre. Z Gastroenterol 2014;52:35–42.

[42] Li J, Girotti P, Konigsrainer I, Ladurner R, Konigsrainer A, Nadalin S: ALPPS in right trisectionectomy: a safe procedure to avoid postoperative liver failure? J Gastrointest Surg 2013;17:956–961.

[43] Adam R, Laurent A, Azoulay D, Castaing D, Bismuth H: Two-stage hepatectomy: A planned strategy to treat irresectable liver tumors. Ann Surg 2000;232:777–785.

[44] Jaeck D, Oussoultzoglou E, Rosso E, Greget M, Weber JC, Bachellier P: A two-stage hepatectomy procedure combined with portal vein embolization to achieve curative resection for initially unresectable multiple and bilobar colorectal liver metastases. Ann Surg 2004;240:1037–1049.

[45] Faitot F, Soubrane O, Wendum D, Sandrini J, Afchain P, Balladur P, De GA, Scatton O: Feasibility and survival of 2-stage hepatectomy for colorectal metastases: definition of a simple and early clinicopathologic predicting score. Surgery 2015;157:444–453.

[46] Adam R, Avisar E, Ariche A, Giachetti S, Azoulay D, Castaing D, Kunstlinger F, Levi F, Bismuth F: Five-year survival following hepatic resection after neoadjuvant therapy for nonresectable colorectal. Ann Surg Oncol 2001;8:347–353.

[47] Bismuth H, Adam R, Levi F, Farabos C, Waechter F, Castaing D, Majno P, Engerran L: Resection of nonresectable liver metastases from colorectal cancer after neoadjuvant chemotherapy. Ann Surg 1996;224:509–520.

[48] Aloia T, Sebagh M, Plasse M, Karam V, Levi F, Giacchetti S, Azoulay D, Bismuth H, Castaing D, Adam R: Liver histology and surgical outcomes after preoperative chemotherapy with fluorouracil plus oxaliplatin in colorectal cancer liver metastases. J Clin Oncol 2006;24:4983–4990.

[49] Mehta NN, Ravikumar R, Coldham CA, Buckels JA, Hubscher SG, Bramhall SR, Wigmore SJ, Mayer AD, Mirza DF: Effect of preoperative chemotherapy on liver resection for colorectal liver metastases. Eur J Surg Oncol 2008;34:782–786.

[50] Rubbia-Brandt L, Audard V, Sartoretti P, Roth AD, Brezault C, Le CM, Dousset B, Morel P, Soubrane O, Chaussade S, Mentha G, Terris B: Severe hepatic sinusoidal obstruction associated withoxaliplatin-based chemotherapy in patients with metastatic colorectal cancer. Ann Oncol 2004;15:460–466.

[51] Karoui M, Penna C, Amin-Hashem M, Mitry E, Benoist S, Franc B, Rougier P, Nordlinger B: Influence of preoperative chemotherapy on the risk of major hepatectomy for colorectal liver metastases. Ann Surg 2006;243:1–7.

[52] Nakano H, Oussoultzoglou E, Rosso E, Casnedi S, Chenard-Neu MP, Dufour P, Bachellier P, Jaeck D: Sinusoidal injury increases morbidity after major hepatectomy in patients with colorectal liver metastases receiving preoperative chemotherapy. Ann Surg 2008;247:118–124.

[53] Vauthey JN, Pawlik TM, Ribero D, Wu TT, Zorzi D, Hoff PM, Xiong HQ, Eng C, Lauwers GY, Mino-Kenudson M, Risio M, Muratore A, Capussotti L, Curley SA, Abdalla EK: Chemotherapy regimen predicts steatohepatitis and an increase in 90-day mortality after surgery for hepatic colorectal metastases. J Clin Oncol 2006;24:2065–2072.

[54] Benoist S, Brouquet A, Penna C, Julie C, El Hajjam M, Chagnon S, Mitry E, Rougier P, Nordlinger B: Complete response of colorectal liver metastases after chemotherapy: does it mean cure? J Clin Oncol 2006;24:3939–3945.

[55] Elias D, Goere D, Boige V, Kohneh-Sharhi N, Malka D, Tomasic G, Dromain C, Ducreux M: Outcome of posthepatectomy-missing colorectal liver metastases after complete response to chemotherapy: impact of adjuvant intra-arterial hepatic oxaliplatin. Ann Surg Oncol 2007;14:3188–3194.

[56] Adam R, Delvart V, Pascal G, Valeanu A, Castaing D, Azoulay D, Giacchetti S, Paule B, Kunstlinger F, Ghemard O, Levi F, Bismuth H: Rescue surgery for unresectable

colorectal liver metastases downstaged by chemotherapy: a model to predict long-term survival. Ann Surg 2004;240:644–657.

[57] Malik H, Khan AZ, Berry DP, Cameron IC, Pope I, Sherlock D, Helmy S, Byrne B, Thompson M, Pulfer A, Davidson B: Liver resection rate following downsizing chemotherapy with cetuximab in metastatic colorectal cancer: UK retrospective observational study. Eur J Surg Oncol 2015;41:499–505.

[58] Douillard JY, Siena S, Peeters M, Koukakis R, Terwey JH, Tabernero J: Impact of early tumour shrinkage and resection on outcomes in patients with wild-type RAS metastatic colorectal cancer. Eur J Cancer 2015;51:1231–1242.

[59] Modest DP, Laubender RP, Stintzing S, Giessen C, Schulz C, Haas M, Mansmann U, Heinemann V: Early tumor shrinkage in patients with metastatic colorectal cancer receiving first-line treatment with cetuximab combined with either CAPIRI or CAPOX: an analysis of the German AIO KRK 0104 trial. Acta Oncol 2013;52:956–962.

[60] Piessevaux H, Buyse M, Schlichting M, Van CE, Bokemeyer C, Heeger S, Tejpar S: Use of early tumor shrinkage to predict long-term outcome in metastatic colorectal cancer treated with cetuximab. J Clin Oncol 2013;31:3764–3775.

[61] Wang X, Sofocleous CT, Erinjeri JP, Petre EN, Gonen M, Do KG, Brown KT, Covey AM, Brody LA, Alago W, Thornton RH, Kemeny NE, Solomon SB: Margin size is an independent predictor of local tumor progression after ablation of colon cancer liver metastases. Cardiovasc Intervent Radiol 2013;36:166–175.

[62] Evrard S, Poston G, Kissmeyer-Nielsen P, Diallo A, Desolneux G, Brouste V, Lalet C, Mortensen F, Stattner S, Fenwick S, Malik H, Konstantinidis I, DeMatteo R, D'Angelica M, Allen P, Jarnagin W, Mathoulin-Pelissier S, Fong Y: Combined ablation and resection (CARe) as an effective parenchymal sparing treatment for extensive colorectal liver metastases. PLoS One 2014;9:e114404.

[63] Faitot F, Faron M, Adam R, Elias D, Cimino M, Cherqui D, Vibert E, Castaing D, Cunha AS, Goere D: Two-stage hepatectomy versus 1-stage resection combined with radiofrequency for bilobar colorectal metastases: a case-matched analysis of surgical and oncological outcomes. Ann Surg 2014;260:822–827.

[64] Richardson AJ, Laurence JM, Lam VW: Transarterial chemoembolization with irinotecan beads in the treatment of colorectal liver metastases: systematic review. J Vasc Interv Radiol 2013;24:1209–1217.

[65] Martin RC, Scoggins CR, Schreeder M, Rilling WS, Laing CJ, Tatum CM, Kelly LR, Garcia-Monaco RD, Sharma VR, Crocenzi TS, Strasberg SM: Randomized controlled trial of irinotecan drug-eluting beads with simultaneous FOLFOX and bevacizumab for patients with unresectable colorectal liver-limited metastasis. Cancer 2015 Oct 15;121(20):3649–58

[66] Kokudo N, Miki Y, Sugai S, Yanagisawa A, Kato Y, Sakamoto Y, Yamamoto J, Yamaguchi T, Muto T, Makuuchi M: Genetic and histological assessment of surgical margins in

resected liver metastases from colorectal carcinoma: minimum surgical margins for successful resection. Arch Surg 2002;137:833–840.

[67] de Haas RJ, Wicherts DA, Flores E, Azoulay D, Castaing D, Adam R: R1 resection by necessity for colorectal liver metastases: is it still a contraindication to surgery? Ann Surg 2008;248:626–637.

[68] Eveno C, Karoui M, Gayat E, Luciani A, Auriault ML, Kluger MD, Baumgaertner I, Baranes L, Laurent A, Tayar C, Azoulay D, Cherqui D: Liver resection for colorectal liver metastases with peri-operative chemotherapy: oncological results of R1 resections. HPB (Oxford) 2013;15:359–364.

[69] Scheele J, Altendorf-Hofmann A: Surgical treatment of liver metastases; In Blumgart LH, Fong Y, (eds): Surgery of the liver and biliary tract. London, W. B. Saunders, 2000, pp 1475–1502.

[70] Kokudo N, Tada K, Seki M, Ohta H, Azekura K, Ueno M, Matsubara T, Takahashi T, Nakajima T, Muto T: Anatomical major resection versus nonanatomical limited resection for liver metastases from colorectal carcinoma. Am J Surg 2001;181:153–159.

[71] Jarnagin WR, Gonen M, Fong Y, Dematteo RP, Ben-Porat L, Little S, Corvera C, Weber S, Blumgart LH: Improvement in perioperative outcome after hepatic resection: analysis of 1,803 consecutive cases over the past decade. Ann Surg 2002;236:397–406.

[72] Taylor I, Mullee MA, Campbell MJ: Prognostic index for the development of liver metastases in patients with colorectal cancer. Br J Surg 1990;77:499–501.

[73] Topal B, Kaufman L, Aerts R, Penninckx F: Patterns of failure following curative resection of colorectal liver metastases. Eur J SurgOncol 2003;29:248–253.

[74] Alexandrescu S, Diaconescu A, Anghel R, Croitoru A, Boros M, Ionescu M, Popescu I: Surgical treatment of recurrent colorectal cancer metastases; Chirurgia (Bucur) 2008; Suppl. 1: pp S34–S35.

[75] Takahashi M, Hasegawa K, Oba M, Aoki T, Sakamoto Y, Sugawara Y, Kokudo N: Repeat resection leads to long-term survival: analysis of 10-year follow-up of patients with colorectal liver metastases. Am J Surg 2015 Nov;210(5):904–10.

[76] Vigano L, Capussotti L, Lapointe R, Barroso E, Hubert C, Giuliante F, Ijzermans JN, Mirza DF, Elias D, Adam R: Early recurrence after liver resection for colorectal metastases: risk factors, prognosis, and treatment. A LiverMetSurvey-based study of 6,025 patients. Ann Surg Oncol 2014;21:1276–1286.

[77] Finch RJ, Malik HZ, Hamady ZZ, Al-Mukhtar A, Adair R, Prasad KR, Lodge JP, Toogood GJ: Effect of type of resection on outcome of hepatic resection for colorectal metastases. Br J Surg 2007;94:1242–1248.

[78] Takayama T, Makuuchi M: Intraoperative ultrasonography and other techniques for segmental resections. Surg Oncol Clin N Am 1996;5:261–269.

[79] Kuhry E, Schwenk W, Gaupset R, Romild U, Bonjer J: Long-term outcome of laparoscopic surgery for colorectal cancer: a cochrane systematic review of randomised controlled trials. Cancer Treat Rev 2008;34:498–504.

[80] Hoekstra LT, Busch OR, Bemelman WA, van Gulik TM, Tanis PJ: Initial experiences of simultaneous laparoscopic resection of colorectal cancer and liver metastases. HPB Surg 2012;2012:893956.

[81] Stanciulea O, Eftimie M, David L, Tomulescu V, Vasilescu C, Popescu I: Robotic surgery for rectal cancer: a single center experience of 100 consecutive cases. Chirurgia (Bucur) 2013;108:143–151.

[82] Alexandrescu S, Diaconescu A, Grigorie R, Ionel Z, Hrehoret D, Brasoveanu V, Ionescu M, Popescu I: Surgical treatment of colorectal liver metastases—a single center experience over 20 years. J Transl Med Res 2015;20:222–232.

[83] Simillis C, Constantinides VA, Tekkis PP, Darzi A, Lovegrove R, Jiao L, Antoniou A: Laparoscopic versus open hepatic resections for benign and malignant neoplasms—a meta-analysis. Surgery 2007;141:203–211.

[84] Topal B, Fieuws S, Aerts R, Vandeweyer H, Penninckx F: Laparoscopic versus open liver resection of hepatic neoplasms: comparative analysis of short-term results. Surg Endosc 2008;22:2208–2213.

[85] Cai XJ, Yang J, Yu H, Liang X, Wang YF, Zhu ZY, Peng SY: Clinical study of laparoscopic versus open hepatectomy for malignant liver tumors. Surg Endosc 2008;22:2350–2356.

[86] Nguyen KT, Gamblin TC, Geller DA: World review of laparoscopic liver resection-2,804 patients. Ann Surg 2009;250:831–841.

[87] Robles R, Marin C, Parrilla P: Laparoscopic liver resection for metastatic disease. Minerva Chir 2008;63:441–453.

[88] Vibert E, Perniceni T, Levard H, Denet C, Shahri NK, Gayet B: Laparoscopic liver resection. Br J Surg 2006;93:67–72.

[89] Geiger TM, Tebb ZD, Sato E, Miedema BW, Awad ZT: Laparoscopic resection of colon cancer and synchronous liver metastasis. J Laparoendosc Adv Surg Tech A 2006;16:51–53.

[90] Hayashi M, Komeda K, Inoue Y, Shimizu T, Asakuma M, Hirokawa F, Okuda J, Tanaka K, Kondo K, Tanigawa N: Simultaneous laparoscopic resection of colorectal cancer and synchronous metastatic liver tumor. Int Surg 2011;96:74–81.

[91] Antoniou A, Lovegrove RE, Tilney HS, Heriot AG, John TG, Rees M, Tekkis PP, Welsh FK: Meta-analysis of clinical outcome after first and second liver resection for colorectal metastases. Surgery 2007;141:9–18.

http://dx.doi.org/10.5772/65223

[92] Chok KS, Cheung TT, Chan AC, Dai WC, Chan SC, Fan ST, Poon RT, Lo CM: Survival outcome of re-resection for recurrent liver metastases of colorectal cancer: a retrospective study. ANZ J Surg 2014;84:545–549.

[93] Wicherts DA, de Haas RJ, Salloum C, Andreani P, Pascal G, Sotirov D, Adam R, Castaing D, Azoulay D: Repeat hepatectomy for recurrent colorectal metastases. Br J Surg 2013;100:808–818.

[94] Carpizo DR, Are C, Jarnagin W, DeMatteo R, Fong Y, Gonen M, Blumgart L, D'Angelica M: Liver resection for metastatic colorectal cancer in patients with concurrent extrahepatic disease: results in 127 patients treated at a single center. Ann Surg Oncol 2009;16:2138–2146.

[95] Elias D, Ouellet JF, Bellon N, Pignon JP, Pocard M, Lasser P: Extrahepatic disease does not contraindicate hepatectomy for colorectal liver metastases. Br J Surg 2003;90:567–574.

[96] Elias D, Gilly F, Boutitie F, Quenet F, Bereder JM, Mansvelt B, Lorimier G, Dube P, Glehen O: Peritoneal colorectal carcinomatosis treated with surgery and perioperative intraperitoneal chemotherapy: retrospective analysis of 523 patients from a multicentric French study. J Clin Oncol 2010;28:63–68.

[97] Mohamed F, Cecil T, Moran B, Sugarbaker P: A new standard of care for the management of peritoneal surface malignancy. Curr Oncol 2011;18:e84–e96.

[98] Adam R, de Haas RJ, Wicherts DA, Vibert E, Salloum C, Azoulay D, Castaing D: Concomitant extrahepatic disease in patients with colorectal liver metastases: when is there a place for surgery? Ann Surg 2011;253:349–359.

Chapter 8

Minimally Invasive Treatments for Liver Cancer

Nicolas Cardenas, Rahul Sheth and Joshua Kuban

Additional information is available at the end of the chapter

http://dx.doi.org/10.5772/65107

Abstract

While surgical resection and chemotherapy have remained mainstays in the treatment of both primary and metastatic liver cancers, various minimally invasive techniques have been developed to treat patients for whom traditional approaches either are not available or have failed. Percutaneous ablation techniques such as radiofrequency, microwave, cryoablation, and irreversible electroporation are considered as potentially curative treatments in patients with hepatocellular carcinoma with early-stage tumors. Transarterial chemoembolization (TACE) and radioembolization with yttrium-90 (Y-90) are palliative treatments that have improved survival in patients with unresectable disease. In this chapter, we discuss these minimally invasive techniques, the criteria for selecting appropriate candidates for treatment, and potential limitations to their use.

Keywords: chemoembolization, percutaneous ablation, radioembolization, minimally invasive therapies, liver cancer

1. Introduction

While surgical resection and chemotherapy have remained mainstays in the treatment of both primary and metastatic liver cancers, a variety of minimally invasive techniques have been developed to treat patients for whom traditional approaches are either not available or have failed. Percutaneous ablation techniques, such as radiofrequency, microwave, cryoablation, and irreversible electroporation, are considered potentially curative treatments in patients with hepatocellular carcinoma with early-stage tumors. Transarterial chemoembolization (TACE) and radioembolization with yttrium-90 (Y-90) are palliative treatments that have improved survival in patients with unresectable disease. In this chapter, we discuss these minimally invasive techniques, the criteria for selecting appropriate candidates for treatment, and potential limitations to their use.

2. Transarterial chemoembolization

Transarterial chemoembolization (TACE) is a minimally invasive technique used to treat liver tumors, predominantly hepatocellular carcinoma (HCC). In the early 1970s, interventional radiologists (IRs) began utilizing embolization agents to effectively block the vascular supply of hepatic tumors, pioneering the technique known as trans-catheter arterial embolization (TAE) or bland embolization. TACE evolved from TAE 10 years later, when IRs began to perform intra-arterial injections of chemotherapeutic agents prior to the delivery of embolization agents [1].

TACE derives its therapeutic effects through two synergistic methods. Selective arterial occlusion induces ischemic tumor necrosis by limiting blood flow to the tumor. Concomitant administration of regional chemotherapy allows the drug to remain in the tumor for an extended period of time, enhancing its therapeutic effects and diminishing adverse systemic side effects [2].

The rationale for using arterial embolization as a treatment for hepatocellular carcinoma is based on the unique blood supply of both the liver and the tumor itself. Due to the liver's dual blood supply, IRs are able to embolize hepatic arteries without causing significant hepatic necrosis. Normal liver parenchyma receives two-thirds of its blood supply from the portal vein and the remaining one-third from the hepatic artery [2]. In contrast, Breedis and Young [3] found that hepatic neoplasms almost exclusively receive their blood supply from the hepatic artery. TACE takes advantage of these characteristics by selectively embolizing branches of the hepatic artery, successfully sparing normal hepatic tissue and targeting the neoplasm.

2.1. Components of TACE

Modern TACE can be segregated into two technical approaches: conventional TACE (cTACE) and drug-eluting bead TACE (DEB-TACE). cTACE bears the closest resemblance to the techniques used in the landmark trials that demonstrated a survival benefit with TACE [4, 5] and typically involves the administration of a mixture composed of a chemotherapeutic agent and ethiodized oil (Lipiodol, Guerbet, Paris, France). The chemotherapy component can be administered either as a mono-drug regimen or combination chemotherapy. The most commonly used single drug agents are doxorubicin and cisplatin. Some physicians prefer to use combination chemotherapy based on the notion that the mixture of agents leads to a synergistic effect and a better outcome. The most common drug combination includes cisplatin, doxorubicin, and mitomycin C. However, there is no established improvement in survival between any one mono-drug therapy vs. other drugs [6, 7] or mono-drug therapy vs. combination chemotherapy [8].

http://dx.doi.org/10.5772/65107

Lipiodol is an oily contrast media derived from poppy seeds that serves three important roles: drug delivery vehicle, microembolic material, and radio-opaque contrast agent [9]. Lipiodol's oily consistency allows for embolization of both arterial and portal vessels. This dual embolization is clinically relevant because high-grade tumors may receive a portion of their blood supply from both the hepatic artery and portal vein [10]. Embolization of both vascular systems enhances the antitumor properties of the procedure in such cases [11].

The majority of cytotoxic molecules used in TACE are hydrophilic and are therefore emulsified in oil droplets when mixed with lipiodol. When injected into a tumor-supplying vessel, the emulsified lipiodol and drug mixture preferentially stays within the tumor vasculature for several weeks to over a year [2]. The reason for the selective and prolonged uptake of lipiodol by hepatocellular carcinoma continues to be debated. One possible explanation is the dense hypervascularity of HCC. Another explanation is the complete absence of a reticuloendothelial system in tumor vasculature, leading to the absence of Kupffer cells, which would normally phagocytize the oil [9].

A variety of embolic agents can be used for further embolization during cTACE, the most common being gelatin sponge, polyvinyl alcohol, and ethanol [12]. The literature has failed to reveal clear superiority of one agent over the other, leading to variability of use among providers [12].

In recent years, efforts have been directed at improving the drug delivery system used in TACE. Drug-eluting beads (DEB) are embolic microspheres loaded with chemotherapeutic agents, most commonly doxorubicin, which ensure slow drug release and decrease systemic spread. In theory, this "reservoir effect" permits deeper diffusion of the drug beyond the perivascular space and into the tumor. Moreover, by coupling chemotherapeutics with calibrated microspheres of reproducible size, the execution of TACE can be standardized to facilitate interpretation of outcomes across patients and institutions with less concern for biases based upon technical variability.

Several trials have investigated the efficacy of cTACE versus DEB-TACE. PRECISION V [13] was a phase II study that showed nonsignificantly higher complete response rates in the DEB-TACE arm; subset analyses, however, showed a significant improvement in response rates with DEB-TACE in patients with Childs-Pugh score B and in patients with bilobar disease. Additionally, systemic toxicities of doxorubicin, including cardiovascular dysfunction and alopecia, as well as liver toxicity, were lower in the DEB-TACE arm.

2.2. Patient selection and indications for TACE

A multidisciplinary evaluation, including oncologists, hepatologists, and IRs, is essential for identifying appropriate candidates for TACE. TACE is considered the standard of care for patients with asymptomatic, unresectable HCC without macrovascular invasion, or extrahepatic metastasis. Four studies, including two randomized trials by Lo et al. [5] and Llovet et al. [14] and two meta analyses by Cammà et al. [15] and Llovet and Bruix [4], established level I evidence showing improved 2-year survival with TACE when compared to symptomatic treatment alone.

The primary indication for TACE is a Barcelona Clinic Liver Cancer (BCLC) stage B HCC that is not amendable to resection. The BCLC is a staging system (**Table 1**) that integrates tumor characteristics and performance status with liver function (Child-Pugh Score) and links them to evidence-based therapeutic options. The BCLC is now established as the basis for American and European HCC management guidelines.

Stage	Performance status	Tumor stage, cancer symptoms	Hepatic function	Treatment
0 (very early)	0	Single nodule <5 cm	Child-Pugh A, normal portal pressure/bilirubin	Resection
A (early)	0	Single nodule <5 cm 3 nodules each <3 cm	Child-Pugh A, elevated portal pressure and/or bilirubin	Liver transplantation or ablation
B (intermediate)	0	Large, multinodular, no cancer symptoms	Child-Pugh A-B	TACE
C (advanced)	1–2	Portal invasion, extrahepatic disease, or cancer symptoms	Child-Pugh A-B	Systemic therapy
D (terminal)	>2	Any	Child-Pugh C	Symptomatic treatment

Table 1. Barcelona clinic liver cancer staging system.

Secondary indications for TACE include decreasing tumor size to facilitate resection or to meet transplantation size criteria [16]. TACE may also be used to extend patients' eligibility for a liver transplant by preventing them from exceeding the Milan liver transplantation criteria (one tumor less than 5 cm, or up to three tumors, each less than 3 cm).

2.3. Contraindications: absolute and relative

The primary indications for TACE encompass a large, heterogenous patient population. This population includes patients with varying tumor burden, underlying etiologies, and liver function. It is the physician's responsibility to select patients for whom TACE is likely to improve their quality of life. Furthermore, it is critical to identify patients at high risk for serious complications that outweigh the potential benefits of the procedure.

Absolute contraindications include poorly compensated advanced liver disease (Child Pugh C). This includes patients with refractory clinical encephalopathy, persistent ascites, jaundice, and hepatorenal syndrome [17]. Other absolute contraindications consist of extensive tumor burden involving both hepatic lobes, uncorrectable bleeding diathesis, renal insufficiency (creatinine $\geq$ 2 mg/dL or creatinine clearance $\leq$ 30 ml/min), anatomical issues involving untreated arteriovenous fistulas, and active infection [17, 18].

Relative contraindications include untreated esophageal varices at risk of bleeding, a tumor size greater than 10 cm, anaphylactic reactions to contrast (gadolinium or carbon dioxide can be used as a substitute) or chemotherapeutic agents (bland embolization may be an alternative), hyperbilirubinemia, incompetent papilla with aerobilia, biliary dilatation, and impaired portal vein blood flow due to portal vein thrombosis (PVT) or hepatofugal blood flow [18]. Patients with PVT may still be eligible for TACE if selective or super selective chemoembolization is performed and the patient is Child-Pugh A [19].

2.4. Pre-procedure preparations

A consent form must be signed by the patient after an explanation of the procedure, risks, and benefits, and reasonable expectations are carefully explained, ideally in the outpatient IR clinic. Laboratory studies are ordered prior to the procedure and include complete blood count, metabolic panel with liver function tests, and coagulation profile. Obtaining abdominal triple-phase computed tomography (CT) or magnetic resonance imaging (MRI) is valuable prior to TACE to localize liver tumors, assess portal vein patency, observe for other conditions such as bile duct obstruction which would require decompression, and to assess arterial anatomy for treatment planning [20]. A patient is placed nil per os a minimum of 8 hours before the procedure, and intravenous fluids are started to maintain the patient well hydrated and avoid kidney damage due to contrast or tumor lysis syndrome. Medications to be administered prior to the procedure include antiemetics and anti-inflammatories to reduce the risk of post-embolization syndrome (discussed below) [20]. Prophylactic antibiotics are usually not given before or after the procedure unless the patient has risk factors for infection, such as a disrupted sphincter of Oddi [20].

2.5. Procedure

Most TACE procedures can be performed with moderate sedation and do not require a general anesthetic. Once appropriate sedation is achieved, the performing physician begins by gaining arterial access, typically from the common femoral artery or radial artery. An abdominal aortogram may be performed to visualize the visceral anatomy and identify any vessels supplying the tumor, such as the intercostal, phrenic, or lumbar arteries [20]. A superior mesenteric arteriogram is conducted to identify any variant anatomy and to assess portal vein patency. The celiac artery is then selected and an arteriogram is performed to study the arterial supply of the tumor and normal viscera. Particular attention is payed to identify vessels that should not be embolized, such as vessels feeding the stomach, intestines, and gallbladder.

Once the major vessels supplying the tumor are identified, a catheter—oftentimes a coaxial microcatheter—is advanced toward the tumor. The goal is to place the chemoembolizing solution as distal as possible to preserve normal liver parenchyma, but proximal enough to treat the entire tumor. With recent advances in imaging as well as catheter technology, "superselective" catheterization of the small subsegmental arteries supplying the tumor can be achieved, thus maximizing therapeutic efficacy while minimizing collateral parenchymal injury. The embolizing solution is then injected directly into the targeted vessel under continuous fluoroscopic visualization in order to prevent inadvertent embolization of vessels feeding normal parenchyma (**Figure 1**).

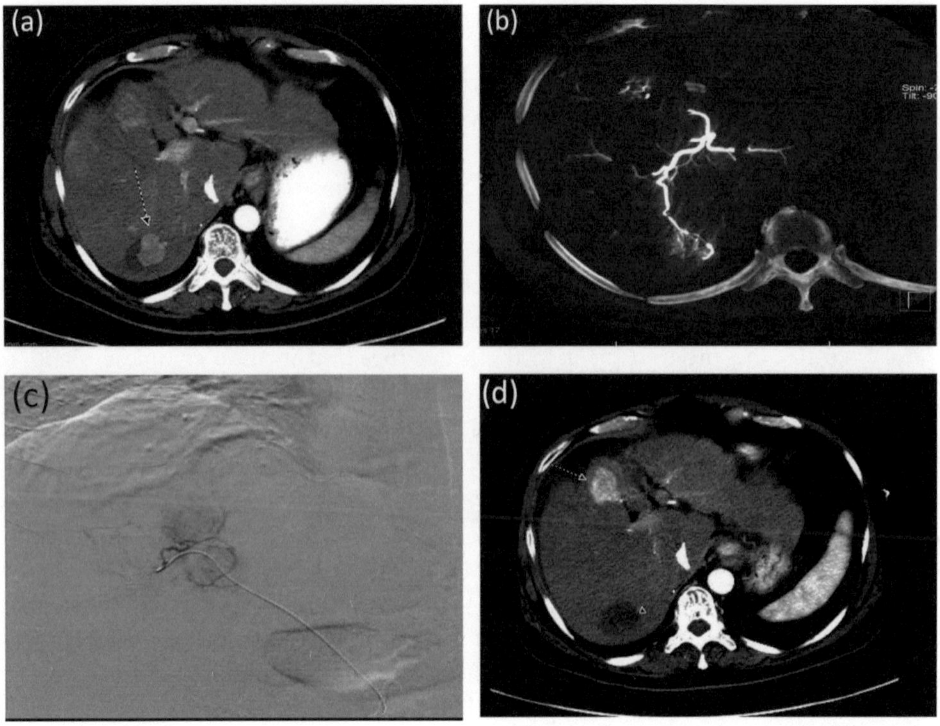

Figure 1. Chemoembolization of HCC. (a) Arterial phase contrast enhanced diagnostic CT of the abdomen showing hypervascular tumor in segment 7 consistent with HCC. (b) Intraoperative cone beam CT angiogram showing the vascular supply to the segment 7 HCC. (c) Digital subtraction angiogram from microcatheter in the feeding artery showing tumor "blush" and no collateral parenchymal supply. (d) Eight-week follow-up scan shows complete response with no arterial enhancement of the treated lesion in segment 7 (arrowhead). There is increased enhancement in a new segment 8 lesion seen anteriorly (arrow).

2.6. Post-procedure management and complications

Post-TACE patients are usually discharged from the hospital within 24 hours of the procedure. Patients are allowed to go home once their pain is controlled, they are tolerating PO intake, ambulating, and producing adequate amount of urine. A noncontrast CT of the abdomen is often performed the day after cTACE involving lipiodol embolization in order to visualize the distribution of the embolizing mixture.

A variety of complications may arise after transarterial chemoembolization, most of which are due to underlying causative factors present before the procedure. Post-embolization syndrome is the most common complication, occurring in 60–80% of patients [2]. The syndrome consists of transient abdominal pain, fever, and elevated liver enzymes. Many argue post-embolization syndrome is not a complication, but rather the body's reaction to necrosis, which was the objective of the procedure. If symptoms are severe enough, an extended hospital stay may be required. In the majority of patients, post-embolization syndrome is self-limiting and resolves in 3–4 days [2].

The most serious complications are fulminant hepatic failure, encephalopathy, and death. Pre-procedural risk factors include a Child-Pugh C, total bilirubin ≥ 4 mg/dL, albumin ≤ 2 mg/dL, major portal vein obstruction, refractory ascites, prolonged prothrombin time, and poor performance status. The incidence of TACE-induced hepatic failure varies widely, ranging from 0 to 49% with a median incidence of 8% [8]. Studies define TACE-induced hepatic failure using different criteria thus leading to the wide variation in incidence. The majority of patients return to pretreatment liver function before the next session of TACE, with only 3% of patients experiencing irreversible hepatic decompensation [8].

Additional TACE-related complications include hepatic abscess, biliary stricture, acute variceal bleed, pulmonary embolism, non-target embolization, and acute renal failure. Song et al. [21] reviewed over 6000 TACE patients and found a 0.2% incidence rate of liver abscess linked to previous intervention in the biliary system and with a compromised sphincter of Oddi.

2.7. Outcomes

The clinical significance of TACE was established following the publication of two pivotal trials in 2002. Llovet et al. [14] performed a randomized controlled trial to assess the survival benefit of frequently repeated chemoembolization (gelatin sponge plus doxorubicin) or arterial embolization (gelatin sponge) alone compared with conservative treatment. The trial was terminated early because chemoembolization provided a statistically significant survival benefit. One- and two-year survival for embolization was 75 and 50%, respectively. One- and two-year survival for chemoembolization was 82 and 63%, respectively, whereas the 1- and 2-year survival for conservative care was 63 and 27%, respectively.

Lo et al. [5] published a randomized trial in 2002 assessing the efficacy of transarterial chemo-embolization with a mixture of cisplatin, lipiodol, and gelatin sponge particles vs. symptomatic treatment. Chemoembolization resulted in significant tumor response and markedly improved survival (1 year, 57%; 2 years, 31%; 3 years, 26%) when compared to the control group (1 year, 32%; 2 years, 11%; 3 years, 3%).

A meta analysis conducted by Cammà et al. [15] concluded that TACE significantly reduced 2-year mortality in patients with unresectable HCC (odds ratio (OR), 0.54; 95% CI, 0.33–0.89; P = 0.015). Another meta-analysis performed by Llovet and Bruix [4] also showed decreased 2-year mortality in patients treated with TACE (odds ratio, 0.53; 95% CI, 0.32–0.89; P = 0.017).

3. Radioembolization

Radioembolization (Y90) is a form of intra-arterial brachytherapy conceptually similar to TACE in its application. However, rather than injecting chemotherapeutic agents, microspheres are embedded with a beta-emitting isotope known as yttrium-90. Highly localized internal radiation therapy is required rather than external beam radiotherapy because the liver is highly sensitive to radiation. The amount of radiation required to destroy tumor tissue is estimated at ≥ 70 Gray (Gy), well above the 35 Gy tolerance dose of normal parenchyma [22]. The intra-arterial approach allows IRs to selectively deposit microspheres in tumor feeding vessels, focusing the radiation dose on tumor tissue while sparing normal parenchyma.

3.1. Components of Y-90

Yttrium-90 is a pure beta emitter with a half-life of 64.1 hours, an average energy emission of 0.9367 MeV, and mean tissue penetration of 2.5 mm with a maximum of 10 mm [23]. Y-90 is embedded in either glass or resin microspheres, facilitating delivery to the target tissue. Glass microspheres, also known as Theraspheres, are approved by the FDA for treatment of unresectable HCC under a "humanitarian device exemption." Resin microspheres, also known as SIR-Spheres, have received FDA premarket approval for treating hepatic metastases from colorectal cancer, coadministered with fluorodeoxyuridine (FUDR) [22]. The activity load of a single glass microsphere is 2500 Bq, whereas the activity load of resin microspheres is 50 Bq. The notable difference in activity load requires larger volumes of resin microspheres to be injected for a desired dose compared to glass microspheres [24].

3.2. Patient selection and indication for Y-90

Patients with HCC, if detected early, may be candidates for curative treatments such as resection and transplantation. Unfortunately, only 10–15% of HCC patients are eligible at the time of presentation [25]. The majority of patients are left with palliative treatment options, such as TACE, Y-90, or symptomatic treatment.

An interdisciplinary team consisting of IRs, surgical oncologists, nuclear medicine, hepatologists, and radiation safety personnel is required to properly evaluate patients for Y-90. Radioembolization is not currently included as a therapeutic option in any HCC treatment guidelines, but there is growing interest and experience in the use of this therapy for early, intermediate, and late-stage HCC [22]. Pretreatment evaluation includes serum chemistries, appropriate tumor markers (CEA, AFP), liver function tests, cross-sectional imaging with CT/MRI/PET scan, meticulous angiography, and ^{99m}Tc macro-aggregated albumin (MAA) scan. Patient characteristics are incorporated into staging systems; the most accepted being Barcelona Clinic Liver Cancer (BCLC) and Eastern Cooperative Oncology Group (ECOG) [26]. Usually, patients with an ECOG performance status between 0 and 2 are eligible for treatment.

3.3. Contraindications: absolute and relative

An absolute contraindication for radioembolization is substantial intratumoral arteriovenous shunting resulting in systemic or pulmonary delivery of the radioactive microspheres. For this reason, a pretreatment angiogram and nuclear medicine study involving the intra-arterial administration of technetium-99-labeled macroaggregated albumin (^{99m}Tc MAA) is performed. From the subsequent scintigraphic imaging, the degree of intratumoral shunting is estimated by quantifying the radioactivity trapped within the lungs. If there is a potential for greater than 30 Gy radiation exposure to the lungs, radioembolization is not performed due to the risk of radiation pneumonitis [19]. The MAA scan may also predict large amounts of radiation

http://dx.doi.org/10.5772/65107

exposure to the gastric circulation via reflux through visceral branches, including the gastroduodenal and right gastric arteries. If the IR is unable to prophylactically embolize the appropriate arteries, the patient's visceral circulation may be exposed to large amounts of radiation, which can lead to severe ulceration, gastrointestinal bleeding, or pancreatitis [26]. Other absolute contraindications include severe renal insufficiency, uncorrectable coagulopathy, and a history of anaphylactoid reaction to iodinated contrast agents.

Relative contraindications include limited hepatic reserve, elevated total bilirubin level (>2 mg/dL) in the absence of a reversible cause, an ECOG score >2, prior radiation therapy involving the liver, and a main PVT with Child-Pugh B or C.

3.4. Pre-procedure preparations

A meticulous preliminary angiographic evaluation is essential in order to document visceral anatomy, localize anatomic variants, identify the hepatic circulation, and evaluate extrahepatic arteries that may require prophylactic embolization [19]. The importance of detailed angiography is augmented by HCC's high propensity to form aberrant vascular anatomy that, if present, requires identification prior to the procedure.

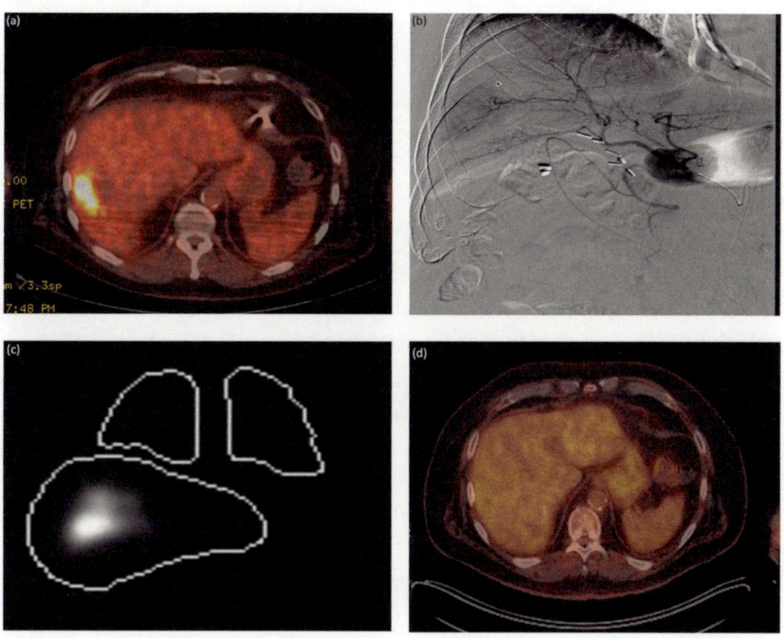

Figure 2. Radioembolization of liver metastasis. (a) 5 cm FDG avid metastatic colorectal lesion in the right liver. (b) Digital subtraction angiogram from a microcatheter in the common hepatic artery showing tumor hypervascularity (arrow) and visceral blood supply. (c) Scintigraphic scan obtained after injecting MAA into vessel supplying tumor with regions of interest (ROI) showing the liver and lungs. No significant counts are seen in the lung ROIs. The patient was therefore eligible for Y-90 treatment. (d) Eight-week follow-up PET/CT showing complete response after Y-90 treatment with no residual abnormal FDG activity.

Pretreatment arteriography involves evaluating the celiac, superior mesenteric, left gastric, gastroduodenal, proper hepatic, and right/left hepatic arteries. In the interest of redistributing blood flow away from the gastrointestinal tract, embolization of the gastroduodenal artery or any additional gastric artery may be required, most commonly the right gastric artery [19]. Other arteries that may necessitate embolization include the falciform, supraduodenal, retroduodenal, left inferior phrenic, accessory left gastric, and inferior esophageal. The objective is to prevent exposing the gastrointestinal tract to radiation, which can result in serious complications.

Selective arteriography is performed in the area where the yttrium-90 will be administered. This allows for dosimetry calculations to be based on the volume of the target vascular bed (liver segments) supplied by the artery to be catheterized [26].

Once the vascular anatomy has been established and prophylactic embolization of nontarget arteries complete, a ^{99m}Tc MAA scan is performed (**Figure 2**). Once injected, the distribution of the tagged albumin is visualized using planar or single photon emission CT (SPECT) γ cameras.

The lung shunt fraction (LSH) is used to assess the degree of shunting to the lungs and gastrointestinal tract. It describes the fraction of ^{99m}Tc MAA observed in the lungs or GI tract relative to the total ^{99m}Tc MAA activity observed. The lungs are able to tolerate 30 Gy per treatment session and a cumulative 50 Gy [27]. Patients are cleared for treatment if their cumulative pulmonary dose does not exceed 50 Gy and no pre-existing pulmonary pathology is present.

3.5. Post-procedure management

Radioembolization is a relatively safe procedure that can be typically performed on an outpatient basis. Patients are placed on a 7–10 day course of a proton pump inhibitor to prevent gastric ulceration. A 7–10 day course of a fluoroquinolone may also be prescribed if the entire right lobe is treated with the gallbladder present. Steroids may also be given after the procedure to decrease fatigue and systemic response to therapy.

A clinic appointment should be scheduled post procedure in order to evaluate the patient's tolerance of the treatment, ECOG performance status, and other adverse sequelae. The timing of the appointment is important because the majority of microsphere radioactivity decays by 12 days (4 half-lives) [26], allowing for an assessment of a patient when peak therapeutic response is achieved.

Cross-sectional imaging is performed 4–6 weeks after the procedure. It is important to note, however, that conventional imaging response criteria are poor predictors of response to radioembolization, particularly at early time points [26]. MRI diffusion-weighted imaging may provide a more accurate assessment of treatment efficacy. An FDG-PET scan may also be performed when appropriate.

In cases where bilobar disease is present, treatment of the second lobe is performed shortly after the assessment of response for the first treatment is complete. The process is repeated until all tumor foci have been treated.

3.6. Complications

Complications associated with radioembolization include post-radioembolization syndrome (PRS), hepatic dysfunction, biliary sequelae, GI ulcerations, radiation pneumonitis, vascular injury, and lymphopenia [28].

The incidence of PRS ranges from 20% to 55% [28]. Symptoms include fatigue, abdominal pain, nausea, vomiting, and fever. The duration of symptoms varies among patients, and hospitalization is usually not required. PRS is managed conservatively with hydration and over-the-counter analgesics. Post-embolization syndrome appears less frequently following Y-90 when compared to TACE because the radioembolization microspheres typically do not cause complete occlusion of the feeding artery [24].

Radiation-induced liver disease (RILD) occurs when normal liver parenchyma is exposed to high doses of radiation. The incidence reported in the literature ranges between 0% and 4% [28]. Hepatic dysfunction is characterized by elevated alanine aminotransferase, aspartate aminotransferase, bilirubin, alkaline phosphatase, and decreased albumin. Supportive care is recommended with close monitoring of patients with pre-existing poor hepatic reserve.

The incidence of biliary sequelae is less than 10% [28]. Damage to the biliary tree is induced by exposure to high doses of radiation or by the microembolic effects of microspheres. Patients are usually asymptomatic and recover with supportive care. Radiation cholecystitis requiring surgical intervention occurs in less than 1% of cases [29].

Radiation pneumonitis is caused by arteriovenous malformations shunting high doses of radiation to the lungs. With the use of standard dosimetry models and an accurate ^{99m}Tc MAA scan, the incidence of pneumonitis is well below 1% [30, 31]. The complication results in restrictive pulmonary dysfunction with a bat-wing appearance on chest CT [28].

Gastric ulceration may be caused when radioembolic microspheres enter the gastrointestinal circulation, becoming embedded in the lining of the GI tract. The incidence is less than 5% when accurate preliminary angiography and prophylactic embolization are performed [32–34]. Early management of severe epigastric pain is vital in preventing serious complications from developing.

3.7. Outcomes

A systematic review and meta-analysis was conducted by Facciorusso et al. [35] comparing the efficacy and safety of Y-90 radioembolization and TACE for treating unresectable HCC. Survival rates assessed at 1 year revealed no significant difference between the two treatment groups (OR = 1.01; 95% CI, 0.78–1.31; P= 0.93). The study revealed similar effects in terms of survival, response rate, and safety profile [35]. A study conducted by Salem et al. [36] concluded that Y-90 patients experienced a more desirable quality of life in terms of social and functional well-being than those treated with TACE. The lower toxicity of radioembolization, its ability to be performed as an outpatient procedure, and the decreased incidence of post-embolization syndrome all contribute to improving the quality of life for patients. Patients with portal vein thrombosis, a relative contraindication for TACE, can be safely treated with Y-90, yielding median survival of 8–14 months [37].

4. Percutaneous tumor ablation

Image-guided percutaneous tumor ablation describes the utilization of needle-like devices to directly administer cytotoxic chemicals or energy to a target tissue. Chemical ablation is most commonly performed using ethanol or acetic acid, whereas energy ablation can be divided into thermal and nonthermal techniques. The most widely applied thermal ablation modalities include radiofrequency (RF), microwave (MW), cryoablation, laser, and high intensity focused ultrasonography (US). Irreversible electroporation (IRE) is considered as a form of nonthermal ablation, although high temperatures may be achieved.

4.1. Ablation types

Understanding the advantages, disadvantages, and mechanisms of action of each ablative technique, along with patient and tumor characteristics, is essential in choosing the modality with the greatest efficacy and safety.

Ethanol ablation is a type of chemical ablation that utilizes 95% ethanol to induce coagulative necrosis through cellular dehydration, protein denaturation, and blood vessel thrombosis. Chemical ablation has largely been replaced by thermal ablation due to the former's variable and unpredictable distribution to surrounding tissue, leading to a high rate of tumor recurrence. However, there are certain situations where chemical ablation remains a viable option. Patients with HCC are good candidates because the fibrosed cirrhotic liver around the tumor can act like a capsule that limits the diffusion of ethanol to the surrounding parenchyma [38]. Patients with metastatic liver disease are not considered good candidates due to the normal parenchyma surrounding the tumor. Chemical ablation may be preferred or used in conjunction with thermal ablation in situations where the tumor is in close proximity to delicate structures or in areas of high perfusion-mediated tissue cooling [38].

Radiofrequency ablation (RFA) is the most commonly used modality for treating HCC and metastatic colorectal carcinoma to the liver. This heat-based ablation technique involves the formation of a closed electrical circuit between an applicator that acts like a cathode and grounding pads applied to the patients' skin that act as the anode. An alternating current is conducted through the applicator causing surrounding ions to vibrate as they try to align with the current. The agitated ions generate heat leading to coagulative necrosis of surrounding tumor. RFA has proven effective in treating tumors less than 3 cm, with a significant drop-off in success noted in tumors greater than 3 cm. The reason for the decrease in effectiveness is likely due to RFA's poor conductive heating and limited ability to overcome perfusion-mediated tissue cooling [38]. The flowing blood in highly vascularized tissue acts like a heat sink, not allowing the temperature to reach cytotoxic levels.

Microwave ablation (MWA) utilizes an antenna that emits electromagnetic waves producing an oscillating electrical field. Surrounding water molecules attempt to align with the changing field leading to the production of kinetic energy, which is converted to heat. Higher temperatures and larger ablations are possible with MWA when compared to RFA. The increase in power allows MWA to overcome perfusion-mediated tissue cooling and rely less on conduction heating. The increase in strength of MWA may lead to higher complications such as portal vein thrombosis, especially in cirrhotic patients where portal venous flow rate is reduced [39].

Cryoablation utilizes the Joule-Thompson principle of thermodynamics to effectively ablate a tumor through multiple freeze/thaw cycles. The process involves pumping high-pressure argon down an insulated narrow tube. A small opening at the end of the tube allows the argon to escape into an expansion chamber. The rapid expansion of the gas results in intense cooling leading to the formation of an ice ball. Similarly, high-pressure helium is forced down the hollow pipe, escaping through the opening, and into the expansion chamber. Rather than rapid cooling, helium causes rapid heating on expansion, effectively thawing the ice ball. The freeze/thaw cycle is repeated multiple times leading to tumor cell death. The formation of intracellular ice crystals causes mechanical disruption of cell membranes, while extracellular crystals create osmotic shifts and local hypertonicity. The low temperatures also cause apoptosis through interruption of cellular metabolism and vascular thrombosis leading to ischemia. An advantage of cryoablation over other ablative techniques is the ability to visualize the ice ball with imaging during the procedure. This allows the physician to assess if an adequate ablation is achieved or if more cycles are needed. Cryoablation is associated with minimal pain, allowing patients who are not good candidates for general anesthesia to undergo the procedure.

Irreversible electroporation (IRE) is the only nonthermal ablative technique available at this time. The procedure involves delivering short bursts of high voltage electrical impulses between two parallel electrodes [40]. The impulses form large pores in cell membranes resulting in cell death. Cytotoxic temperatures may be achieved in certain IRE ablations depending on the parameters of the case. The non-thermal mechanism of IRE makes it a preferable option for tumors in close proximity to critical structures, such as the bile ducts.

4.2. Patient selection and indications for ablation

The American Association for the Study of Liver Disease (AASLD) and the European Association for the Study of the Liver (EASL) have adopted the Barcelona Clinic Liver Cancer (BCLC) staging system for the management of HCC. Tumor ablation, particularly radiofrequency ablation, is considered curative and the treatment of choice for patients with *very early* and *early stage* HCC not amendable to surgical resection or transplantation [41, 42]. *Very early stage* includes patients with a performance status of 0, Child-Pugh A, and a single HCC < 2 cm. An *early stage* HCC is a patient with a performance status of 0, Child-Pugh A-B, single HCC <5 cm or 3 nodules <3 cm each.

4.3. Contraindications: absolute and relative

Absolute contraindications for percutaneous tumor ablation include tumor located less than 1 cm from the main biliary duct, intrahepatic bile duct dilatation, anterior exophytic location of the tumor due to risk of tumor seeding, untreatable coagulopathy, and unmanageable liver failure [43].

The number of hepatic lesions, usually greater than 5, should be considered a relative contraindication if all tumor foci cannot be effectively treated. If the extent of liver metastasis is too great, percutaneous ablation is not indicated. The majority of treatment centers prefer to treat patients with five or fewer lesions. The highest rate of treatment success has been established in tumors 3 cm or less along their longest axis. Tumors larger than 3 cm are considered a relative contraindication. Tumors located superficially or near any high-risk structures, such as the gastrointestinal tract, gallbladder, or biliary tree, are considered relative contraindications.

4.4. Pre-procedure preparations

Once a patient has been thoroughly evaluated and considered a candidate for percutaneous ablation, the pre-procedure preparations begin. Laboratory studies, such as complete blood count, creatinine, prothrombin time/INR, liver function tests, and tumor markers (alpha-fetoprotein), are ordered prior to the procedure in order to establish baseline measurements. Pre-procedure calculations of the patient's ECOG performance status and tumor markers are especially important for monitoring hepatic complications and treatment success post procedure.

Multidetector spiral computed tomography (CT) or dynamic magnetic resonance (MR) imaging should be obtained in order to carefully define the location of each tumor and their respective surrounding anatomy. Accurate imaging is essential for selecting the most appropriate ablative modality with the highest efficacy and lowest risk of complications.

Tumors in close proximity to structures, such as the biliary system, gastrointestinal tract, and major blood vessels, require careful consideration. Although radiofrequency ablation is the gold standard modality, if the risk for thermal injury is too great, other techniques should be considered. Ethanol ablation in conjunction with radiofrequency may decrease the risk for thermal injury and effectively treat the tumor [44]. Other nonablative modalities such as TACE or radioembolization may be indicated if the risk of complications with ablation is too high.

Superficial tumors whose margins abut adjacent structures, such as bowel, gallbladder, pancreas, or abdominal wall, require careful pre-procedure planning in regard to patient position, needle leverage maneuvers, and the potential need for hydrodissection or pneumodissection [44]. Hydrodissection involves the creation of artificial ascites by injecting a solution of 5% dextrose and 2% contrast into the peritoneum. The fluid displaces the at-risk structures, allowing for thermal ablation to be performed. Analogously, displacement of anterior structures can be performed with pneumodissection using carbon dioxide gas (**Figure 3**).

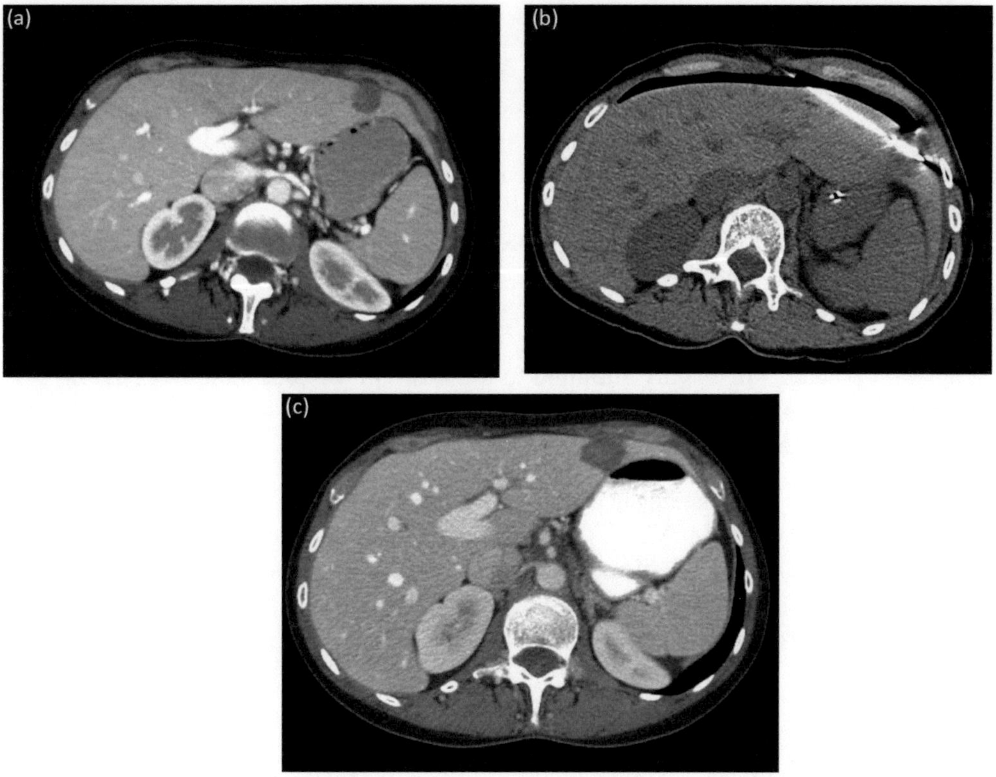

Figure 3. Thermal ablation of hepatic metastasis using pneumodissection. (a) A 59-year-old female with metastatic leiomyosarcoma to the left hepatic lobe. The tumor extends to the anterior liver border. (b) Microwave ablation of the metastasis was performed. To allow for the ablation margin to extend to the anterior liver border without injuring the peritoneal lining and abdominal wall, pneumodissection was performed by delivering carbon dioxide gas anterior to the liver, thus displacing the liver from the peritoneum. (c) Post-procedure CT demonstrates complete response of the metastasis.

4.5. Procedure

Tumor ablation may be performed under general anesthesia or conscious sedation with local anesthesia. Once appropriate sedation is achieved, the performing physician localizes the tumor under ultrasound or CT guidance. Ultrasound is most often used for initial needle placement due to the ability to visualize the needle in real time. Once the needle is in place, CT may be used to evaluate placement relative to surrounding critical structures.

Radiofrequency ablation utilizes thermal energy to cause cell death. The amount of tissue damage depends on the temperature achieved and duration of heating. Permanent cellular damage is attained when tissue temperature exceeds 50°C for 4–6 minutes. Temperatures above 100°C are not recommended due to tissue vaporization and carbonization leading to the production of gas which acts as an insulator. The gas production makes establishing a large enough ablation zone difficult. With this in mind, the objective is to maintain a temperature between 50°C and 100°C throughout the entire target tissue for at least 4–6 minutes. Depending on the size of the lesion, multiple electrodes are usually required to achieve the target temperature.

In order to ensure low rates of local tumor recurrence, appropriate ablation margins need to be achieved. According to Crocetti et al., [43] the ablation must extend 1–2 cm beyond the tumor margin in order to treat possible microscopic satellite lesions. Repeat CT scans are performed throughout the procedure to assess achievement of adequate tumor margins and monitor potential surrounding tissue damage.

4.6. Post-procedure management

Post-ablation patients are usually admitted to the hospital for overnight observation. If vital signs and laboratory results remain within normal limits, patients are discharged home the day after the procedure.

A consensus has yet to be established on the optimal interval or frequency of post-ablation imaging. According to Crocetti et al., [45] imaging 4–8 weeks after the procedure is recommended. A successful ablation will appear as a nonenhancing area with or without a peripheral enhancing rim. Routine follow-up imaging along with tumor marker measurements is important to detect recurrence in the future.

4.7. Complications

The rate of major complications post ablation ranges between 2.2% and 3.1% and include intraperitoneal hemorrhage, liver abscess formation, bowel perforation, tumor seeding, bile duct stenosis, pneumothorax/hemothorax, and skin burns [46].

According to a multicenter study by Livraghi et al., [46] the incidence of intraperitoneal hemorrhage requiring therapy is 0.5%. An INR < 1.5 and a platelet count above 50,000 per μL are required to maintain a low risk of bleeding during or after the procedure. Tract cauterization when removing the needle also decreases the incidence of bleeding.

With the use of proper sterile technique, the incidence of intrahepatic abscess is maintained low at 0.3% [46]. Patients with risk factors such as biliary enteric anastomosis or altered bile ducts should be placed on a 10-day course of antibiotics post procedure.

The incidence of intestinal perforation and bile duct stenosis is 0.3% and 0.1%, respectively [46]. Accurate imaging, careful pre-procedural planning, and the use of hydrodissection if needed are important in avoiding thermal damage to these structures.

The incidence of tumor seeding is 0.5% [46]. Performing needle tract ablation and avoiding direct puncture of peripheral liver tumors help to keep the incidence of seeding low.

The incidence of minor complications ranges from 4.7% to 8.9% and include pain, fever, self-limiting intraperitoneal bleed, and minor skin burns. The mortality rate of patients undergoing ablation ranges from 0.1% to 0.5% and is most commonly caused by sepsis, hepatic failure, colon perforation, and portal vein thrombosis.

http://dx.doi.org/10.5772/65107

4.8. Outcomes

According to Livraghi et al. [47], the complete response rates of patients with *very early stage* HCC (<2 cm) treated with radiofrequency ablation approach 97%, with 5-year survival rates of 68%. A study conducted by Cho et al. [48] in 2010 concluded that radiofrequency ablation is just as effective in treating *very early stage* HCC when compared to surgical resection. Despite similar success rates, patient characteristics and tumor location may indicate the use of one treatment over the other. For example, lesions in a subcapsular location or adjacent to the gallbladder may be better treated with surgical resection instead of RF ablation.

A study conducted by Lencioni et al. [49] revealed that patients with *early stage* HCC (single tumor ≤ 5 cm, or fewer than three tumors each ≤ 3 cm) treated with radiofrequency ablation exhibited 5-year survival rates ranging between 51% and 64%. Surgical resection remains the most effective treatment in patients with *early stage* HCC.

A randomized controlled trial was conducted by Morimoto et al. [50] determining the efficacy of radiofrequency ablation combined with transcatheter arterial embolization. The study concluded that patients with intermediate sized (3.1–5 cm) HCC treated with combination TACE-RF ablation exhibited better outcomes and tumor control when compared to RF only. TACE-RF ablation patients had 6% local tumor progression compared to 39% in the RF only patients.

Author details

Nicolas Cardenas, Rahul Sheth and Joshua Kuban*

*Address all correspondence to: JDKuban@mdanderson.org

Division of Diagnostic Imaging, Department of Interventional Radiology, MD Anderson Cancer Center, Houston, TX, USA

References

[1] Guan Y-S, He Q, Wang M-Q, Guan Y-S, He Q, Wang M-Q. Transcatheter arterial chemoembolization: history for more than 30 years. Int Sch Res Not 2012, 2012:e480650.

[2] Shin SW. The current practice of transarterial chemoembolization for the treatment of hepatocellular carcinoma. Korean J Radiol 2009;10(5):425–434.

[3] Breedis C, Young G. The blood supply of neoplasms in the liver. Am J Pathol 1954;30(5): 969–985.

[4] Llovet JM, Bruix J. Systematic review of randomized trials for unresectable hepatocellular carcinoma: Chemoembolization improves survival. Hepatology 2003;37(2):429–442.

[5] Lo C-M, Ngan H, Tso W-K, et al. Randomized controlled trial of transarterial lipiodol chemoembolization for unresectable hepatocellular carcinoma. Hepatology 2002;35(5): 1164–1171.

[6] Kawai S, Tani M, Okamura J, et al. Prospective and randomized trial of lipiodol-transcatheter arterial chemoembolization for treatment of hepatocellular carcinoma: a comparison of epirubicin and doxorubicin (second cooperative study). The Cooperative Study Group for Liver Cancer Treatment of Japan. Semin Oncol 1997;24(2 Suppl 6):S6–38–S6–45.

[7] Watanabe S, Nishioka M, Ohta Y, Ogawa N, Ito S, Yamamoto Y. Prospective and randomized controlled study of chemoembolization therapy in patients with advanced hepatocellular carcinoma. Cooperative Study Group for Liver Cancer Treatment in Shikoku area. Cancer Chemother Pharmacol 1994;33 Suppl:S93–S96.

[8] Marelli L, Stigliano R, Triantos C, et al. Transarterial therapy for hepatocellular carcinoma: which technique is more effective? A systematic review of cohort and randomized studies. Cardiovasc Intervent Radiol 2006;30(1):6–25.

[9] Idée J-M, Guiu B. Use of Lipiodol as a drug-delivery system for transcatheter arterial chemoembolization of hepatocellular carcinoma: A review. Crit Rev Oncol Hematol 2013;88(3):530–549.

[10] Takayasu K, Shima Y, Muramatsu Y, et al. Hepatocellular carcinoma: treatment with intraarterial iodized oil with and without chemotherapeutic agents. Radiology 1987;163(2):345–351.

[11] Sasaki Y, Imaoka S, Kasugai H, et al. A new approach to chemoembolization therapy for hepatoma using ethiodized oil, cisplatin, and gelatin sponge. Cancer 1987;60(6): 1194–1203.

[12] Coldwell DM, Stokes KR, Yakes WF. Embolotherapy: agents, clinical applications, and techniques. RadioGraphics 1994;14(3):623–643.

[13] Lammer J, Malagari K, Vogl T, et al. Prospective randomized study of doxorubicin-eluting-bead embolization in the treatment of hepatocellular carcinoma: results of the PRECISION V study. Cardiovasc Intervent Radiol 2010;33(1):41–52.

[14] Llovet JM, Real MI, Montaña X, et al. Arterial embolisation or chemoembolisation versus symptomatic treatment in patients with unresectable hepatocellular carcinoma: a randomised controlled trial. Lancet Lond Engl 2002;359(9319):1734–1739.

[15] Cammà C, Schepis F, Orlando A, et al. Transarterial chemoembolization for unresectable hepatocellular carcinoma: meta-analysis of randomized controlled trials. Radiology 2002;224(1):47–54.

[16] Chapman WC, Majella Doyle MB, Stuart JE, et al. Outcomes of neoadjuvant transarterial chemoembolization to downstage hepatocellular carcinoma before liver transplantation. Ann Surg 2008;248(4):617–625.

[17] Lencioni R, Petruzzi P, Crocetti L. Chemoembolization of hepatocellular carcinoma. Semin Interv Radiol 2013;30(1):3–11.

[18] Sieghart W, Hucke F, Peck-Radosavljevic M. Transarterial chemoembolization: modalities, indication, and patient selection. J Hepatol 2015;62(5):1187–1195.

[19] RMBD.pdf [Internet] [Cited 2016 July 9]. Available from: http://www.acr.org/~/media/ACR/Documents/PGTS/guidelines/RMBD.pdf

[20] Van Ha TG. Transarterial chemoembolization for hepatocellular carcinoma. Semin Interv Radiol 2009;26(3):270–275.

[21] Song SY, Chung JW, Han JK, et al. Liver abscess after transcatheter oily chemoembolization for hepatic tumors: incidence, predisposing factors, and clinical outcome. J Vasc Interv Radiol JVIR 2001;12(3):313–320.

[22] Kennedy A, Nag S, Salem R, et al. Recommendations for radioembolization of hepatic malignancies using yttrium-90 microsphere brachytherapy: A Consensus Panel Report from the Radioembolization Brachytherapy Oncology Consortium. Int J Radiat Oncol 2007;68(1):13–23.

[23] Salem R, Lewandowski RJ, Atassi B, et al. Treatment of unresectable hepatocellular carcinoma with use of 90Y microspheres (TheraSphere): safety, tumor response, and survival. J Vasc Interv Radiol 2005;16(12):1627–1639.

[24] Edeline J, Gilabert M, Garin E, Boucher E, Raoul J-L. Yttrium-90 microsphere radioembolization for hepatocellular carcinoma. Liver Cancer 2015;4(1):16–25.

[25] Llovet JM. Treatment of hepatocellular carcinoma. Curr Treat Options Gastroenterol 2004;7(6):431–441.

[26] Salem R, Thurston KG. Radioembolization with 90Yttrium microspheres: a state-of-the-art brachytherapy treatment for primary and secondary liver malignancies. Part 1: technical and methodologic considerations. J Vasc Interv Radiol 2006;17(8):1251–1278.

[27] Ho S, Lau WY, Leung TW, Chan M, Johnson PJ, Li AK. Clinical evaluation of the partition model for estimating radiation doses from yttrium-90 microspheres in the treatment of hepatic cancer. Eur J Nucl Med 1997;24(3):293–298.

[28] Riaz A, Lewandowski RJ, Kulik LM, et al. Complications following radioembolization with yttrium-90 microspheres: a comprehensive literature review. J Vasc Interv Radiol 2009;20(9):1121–1130.

[29] Rhee TK, Naik NK, Deng J, et al. Tumor response after yttrium-90 radioembolization for hepatocellular carcinoma: comparison of diffusion-weighted functional MR imaging with anatomic MR imaging. J Vasc Interv Radiol JVIR 2008;19(8):1180–1186.

[30] Leung TW, Lau WY, Ho SK, et al. Radiation pneumonitis after selective internal radiation treatment with intraarterial 90yttrium-microspheres for inoperable hepatic tumors. Int J Radiat Oncol Biol Phys 1995;33(4):919–924.

[31] Salem R, Parikh P, Atassi B, et al. Incidence of radiation pneumonitis after hepatic intra-arterial radiotherapy with yttrium-90 microspheres assuming uniform lung distribution. Am J Clin Oncol 2008;31(5):431–438.

[32] Murthy R, Brown DB, Salem R, et al. Gastrointestinal complications associated with hepatic arterial Yttrium-90 microsphere therapy. J Vasc Interv Radiol JVIR 2007;18(4): 553–561; quiz 562.

[33] Mallach S, Ramp U, Erhardt A, Schmitt M, Häussinger D. An uncommon cause of gastro-duodenal ulceration. World J Gastroenterol 2008;14(16):2593–2595.

[34] Szyszko T, Al-Nahhas A, Tait P, et al. Management and prevention of adverse effects related to treatment of liver tumours with 90Y microspheres. Nucl Med Commun 2007;28(1):21–24.

[35] Facciorusso A, Serviddio G, Muscatiello N. Transarterial radioembolization vs chemo-embolization for hepatocarcinoma patients: a systematic review and meta-analysis. World J Hepatol 2016;8(18):770–778.

[36] Salem R, Gilbertsen M, Butt Z, et al. Increased quality of life among hepatocellular carcinoma patients treated with radioembolization, compared with chemoembolization. Clin Gastroenterol Hepatol 2013;11(10):1358–1365.e1.

[37] Kulik LM, Carr BI, Mulcahy MF, et al. Safety and efficacy of 90Y radiotherapy for hepatocellular carcinoma with and without portal vein thrombosis. Hepatol Baltim Md 2008;47(1):71–81.

[38] Wells SA, Hinshaw JL, Lubner MG, Ziemlewicz TJ, Brace CL, Lee Jr. FT. Liver ablation: best practice. Radiol Clin North Am 2015;53(5):933–971.

[39] Livraghi T, Meloni F, Solbiati L, Zanus G, System F; CIG using AMICA system. Complications of microwave ablation for liver tumors: results of a multicenter study. Cardiovasc Intervent Radiol 2011;35(4):868–874.

[40] Golberg A, Yarmush ML. Nonthermal irreversible electroporation: fundamentals, applications, and challenges. IEEE Trans Biomed Eng 2013;60(3):707–714.

[41] Bruix J, Sherman M. Management of hepatocellular carcinoma: an update. Hepatol Baltim Md 2011;53(3):1020–1022.

[42] European Association for the Study of the Liver; European Organisation for Research and Treatment of Cancer. EASL–EORTC Clinical Practice Guidelines: management of hepatocellular carcinoma. J Hepatol 2012;56(4):908–943.

[43] Crocetti L, de Baere T, Lencioni R. Quality improvement guidelines for radiofrequency ablation of liver tumours. Cardiovasc Intervent Radiol 2010;33(1):11–17.

[44] Ziemlewicz TJ, Wells SA, Lubner MG, Brace CL, Lee FT, Hinshaw JL. Hepatic tumor ablation. Surg Clin North Am 2016;96(2):315–339.

[45] Crocetti L, Della Pina C, Cioni D, Lencioni R. Peri-intraprocedural imaging: US, CT, and MRI. Abdom Imaging 2011;36(6):648–660.

[46] Livraghi T, Solbiati L, Meloni MF, Gazelle GS, Halpern EF, Goldberg SN. Treatment of focal liver tumors with percutaneous radio-frequency ablation: complications encountered in a multicenter study. Radiology 2003;226(2):441–451.

[47] Livraghi T, Meloni F, Di Stasi M, et al. Sustained complete response and complications rates after radiofrequency ablation of very early hepatocellular carcinoma in cirrhosis: Is resection still the treatment of choice? Hepatology 2008;47(1):82–89.

[48] Cho YK, Kim JK, Kim WT, Chung JW. Hepatic resection versus radiofrequency ablation for very early stage hepatocellular carcinoma: a Markov model analysis. Hepatol Baltim Md 2010;51(4):1284–1290.

[49] Lencioni R, Crocetti L. Local-regional treatment of hepatocellular carcinoma. Radiology 2012;262(1):43–58.

[50] Morimoto M, Numata K, Kondou M, Nozaki A, Morita S, Tanaka K. Midterm outcomes in patients with intermediate-sized hepatocellular carcinoma: a randomized controlled trial for determining the efficacy of radiofrequency ablation combined with transcatheter arterial chemoembolization. Cancer 2010;116(23):5452–5460.

Chapter 9

Assessment and Optimization of the Future Liver Remnant

Mandivavarira Maundura and Jonathan B Koea

Additional information is available at the end of the chapter

http://dx.doi.org/10.5772/66139

Abstract

Safe liver resection is a vital element in the management of primary and secondary hepatic malignancies. The indications for resection have evolved Over time, and this has in part been due to the ability to improve the future liver remnant (FLR). This chapter reviews the current and future methods used for assessing the future liver remnant volume and function in order to minimize the risk of post-hepatectomy liver failure (PHLF). Current and evolving methods used in augmenting the future liver remnant are also considered. Since its introduction in the 1990s, portal venous embolization (PVE) has become the most widely used method of augmenting the FLR. The factors that affect hypertrophy following embolization as well as techniques used in portal venous embolization will be reviewed. Other methods of augmentation discussed include portal vein ligation (PVL) and the emerging method of associating liver partition and portal vein ligation for staged hepatectomy (ALPPS). The chapter also considers the various methods in the context of limiting tumour progression in the future liver remnant and attempts to integrate newer techniques such as ALPPS into current treatment algorithms.

Keywords: future liver remnant, volume, portal venous embolization, hypertrophy, liver function measurement, resectability

1. Introduction

Safe liver resection is a vital element in the curative management of primary and secondary hepatic malignancies. The ability to perform major liver resections relies on the capacity of the future liver remnant (FLR) to maintain normal liver function. The quality of the FLR may also be influenced by pre-existing liver disease and/or prior chemotherapy, thereby limiting the size of resection possible. Various methods have been utilized to assess the size and functionality of the

Characteristics	Historical indications	Current indications
Tumour number	<4 lesions	Any
Lobes involved	Unilobar	Bilobar or unilobar
Size of tumour	<5 cm	Any
Extrahepatic disease	None	Treatable extrahepatic disease
Functional Liver Remnant	Adequate	Adequate or amenable to augmentation
Lymph node involvement	No hepatic pedicle nodes	No coeliac node involvement
Synchronicity	Metachronous	Metachronous or synchronous
Venous involvement	No vena caval or hepatic venous involvement	Venous resection or reconstruction

Adapted from Sherman and Mahvi [2].

Table 1. Indications for surgical resection of liver metastases.

future liver remnant to avoid post-hepatectomy liver failure and, when major liver resections are being considered, techniques are available to increase the volume of the FLR.

The commonest indication worldwide for hepatic resection is to treat colorectal cancer metastatic to the liver, and overtime the criteria for surgical resectability of colorectal liver metastases has evolved (**Table 1**). Initially, surgically resectable colorectal liver metastases included low volume, unilobar disease of 1–3 metastases which could be resected with a 1 cm macroscopic margin and no evidence of extrahepatic disease [1]. More recently, the number or bilaterality of metastases is not in itself a contraindication provided they can be resected with a macroscopic margin with an adequate FLR [2], and increasingly the presence of localized extrahepatic disease [2] is not an absolute contraindication to resection. However, the response of metastases to chemotherapy has emerged as an important prognostic factor for disease-free survival [3], and consequently, most patients now receive neoadjuvant treatment prior to resection. These factors and a globally more aggressive policy of resection have increased the numbers of patients eligible for potentially curative therapy but placed new emphasis on the importance of accurate assessment of the volume and function of the FLR.

The aim of this chapter is to review currently available methods to assess the quality and volume of the FLR pre-operatively as well as summarizing the methods used to improve the FLR including pre-operative portal venous embolization (PVE) and associating liver partition and portal vein ligation for staged hepatectomy (ALPPS).

2. Pre-operative assessment of liver function

Whether the indication for liver resection is a primary or secondary liver malignancy in order for surgery to be successful, the patient must be able to tolerate the physical and psychological challenges of surgery and the FLR must be able to sustain liver function. A thorough history and examination should identify presence and extent of comorbidities [4]. The assessment should also include assessment of liver function tests, coagulation status, full blood count and platelet count, relevant tumour markers and cross-sectional radiology [4]. All radiology and clinical information should be reviewed in a multidisciplinary meeting and early input obtained from specialist services such as hepatology, interventional radiology and medical oncology.

2.1. Assessing liver function

2.1.1. Liver function tests

The assessment of liver function is complex and largely reliant on surrogate markers. Initial clinical assessment involves assessment for signs of overt liver disease such as jaundice, spider naevi and palmar erythema. An initial set of liver function tests including measurement of plasma bilirubin, transaminases, γ-glutamyl transferase and alkaline phosphatase as well as albumin and prothrombin time should be performed [5]. Two commonly used scoring systems have been developed using these parameters to assess liver function and associated surgical risk.

2.1.2. Scoring systems

The Child-Pugh (CP) and Model for End-Stage Liver Disease (MELD) scores are the most widely used stratification scores used in making decisions regarding surgery in cirrhotic patient (**Tables 2** and **3**).

Factor	1 point	2 points	3 points
Bilirubin (μmol/L)	<34	34–50	>50
Albumin (g/L)	>35	28–35	<28
INR	<1.7	1.7–2.2	>2.2
Ascites	None	Diuretic controlled	Refractory
Encephalopathy	None	Grade I-II (medication controlled)	Grade III-IV (refractory)

Class A = 5–6 points, Class B = 7–9 points, Class C = 10–15 points.
INR; international normalized ratio.
Modified from Hanje and Patel [10].

Table 2. Child-Pugh score.

MELD = 3.78 × ln[serum bilirubin (mg/dL)] + 11.2 × ln[INR] + 9.57 × ln[serum creatinine (mg/dL)] + 6.43
Predicts development post-operative liver failure post-hepatectomy for hepatocellular carcinoma where a score >11 is predictive of worse outcome. Maximum creatinine is 4.0 mg/dL. Patients dialysing twice within the last week are assigned the maximum creatinine.
Adapted from Hanje and Patel 2007 [10] and Cha 2012 [39].

Table 3. MELD score.

The CP score has been in clinical use for several decades and is based on the patient's albumin, bilirubin, coagulation studies, severity of ascites and encephalopathy [6]. Individuals are stratified to Child A, B and C, and these correspond to increasing risk of perioperative mortality as well as post-operative complications such as bleeding, infection, ascites, renal failure and hepatic failure [6] (**Figure 1**).

The MELD score originally used to predict mortality following transjugular intrahepatic portosystemic shunt (TIPS) has since been extrapolated to stratifying liver transplant patients as well predicting perioperative mortality [6] (**Figure 1**).

2.2. Dynamic tests of liver function

These tests are based on complete hepatic clearance or metabolism of a substrate following intravenous administration and include indocyanine green (ICG) clearance as well as nuclear medicine techniques.

2.2.1. Indocyanine green clearance

ICG is the most widely discussed pre-operative test to assess liver function. Historically, the test entails intravenous administration of ICG with multiple blood samples taken at 15-min intervals to determine plasma clearance but has become easier to perform with the availability of non-invasive bedside monitors [7]. ICG is a water soluble, inert tricarbocyanine with a hepatic extraction rate above 70%, and is almost completely excreted in its unchanged form by the liver [7].

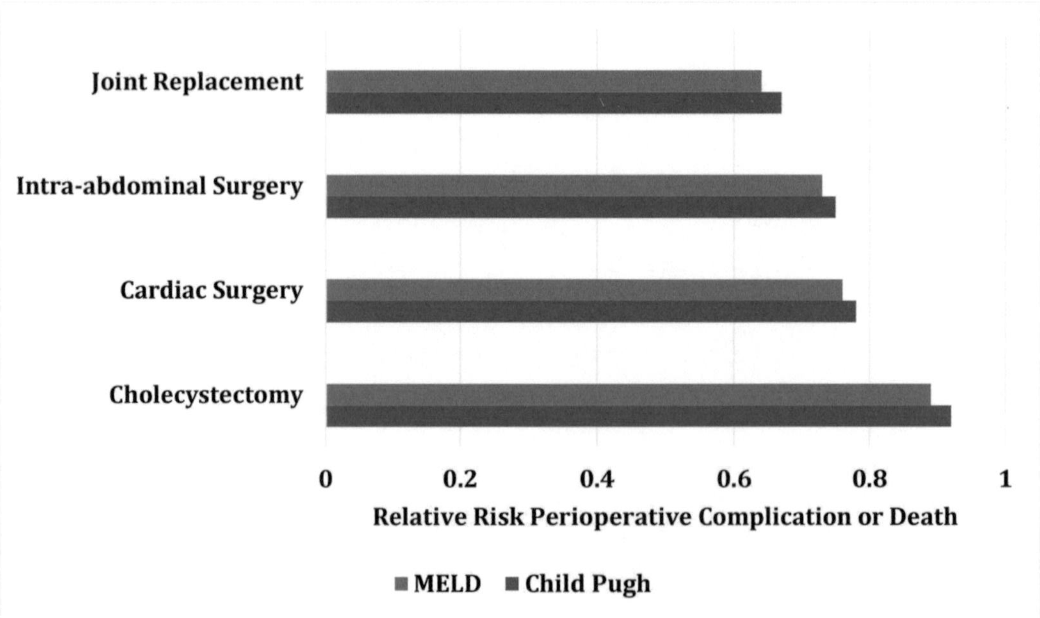

Figure 1. Relative risk of perioperative complication or death with increasing Child-Pugh and MELD scores. Adapted from Hanje and Patel [10].

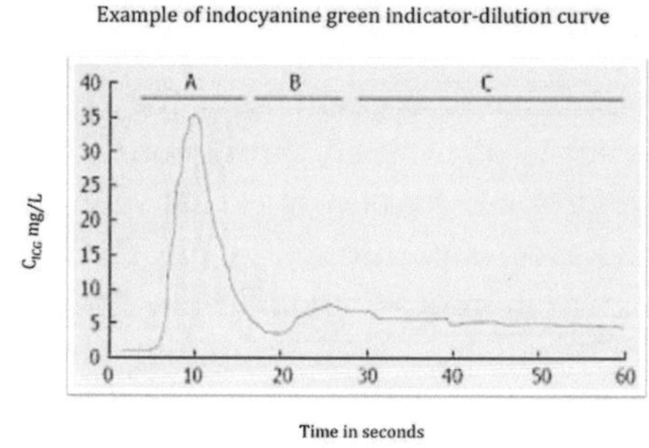

Figure 2. Indocyanine green plasma clearance curve obtained from serial blood sampling or optical pulse spectrophotometry. Retention at 15 min (arrow) is commonly used to assess liver function. Modified from Cha *et al.* [39].

Test results are most commonly expressed as percentage of ICG retained after 15 min (ICG-R15), and however, they can also be reported as the plasma disappearance rate (ICG PDR) or as the ICG elimination rate constant [8] (**Figure 2**). The safety limit when expressed as ICG-R15 varies from 14 to 20% [8].

The use of ICG is limited in the presence of hyperbilirubinaemia since uptake is by the same hepatic transporters [8] and will therefore artificially decrease ICG clearance. The test is also dependent on overall liver blood flow and is less reliable in those with non-flow-dependent liver diseases [8].

2.2.2. *Nuclear Medicine*

Scintigraphy has been used to provide quantitative information on total and regional liver function using a variety of radiolabelled probes.

2.2.2.1. *^{99m}Tc-Mebrofenin*

Mebrofenin is the iminodiacetic acid (IDA) analogue with the highest specificity for hepatocytes [8, 9]. It is absorbed by hepatocytes and eliminated in the bile without biotransformation in a similar fashion to bilirubin [8, 9]. The rate of hepatocyte uptake of technicium-labelled mebrofenin can be quantitatively assessed using scintigraphy and rate of biliary excretion determined.

2.2.2.2. *^{99m}Tc-GSA*

(99m)Tc-DTPA-galactosyl serum albumin (where DTPA is diethylenetriaminepentaacetic acid) binds to the asialoglycoprotein receptor found on the sinusoidal surface of the hepatocyte[8]. ^{99m}Tc-GSA is an asialoglycoprotein analogue that is taken up only in the liver [8]. The uptake of this agent is not affected by hyperbilirubinaemia and can therefore still be used for liver function assessment in the cholestatic patient [8]. Scintigraphy permits assessment of hepatic uptake as measure of function, and ^{99m}Tc-GSA remains trapped in the liver which permits further assessment of liver volume. However, this agent is not widely available outside of Japan.

2.2.3. ^{13}C-Methacetin Breath Test (LiMax)

The ^{13}C-methacetin breath test is based on activity of the cytochrome P450 1A2 (CYP1A2) enzyme system [8]. The system is distributed throughout the liver and is not affected by drugs or genetic variation [8]. ^{13}C-methacetin is exclusively metabolized by CYP1A2 into paracetamol and $^{13}CO_2$ [10]. The test is performed by measuring $^{13}CO_2/^{12}CO_2$ ratio in expired breath before and after administration of ^{13}C-methacetin. The result is expressed in μg/kg/h and gives total liver function. If combined with computed tomographic (CT) scan, it may be used to approximate the function of a section of liver, and however, this assumes uniform distribution of hepatic function, and it is known that this may vary between segments [8].

3. Radiological measurement of liver volume

Multiple cross-sectional imaging modalities are available for imaging the liver and include ultrasound, CT and magnetic resonance imaging (MRI). Data obtained with these investigations can be used to volumetrically assess the FLR as well as define the presence and position of hepatic tumours and the presence of chronic liver disease.

3.1. Ultrasound

Transabdominal ultrasound is widely available, non-invasive and low cost. However, it is operator independent, and its accuracy may be affected by body habitus, the presence of ileus or ascites as well as the presence of diffuse hepatic disease and steatosis which may be seen following chemotherapy [11].

In patients with colorectal liver metastases, the sensitivity of lesion-by-lesion analysis ranges from 60.9 to 64.9%. The specificity ranges from 50 to 60%, and the range increases from 76.7 to 83.3% with the use of contrast [11]. The increased sensitivity of contrast-enhanced US (80–90%) makes it useful in guiding the percutaneous biopsies of lesions [11].

Three-dimensional ultrasound probes are available, but the use of transabdominal ultrasound in hepatic volumetry assessment remains limited by the previously stated problems of body habitus and operator expertise [12]. Ultrasound is also routinely used intraoperatively where it may identify occult liver metastases denoting unresectable disease in up to 25% of patients [13] but currently has no role in assessing FLR volume.

3.2. Computed tomography (CT)

CT has become widely available and is relatively inexpensive. It offers the ability not only to detect lesions, but also to detect accurately localize lesions as well as their vascular and biliary relations [11]. It does involve exposure to ionizing radiation and the risk of allergic reactions to iodinated contrast [11]. The lesion-by-lesion sensitivity is up to 75% [11] although the rate of detection decreases with size of the lesion with a 16% detection rate for lesions smaller than 10mm in diameter [11]. The ability to construct three-dimensional (3D) models from the images allows for more accurate planning of surgical resection and appreciation of intrahepatic vascular anatomy prior to resection [14].

CT scan is also commonly used to estimate the volume of the FLR by directly quantifying the volume from scan acquired data. The FLR volume is measured by CT and then standardized to the total estimated liver volume (TELV) [15].

$$\text{TELV}\,(\text{cm}^3) = -794.41 + 1267.28 \times \text{BSA}(\text{m}^2)$$

The ratio of the CT measured FLR volume to the TELV is known as the standardized FLR (sFLR) that allows a uniform comparison of FLR volume before and after PVE [15]. More commonly, total liver volume can be measured using data acquired in the CT scan, and comparison is made with the directly measured volume of the FLR (**Figure 3**).

3.3. Magnetic resonance imaging (MRI)

MRI is the most accurate of the available modalities in detecting colorectal metastases as well as many other malignancies. It does not make use of ionizing radiation and gadolinium-based extracellular agents or hepatocyte-specific contrast agents such as gadoxetic acid may be used as contrast [11]. Overall, the sensitivity of contrast-enhanced MRI is 94% for colorectal metastases[11] and is superior to CT scan in the detection of small lesions as well as lesions in steatotic livers [11]. MRI is not routinely used clinically to assess hepatic volumetry.

3.4. PET CT

Fluorodeoxyglucose positron emission tomography (^{18}FDG PET) provides metabolic information which when combined with CT provides a metabolic map of glucose uptake [16] that is highly specific for cancer. PET CT is less sensitive in the detection of hepatic lesions than CT or MRI but is more specific and is able to accurately define the presence of extrahepatic disease [16]. PET CT is not currently used to assess hepatic volumetry.

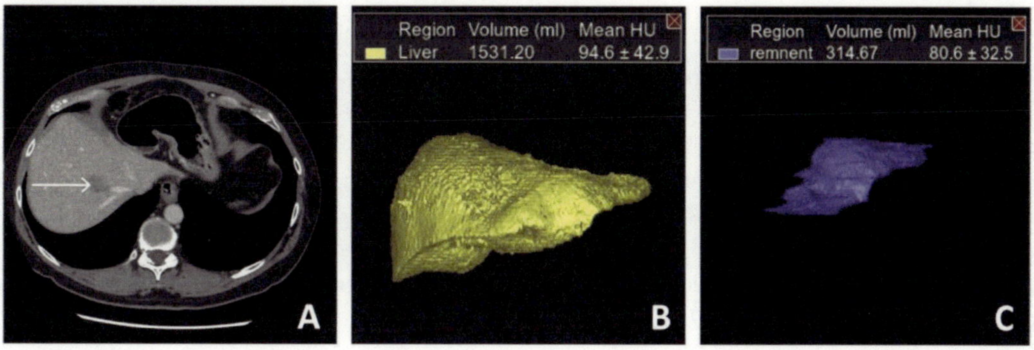

Figure 3. A: Axial CT scan showing solitary colorectal metastasis in segment 8 (arrow) with a congenitally small left lobe. B: Three-dimensional reconstruction and total liver volume (1531.20 ml) measured 6 weeks following right portal vein embolization. C: Three-dimensional reconstruction and total remnant volume (314.67 ml) measured 6 weeks following right portal vein embolization. The left-sided remnant now constitutes 20.5% of the total liver volume and the patient proceeded to right hepatic lobectomy.

4. Combined imaging and dynamic tests

As previously described, available imaging and liver function tests have a number of shortcomings with regard to estimation of function of the future liver remnant. This is important since hepatic volume and hepatic function do not have a linear correlation. A number of groups have attempted to improve predictability of FLR volume and function by combining modalities (**Table 4**).

Group	Modalities	Outcome
Chapelle *et al.* [25]	^{99m}Tc-mebrofenin/FLRV	Predicts future liver function after resection (eFLRF). Cut-off of 2.3%/min/m^2 for eFLRF would have prevented all mortalities related to PHLF
Hwang *et al.* [40]	FRL-kICG (derived ICG and CT volumetry)	Appeared to predict PHLF risk quantitatively
De Graaf *et al.* [41]	^{99m}Tc-mebrofenin/SPECT	No difference between actual FLR and predicted FLR

PHLF, post-hepatectomy liver failure. FRL-kICG is the ICG clearance rate constant (ICG-K) fraction of future remnant liver to total liver volume.

Table 4. Examples of combined modalities in FLR estimation.

5. Definition of an adequate future liver remnant

With regard to the future liver remnant, an FLR ≤20% of total hepatic volume is the strongest predictor of hepatic insufficiency and is thus set as the minimum FLR volume for a healthy non-cirrhotic liver [17]. It has generally been regarded that those who have received chemotherapy for longer than 12 weeks should have an FLR >30% of total hepatic volume and those with fibrosis or cirrhosis an FLR >40–50% of total hepatic volume [17]. However, it must be emphasized that patients with cirrhotic livers, even where FLR is adequate, remain at increased risk of wound breakdown, infection, ascites and fluid retention, as they would be for any major surgery.

The increased FLR requirement for patients who have received chemotherapy is based on the premise that pre-operative chemotherapy may cause liver damage or increase the risk of post-operative complications [18]. Treatment with irinotecan is associated with rates of steatohepatitis as high as 20.2% compared to 4.4% in those not on chemotherapy [19]. Treatment with oxaliplatin is associated with hepatic sinusoidal injury that can result in venoocclusive disease and nodular regenerative hyperplasia [19]. There is greater morbidity following hepatectomy in those with evidence of sinusoidal obstruction syndrome and a greater risk of peri-operative blood transfusion [19].

However, the majority of investigations have shown (**Table 5**) that liver injury in the setting of neoadjuvant therapy does not appear to have significant clinical consequences if chemotherapy is maintained until a response is observed and disease is then resected as early as is feasible [20].

http://dx.doi.org/10.5772/66139

Author	Intervention	No.	Comparison	FLR effect
Goéré *et al.* [42]	PVE	20	≥1 -month interval vs no interval	None
Ribero *et al.* [43]	PVE	112	Chemo vs no chemo	None
Gruenberger *et al.* [44]	Hepatectomy	52		None
Covey *et al.* [45]	PVE	100	Chemo vs no chemo	None
Aussilhou *et al.* [46]	PVE	40	Chemo+bevacizumab/chemo without bevacizumab	Impaired FLR/none
Tanaka *et al.* [47]	PVE/Hepatectomy	60	Chemo vs no chemo	None
Sturesson *et al.* [48]	PVE	26	Chemo vs no chemo	Impaired FLR
Sturesson *et al.* [49]	Hepatectomy	74	Chemo vs no chemo	Impaired FLR
Beal *et al.* [50]	Hepatectomy	72	Chemo vs no chemo >6 cycles vs ≤6 cycles	None
Dello *et al.* [51]	Hepatectomy	72	Chemo vs no chemo >6 cycles vs ≤6 cycles	None
Fischer *et al.* [52]	PVE	64	Chemo vs no chemo	None

PVE, portal vein embolization; FLR, future liver remnant.
Adapted from Simoneau *et al.* [27].

Table 5. Effect of chemotherapy on liver hypertrophy.

6. Augmentation of the future liver remnant

With advances in surgical technique and radiological imaging, more extensive liver resections have become feasible and the challenge remains the ability to maintain liver function post-operatively. Methods have been developed aiming to increase the size of the future liver remnant. These include portal venous embolization, portal vein ligation (PVL) and associating liver partition and portal vein ligation for staged hepatectomy (ALPPS). Augmentation is recommended where FLR is anticipated to be ≤20% for normal, ≤30% for those with chemotherapy associated steatohepatitis and ≤40–50% in those with cirrhosis [21].

6.1. Portal venous embolization

Portal venous embolization was developed to improve the size and function of the FLR in tumour bearing liver by occluding the ipsilateral portal vein, the non-tumour bearing contralateral side, which is to be the FLR, increases in volume by a combination of hypertrophy and hyperplasia [22]. The capacity for regeneration in the otherwise healthy liver is significant, and PVE results in increased FLR volume in roughly 60% of patients with the average increase in volume being 12% [17]. The response is variable, and the size of the FLR prior to PVE may predict the degree of hypertrophy [23]. There is evidence to suggest that the degree of hypertrophy is inversely proportional to the FLR ratio before PVE such that a smaller FLR will have a larger hypertrophy [24]. PVE is contraindicated in the presence of ipsilateral portal vein tumour thrombus or occlusion and in patients with severe portal hypertension [22].

PVE may be performed under general anaesthesia or local anaesthesia with sedation, and the approach may be contralateral or ipsilateral [24]. The procedure is commonly used to occlude the right portal vein and induce left lobe hypertrophy. In the contralateral approach, the left portal vein is punctured to give access for embolization of the right portal vein [24]. The contralateral approach is less technically demanding, and however, it does risk potential injury to the FLR [24]. Where extended right hepatectomy is considered, embolization of portal vein branches to segment IVa and IVb can be undertaken. A short segment (1 cm) of unembolized right portal vein may be left to allow for surgical ligation during resection [25].

Various agents have been used for embolization, and most are associated with adequate hypertrophy rates and acceptable complication profiles (**Table 6**).

The degree of FLR hypertrophy is also influenced by the health of the underlying liver. Non-cirrhotic liver hypertrophies at a rate of about 12–21 cm^3/day at 2 weeks compared to just 9 cm^3/day for a cirrhotic liver [22] and the growth rate can be used to predict the probability of liver failure and major complications [23] (**Figure 4**).

Embolic agent	Authors	No. of patients	Increase FRL %
Gelatin sponge	Fuji *et al.* [53]	30	17.8
	Kusaka *et al.* [54]	18	21.2
	Kazikawa *et al.* [55]	14	23.8
	Nanashima *et al.* [56]	30	29.4
Polyvinyl alcohol + coils or plugs	Covey *et al.* [44]	100	24.3
	Van den Esschert *et al.* [57]	10	26.1
	Libicher *et al.* [58]	10	26.4
N-butyl cyanoacrylate	De Baere *et al.* [59]	107	57.8
	Giraudo *et al.* [60]	146	41.7
	Elias *et al.* [61]	68	59.1
	Broering *et al.* [62]	17	69.4
Fibrin glue	Nagino *et al.* [63]	105	27.4
	Liem *et al.* [64]	15	31.4

Modified from Loffroy *et al.* [24].

Table 6. Hypertrophic response to embolic agents.

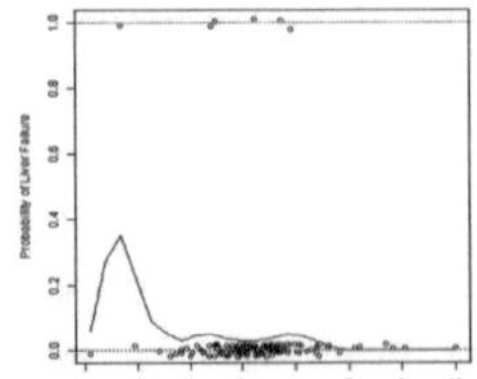

Figure 4. Nonparametric regression of measured future liver remnant growth rate to predict probability of liver failure. Minimal or negative remnant growth rate following portal vein embolization was associated with higher rates of post-resection liver failure. Reproduced from Leung *et al.* [23] with permission.

While PVE is used for its effect on the contralateral lobe of liver, it has also been associated with tumour progression. Liver growth is regulated by a number of growth factors and cytokines the up-regulation of which is known to be involved in multiple tumour pathways [26]. Other factors thought to contribute to tumour progression are the compensatory increased inflow via the hepatic artery and the cellular host response [26]. There are currently no specific therapies available aimed at limiting the effects of these growth factors and cytokines on tumour progression. However, two-stage hepatectomy or ablation can be used where disease in the FLR is resected or ablated prior to PVE or PVL [14].

The timing of definitive resectional surgery following PVE is not formally prescribed, and however, most investigations report repeating imaging (usually CT scan) at 4–6 weeks following PVE and, if sufficient FLR volume has been achieved, undertaking resection soon afterward. Simoneau *et al.* demonstrated an increase of 1-day post-PVE increased the risk of tumour progression by 1% [27]. It has been suggested that earlier surgery such as 2 weeks after PVE may reduce the risk of tumour progression [26].

6.2. Portal vein ligation

PVL is undertaken operatively and often in the setting of staged hepatectomies where small tumours in the FLR are removed or ablated and open ligation of the right portal vein is performed. Pandanaboyana *et al.* in their meta-analysis found that PVE and PVL had a mean percentage increase in FLR volume of 39% and 27%, respectively; however, this did not reach statistical significance [28]. They proposed that this may be explained the observation that the later formation of portoportal collaterals does not impact on liver hypertrophy as this is induced early after portal occlusion [28].

6.3. Associated liver partition and portal vein ligation

ALPPS was first performed in 2007 and was noted to result in significant hepatic hypertrophy with increased resectability in those with large tumours [29]. The procedure was performed during an exploration for hilar cholangiocarcinoma. A left hepaticojejunostomy was performed to reduce cholestasis to the FLR, the liver was divided along the falciform ligament, and the right portal vein was ligated [29]. A CT scan performed 8 days later demonstrated a 94% increase in FLR, and the resection was successfully completed the following day [29].

The classical ALPPS procedure for a large right-sided tumours involves right portal vein ligation, ligation and division of the segment IV portal branches as well as transection of the liver parenchyma along the falciform ligament [29]. Any tumour deposits within the future liver remnant can also be resected or ablated at this time.

Associating liver tourniquet and portal ligation for staged hepatectomy (ALTPS) is a variation in which rather than dividing the liver parenchyma and ligating the portal vein, the effect of occluding portal flow and transection is achieved by use of tourniquet [29] and radiofrequency or microwave ablation may also be combined with portal vein ligation [29]. In an attempt to reduce surgical complications following the initial surgical procedure, a partial ALPPS in which parenchymal transection is not complete has also been described [29].

The advantage ALPPS over two-stage hepatectomy is that it may improve the feasibility of resecting previously unresectable tumours owing to the very high FLR gains seen. The short time between the procedures makes tumour progression unlikely [30].

In 2012, the International ALPPS registry was formed to systematically collect data from multiple centres performing the procedure, and the first analysis was published in 2014 [31]. This analysis which included 202 patients, 70% of whom had an underlying diagnosis colorectal liver metastases, and reported a 90-day mortality of 9% [31] (**Table 7**). Independent risk factors for in hospital severe complications included patient age >60 years, tumours other than colorectal liver metastases as well as 2 markers of complex liver resection (stage 1 ALPPS procedure >5 h and/or the need for intraoperative blood transfusions) [31].

The data in **Table 7** confirm that ALPPS is a physiologically demanding procedure, and there is a paucity of data concerning long-term outcomes. Buac *et al.* [32] recently conducted a survey of 66% of the surgeons contributing to the International ALPPS registry and noted that there was significant variability in the indications for surgery as well as how it is performed. Currently, PVE is widely used while ALPPS is still under investigation. Schadde *et al.* [31] published a head to head comparison of the two procedures (**Table 8**).

6.4. Assessment of liver remnant volume using ICG clearance intraoperatively during vascular exclusion (ALIIVE)

This is a newly reported intraoperative procedure, which may have the advantage of some planned ALPPS procedures occurring as a single-step hepatectomy as well as identifying the need for an ALPPS procedure where one had not been planned [33]. The technique involves non-invasive measurement of ICG PDR at 5 points during resectional surgery. Measurement occurs before anaesthetic induction (ICG 1), following mobilization of FLR (ICG 2), during inflow occlusion of the resection lobe (ICG 3), following parenchymal transection with inflow occlusion (ICG 4) and finally during inflow as well as outflow occlusion following parenchymal transection (ICG 5/ALIIVE) [33].

The aim of this test is to replicate the post-resection state intraoperatively. Lau *et al.* published their initial experience and while their series was too small to deduce an ICG PDR cut-off level, they suggested that as the post-hepatectomy state was replicated, it was likely that previously demonstrated cut-off levels could be applied to the procedure [33]. Previous studies have suggested a PDR >9%/min would likely be safe, while a PDR <7%/min would confer a high risk of insufficiency [33]. Interestingly, the only mortality of the 10 patients had an ALIIVE ICG of 7.1%/min [33].

This procedure will require further validation studies, but could certainly spare some patients a second procedure or allow others the opportunity of an ALPPS procedure if not already planned pre-operatively.

6.5. Transarterial embolization (TAE)

Transarterial chemoembolization (TACE) is based on the concept that blood supply to tumour is generally derived from the hepatic artery [34]. Following portal venous embolization, the

Author	Number of patients	Simultaneous colorectal resection	FLR hypertrophy %	Mean LOS	Morbidity%	Mortality %	Follow-up days	DFS %	OS%
Schnitzbauer *et al.* [65]	25	0	74	nr	68	12	60-776	80	86
Alvarez *et al.* [66]	15	3	78.4	19	53	0	18–410	73	100
Li *et al.* [67]	9	nr	87.2	nr	100	22	nr	nr	nr
Dokmak and Belghiti [68]	8	nr	70	42	90	nr	nr	nr	nr
Machado *et al.* [69]	8	nr	88	nr	nr	0	nr	nr	nr
Donati *et al.* [70]	8	nr	66–200	nr	nr	nr	nr	nr	nr
Adriani *et al.* [71]	2	nr	nr	nr	nr	0	912–1460	0	100
Govil [72]	1	nr	nr	nr	nr	nr	nr	nr	nr
Oldhafer *et al.* [73]	1	0	nr	nr	nr	0	nr	nr	nr
Conrad *et al.* [74]	1	nr	45	nr	0	0	nr	nr	nr
Cavaness *et al.* [75]	1	0	100	13	nr	0	nr	nr	nr

Adapted from Alvarez *et al.* [76].
Nr, not reported; DFS, disease-free survival; OS, overall survival.

Table 7. Overview of hypertrophy, mortality and morbidity following ALPPS for various studies.

Reason for failure	PVE/PVL (n = 83)	ALPPS (n = 48)
Perioperative death (90 days) %	6%	15%
No stage 2 due to tumour progression %	16%	0%
No stage 2 due to failure to grow%	7%	0%
R1 resection %	5%	2%
Failure to reach primary endpoint %	34%	17%

Table 8. Mortality and outcomes of ALPPS v PVE/PVL. Modified from Schadde *et al.* 2014 [31].

hepatic arterial flow is increased and this is thought to preserve viability of the embolized lobe [35]. However, there may still not be adequate hypertrophy of the FLR, and it has been suggested that further interruption of the vascular inflow (arterial occlusion) may result in further hypertrophy [35]. However, the near complete occlusion that occurs with PVE followed by TAE may induce parenchymal infarction, and this sequence currently has few applications [35].

Conversely, TAE followed by PVE has demonstrated safety in case of hepatocellular carcinoma with inadequate FLR [35]. Unfortunately, this has not been useful in management of colorectal metastases as these tumours are generally not fed by an artery [35].

6.6. Radioembolization

Selective internal radiation therapy (SIRT) with Y-90 has generally been used as treatment for locally advanced liver tumours. A transarterial catheter is introduced, and Y-90 microspheres are infused to lodge at the tumour arteriolar level. The radioactive microspheres result in reduced blood flow to the tumour but also deliver Y-90 brachytherapy [36]. The reported rates of response are 42–70% for colorectal liver metastases [36] and, in addition to the local control of tumour, unilateral treatment has been noted to result in hypertrophy of the contralateral liver lobe [37]. The theoretical advantage of SIRT over PVE would then be that tumour progression might not continue unabated while awaiting hypertrophy of the FLR if SIRT were selectively administered. Teo *et al.* [36] in a systematic review found that, while the degree of hypertrophy from SIRT was comparable to that of PVE (26–47% vs 10–46%), the time interval over which growth occurred was much slower than that of PVE (44 days to 9 months vs 2–8 weeks) making it less likely to be clinically useful.

6.7. Associating portal embolization and artery ligation (APEAL)

This procedure combines portal vein embolization and arterial ligation [38]. At the first stage of the procedure, the FLR is surgically mobilized as in the ALPPS procedure. The right portal vein is embolized before being ligated and divided [38]. A right sectoral hepatic artery ligation is performed (either the artery for segments V/VIII or segments VI/VII), and the segment IVb inflow is also interrupted [38]. There is no parenchymal transection. The second, resection stage of the procedure is undertaken 1–2 months later.

Dupre *et al.* [38] published their series of 10 patients who had required two-stage extended right hemihepatectomy for bilobar colorectal metastases. All the patients included had a low FLR volume and/or prolonged pre-operative chemotherapy and the procedure resulted in

http://dx.doi.org/10.5772/66139

FLR hypertrophy of over 100% at day 7 [38]. There were no complications related to hepatic necrosis, and the authors suggest that the avoidance of parenchymal dissection reduces the risk of bile leak and infection. The interval of 1–2 months between stages was chosen to allow for post-operative recovery and to identify those with rapidly progressive disease. Initial results suggest morbidity and mortality rates comparable to ALPPS and PVE, and however, more long-term results and further validation studies are required [38].

7. Conclusion

The indications for liver resection continue to evolve as do the improvements in radiological ability to assess disease extent and accurately measure FLR volume. This information enables surgical teams to precisely calculate perioperative risk and determine resectability—almost to the millimetre. There is an evolving use biochemical markers which, when combined with imaging, may improve the safety of surgery further by allowing not only for estimating the volume but also the function of the future liver remnant.

The development of surgical techniques such as ALPPS, ALIIVE as well as adjuncts to surgery such as PVE/PVL and perhaps SIRT are increasing the number of patients who can be considered to have resectable disease. This would not be possible in the absence of oncological advancements as well as improvement in perioperative care. As our imaging and functional assessment technology improves, current management algorithms will also evolve (**Figure 5**).

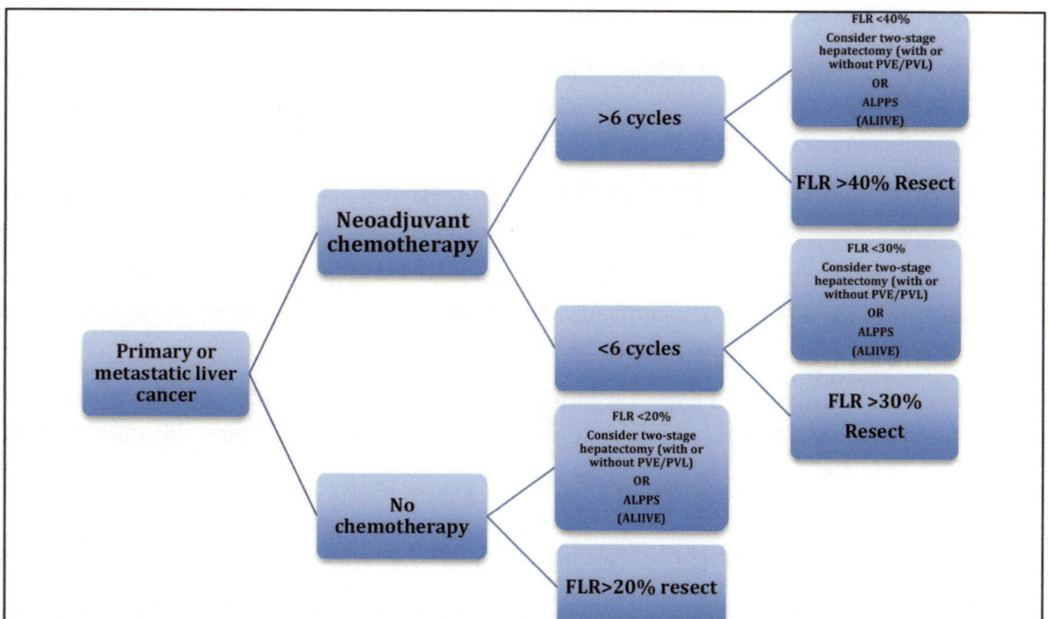

Figure 5. Example of future algorithm. ALIIVE technique could be utilized at the time of first stage hepatectomy or ALPPS to determine whether resection can be completed at first stage.

Author details

Mandivavarira Maundura and Jonathan B Koea*

*Address all correspondence to: jonathan.koea@waitematadhb.govt.nz

Upper Gastrointestinal Unit, Department of Surgery, North Shore Hospital, Auckland, New Zealand

References

[1] Dunne DFJ, Parks RW, Jones RP, Adam R, Poston G. Colorectal liver metastases. In: Garden OJ A Companion to Specialist Surgical Practice: Hepatobiliary and Pancreatic Surgery 5th ed. Elsevier New York; 2014. p. 109–131.

[2] Sherman K, Mahvi D. Liver metastases. In: Niederhuber JE, Armitage JO, Doroshow JH. Karstan MB, Tepper JE. Abeloff's Clinical Oncology 5th ed. Saunders; Philadelphia 2014. p778–793.

[3] Brouquet A, Nordlinger B. Neoadjuvant and adjuvant chemotherapy in relation to surgery for colorectal liver metastases. Scandinavian Journal of Gastroenterology. New York 2012;47:286–295.

[4] Koea J. Cancer of the Bile Ducts: Intrahepatic Cholangiocarcinoma. In: Jamagin W, Blumgart L editors, Blumgart's Surgery of the Liver, Biliary Tract and Pancreas 5th ed. Saunders Philadelphia 2012; p760–770.

[5] Wigmore SJ, Parks RW, Stutchfield BM, Forbes SJ. Liver function and failure. In: Garden OJ editor, A Companion to Specialist Surgical Practice: Hepatobiliary and Pancreatic Surgery 5th ed. Elsevier, New York; 2104. p.1–16.

[6] Friedman L. Surgery in the patient with liver disease. Transactions of the American Clinical and Climatological Association. 2010;121:192–205.

[7] De Gasperi A, Mazza E, Prosperi M. Indocyanine green kinetics to assess liver function: ready for a clinical dynamic assessment in major liver surgery? World Journal of Hepatology. 2016;8:355–367. doi: 10.4254/wjh.v8.i7.355

[8] Cieslak KP, Runge JH, Heger M, Stoker J, Bennink RJ, Van Gulik TM. New perspectives in the assessment of future remnant liver. Digestive Surgery. 2014;31:255–268. doi:10.1159/000364836

[9] Geisel D, Lüdemann L, Hamm B, Denecke T. Imaging-based liver function tests—past, present and future. Fortschr Röntgenstr. 2015;187:863–871.

[10] Hanje AJ, Patel T. Nature Clinical Practice Gastroenterology and Hepatology. Preoperative evaluation of patients with liver disease. 2007;4:266–276.

[11] Matos AP, Altun E, Ramalho M, Velloni F, Alobaidy M, Semelka RC. An overview of imaging techniques for liver metastases management. Expert Review of Gastroenterology and Hepatology. 2015;9:1561–1576.

[12] D'Onofrio M, De Robertis R, Demozzi E, Crosara S, Canestrini S, Mucelli RP. Liver volumetry: is imaging reliable? Personal experience and review of the literature. World Journal of Radiology. 2014;6:62–71. doi:10.4329/wjr.v6.i4.62

[13] Simoneau E, Alanazi R, Alshenaifi J, Molla N, Aljiffry M, Medkhali A, Boucher LM, Asselah J, Metrakos P, Hassanain M. Neoadjuvant chemotherapy does not impair liver regeneration following hepatectomy or portal vein embolisation for colorectal liver metastases. Journal of Surgical Oncology. 2016;113:449–455.

[14] Lamade W, Glombitza G, Fischer L. The impact of 3-dimensional reconstruction on operative planning in liver surgery. Archives of Surgery. 2000;135:1256–1261.

[15] Ribero D, Chun YS, Vauthey JN. Surgery for colorectal metastases. In: Vauthey JN, Hoff PMG, Audisio RA, Poston GJ, Editors. Liver Metastases. 1st ed. Springer. London; 2009. p25–38.

[16] Mattar RE, Al-Alem F, Simoneau E, Hassanain M. Preoperative selection of patients with colorectal cancer liver metastasis for hepatic resection. World Journal of Gastroenterology. 2016;22:567–581. doi:10.3748/wjg.v22.i2.567

[17] Ethun C, Maithel S. Determination of resectability. Surgical Clinics of North America. 2016;96:163–181. doi:10.1016/j.suc.2015.12.002

[18] Brudvik KW, Passot G, Vauthey JN. Colorectal liver metastases: a changing treatment landscape. Journal of Oncology Practice. 2016;12:40–41.

[19] Maor Y, Malnick S. Liver injury by anticancer chemotherapy and radiation therapy. International Journal of Hepatology. 2013; Article ID 815105, 8 pages. Published online 2013, July 17. Doi:10.1155/2013/815105

[20] Nordlinger B, Vauthey JN, Poston G, Benoist S, Rougier P, Van Custem E. The timing of chemotherapy and surgery for the treatment of colorectal liver metastases. Clinical Colorectal Cancer. 2010;9:212–218.

[21] Orcutt ST, Kobayashi K, Sultenfuss M, Hailey BS, Sparks A, Satpathy B, Anaya DA. Portal vein embolization as an oncosurgical strategy prior to major hepatic resection: anatomic, surgical, and technical considerations. Frontiers in Surgery. 2016;3:14. Published online 2016, March 11. doi:10.3389/fsurg.2016.00014

[22] May BJ, Madoff DC. Portal vein embolization: rationale, technique, and current application. Seminars in Interventional Radiology. 2012;29:81–89.

[23] Leung U, Simpson AL, Arajuo RLC, Gönen M, McAuliffe C, Miga MI, Parada EP, Allen PJ, D'Angelica MI, Kingham TP, DeMatteo RP, Fong Y, Jarnagin WR. Remnant growth rate after

portal vein embolization is a good early predictor of post-hepatectomy liver failure. Journal of the American College of Surgeons. 2014;219:620–630. doi:10.1016/j.jamcollsurg.2014.04.022

[24] Loffroy R, Favelier S, Chevallier O, Estivalet L, Genson PY, Pottecher P, Gehin S, Krausé D, Cercueil JP. Preoperative portal vein embolization in liver cancer: indications, techniques and outcomes. Quantitative Imaging in Medicine and Surgery. 2015;5:730–739. doi:10.3978/j.issn.2223-4292.2015.10.04

[25] Chapelle T, Op De Beeck B, Huyghe I, Driessen A, Roeyen G, Ysebaert D, De Greef K. Future remnant liver function estimated by combining liver volumetry on magnetic resonance imaging with total liver function on (99m)Tc-mebrofenin hepatobiliary scintigraphy: can this tool predict post-hepatectomy liver failure? HPB. 2016;18:494–503.

[26] Al-Sharif E, Simoneau E, Hassanain M. Portal vein embolization effect on colorectal cancer liver metastasis progression: lessons learned. World Journal of Clinical Oncology. 2015;6:142–146. doi:10.5306/wjco.v6.i5.142

[27] Simoneau E, Hassanain M, Shaheen M, Aljiffry M, Molla N, Chaudhury P, Anil S, Khashper A, Valenti D, Metrakos P. Portal vein embolization and its effect on tumour progression of colorectal cancer liver metastases. British Journal of Surgery. 2015;102:1240–1249.

[28] Pandanaboyana S, Bell R, Hidalgo E, Toogood G, Prasad KJ, Bartlett A, Lodge JP. A systematic review and meta-analysis of portal vein ligation versus portal vein embolization for elective liver resection. Surgery. 2015;157:690–698. doi:10.1016/j.surg.2014.12.009

[29] Li J, Ewald F, Gulati A, Nashan B. Associating liver partition and portal vein ligation for staged hepatectomy: from technical evolution to oncological benefit. World Journal of Gastrointestinal Surgery. 2016;8:124–133. doi:10.4240/wjgs.v8.i2.12

[30] Vennarecci G, Grazi GL, Sperduti I, Rizzi EB, Felli E, Antonini M, D'Offizi, Ettorre GM. ALPPS for primary and secondary liver tumors. International Journal of Surgery. 2016;30:38–44.

[31] Schadde E, Ardiles V, Slankamenac K, Tschuor C, Sergeant G, Amacker N, Baumgart J, Croome K, Hernandez-Alejandro R, Lang H, de Santibanes E, Clavien PA. ALPPS offers a better chance of complete resection in patients with primarily unresectable liver tumors compared with conventional-staged hepatectomies: results of a multicenter analysis. World Journal of Surgery. 2014;38:1510–1519. doi:10.1007/s00268-014-2513-3

[32] Buac S, Schadde E, Schnitzbauer AA, Vogt K, Hernandez-Alejandro R. The many faces of ALPPS: surgical indications and techniques among surgeons collaborating in the international registry. HPB. 2016;18:442–448.

[33] Lau L, Christophi C, Nikfarjam M, Starkey G, Goodwin M, Weinberg L, Ho Loretta Muralidharan V. Assessment of liver remnant using ICG clearance intraoperatively during vascular exclusion: early experience with the ALIIVE technique. HPB Surgery. 2015;757052. doi:10.1155/2015/757052

[34] Riemsma RP, Bala MM, Wolff R, Kleijnen J. Transarterial (chemo)embolisation versus no intervention or placebo intervention for liver metastases. Cochrane Database of Systematic Reviews.2013;http://onlinelibrary.wiley.com/doi/10.1002/14651858.CD009498.pub3/abstract. Accessed online Dec 2, 2016

[35] Yokoyama Y, Nagino M. Sequential PVE and TAE for biliary tract cancer and liver metastases. In: Madoff DC, Makuuchi M, Mizuno T, Vauthey JN, editors, Venous Embolization of the Liver. Springer-Verlag London 2011. p241–248.

[36] Teo JY, Allen JC, Ng DC, Choo SP, Tai DWM, Chang JPE, Cheah FK, Chow PKH, Goh BKP. A systematic review of contralateral liver lobe hypertrophy after unilobar selective internal radiation therapy with Y90. HPB. 2016;18:7–12. doi:10.1016/j.hpb.2015.07.002

[37] Bester L, Meteling B, Boshell D, Chua TC, Morris DL. Transarterial chemoembolization and radioembolisation for the treatment of primary liver cancer and secondary liver cancer: a review of the literature. Journal of Medical Imaging and Radiation Oncology. 2014;58:341–352.

[38] Dupre A, Hitier M, Peyrat P, Chen Y, Meeus P, Rivoire M. Associating portal embolization and artery ligation to induce rapid liver regeneration in staged hepatectomy. The British Journal of Surgery. 2015;102:1541–1550. doi:10.1002/bjs.9900

[39] Cha C. Assessment of hepatic function. In: Jamagin W, Blumgart L editors, Blumgart's Surgery of the Liver, Biliary Tract and Pancreas 5th ed. Saunders Philadelphia 2012; p58–64.

[40] Hwang S, Ha TY, Song GW, Jung DH, Ahn CS, Moon DB, Kim KH, Lee YJ, Lee SG. Quantified risk assessment for major hepatectomy via the indocyanine green clearance rate and liver volumetry combined with standard liver volume. Journal of Gastrointestinal Surgery. 2015;19:1305–1314.

[41] De Graaf W, van Lienden KP, van Gulik TM, Bennink RJ. 99mTc-mebrofenin hepatobiliary scintigraphy with SPECT for the assessment of hepatic function and liver functional volume before partial hepatectomy. Journal of Nuclear Medicine. 2010;51:229–236.

[42] Goéré D, Farges O, Leporrier J, Sauvanet A, Vilgrain V, Belghiti J. Chemotherapy does not impair hypertrophy of the left liver after right portal vein obstruction. Journal of Gastrointestinal Surgery. 2006;10:365–370.

[43] Ribero D, Abdalla EK, Madoff DC, Donaldon M, Loyer EM, Vauthey JN. Portal vein embolization before major hepatectomy and its effects on regeneration, resectability and outcome. British Journal of Surgery. 2007;94:1386–1394.

[44] Gruenberger B, Tamandl D, Schueller J, Scheithauer W, Zielinski C, Herbst F, Gruenberger T. Bevacizumab, capecitabine, and oxaliplatin as neoadjuvant therapy for patients with potentially curable metastatic colorectal cancer. Journal of Clinical Oncology. 2008;26:1830–1835.

[45] Covey AM, Brown KT, Jarnagin WR, Brody LA, Schwartz L, Tuorto S, Sofocleous CT, D'Angelica M, Getrajdman GI, DeMatteo R, Kemeny NE, Fong Y. Combined portal vein embolization and neoadjuvant chemotherapy as a treatment strategy for resectable hepatic colorectal metastases. Annals of Surgery. 2008;247:451–455.

[46] Aussilhou B, Dokmak S, Faivre S, Paradis V, Vilgrain V, Belghiti J. Preoperative liver hypertrophy induced by portal flow occlusion before major hepatic resection for colorectal metastases can be impaired by bevacizumab. Annals of Surgical Oncology. 2009;16:1553–1559.

[47] Tanaka K, Kumamoto T, Matsuyama R, Takeda K, Nagano Y, Endo I. Influence of chemotherapy on liver regeneration induced by portal vein embolization or first hepatectomy of a staged procedure for colorectal liver metastases. Journal of Gastrointestinal Surgery. 2010;14:359–368.

[48] Sturesson C, Keussen I, Tranberg KG. Prolonged chemotherapy impairs liver regeneration after portal vein occlusion—an audit of 26 patients. European Journal of Surgical Oncology. 2010;36:358–364.

[49] Sturesson C, Nilsson J, Eriksson S, Spelt L, Andersson R. Limiting factors for liver regeneration after a major hepatic resection for colorectal cancer metastases. HPB (Oxford). 2013;15:646–652.

[50] Beal IK, Anthony S, Papadopoulou A, Hutchins R, Fusai G, Begent R, Davies N, Tibballs J, Davidson B. Portal vein embolisation prior to hepatic resection for colorectal liver metastases and the effects of periprocedure chemotherapy. The British Journal of Radiology. 2006;79:473–478.

[51] Dello SAWG, Kele PGS, Porte RJ, van Dam RM, Klaase JM, Verhoef C, van Gulik T, Molenaar Q, Bosscha K, van der Jagt EJ, Dejong CHC, de Boer MT. Influence of preoperative chemotherapy on CT volumetric liver regeneration following right hemihepatectomy. World Journal of Surgery. 2014;38:497–504.

[52] Fischer C, Melstrom LG, Arnaoutakis D, Jarnagin W, Brown K, D'Angelica M, Covey A, DeMatteo R, Allen P, Kingham TP, Tuorto S, Kemeny N, Fong Y. Chemotherapy after portal vein embolization to protect against tumor growth during liver hypertrophy before hepatectomy. JAMA Surgery. 2013;148:1103–1108.

[53] Fujii Y, Shimada H, Endo I, Kamiyama M, Kamimukai N, Tanaka K, Kunisaki C, Sekido H, Togo S, Nagashima Y. Changes in clinicopathological findings after portal vein embolization. Hepatogastroenterology. 2000;47:1560–1563.

[54] Kusaka K, Imamura H, Tomiya T, Makuuchi M. Factors affecting liver regeneration after right portal vein embolization. Hepatogastroenterology. 2004;51:532–535.

[55] Kakizawa H, Toyota N, Arihiro K, Naito A, Fujimura Y, Hieda M, Hirai N, Tachikake T, Matsuura N, Murakami Y, Itamoto T, Ito K. Preoperative portal vein embolization

with a mixture of gelatin sponge and iodized oil: efficacy and safety. Acta Radiologica. 2006;47:1022–1028.

[56] Nanashima A, Sumida Y, Abo T, Nonaka T, Takeshita H, Hidaka S, Sawai T, Yasutake T, Sakamoto I, Nagayasu T. Clinical significance of portal vein embolization before right hepatectomy. Hepatogastroenterology. 2009;56:773–777.

[57] Van den Esschert JW, de Graaf W, van Lienden KP, Busch OR, Heger M, van Delden OM, Gouma DJ, Bennink RJ, Laméris JS, van Gulik TM. Volumetric and functional recovery of the remnant liver after major liver resection with prior portal vein embolization. Journal of Gastrointestinal Surgery. 2009;13:1464–1469.

[58] Libicher M, Herbrik M, Stippel D, Poggenborg J, Bovenschulte H, Schwabe H. Portal vein embolization using the amplatz vascular plug II: preliminary results. Rofo. 2010;182:501–506.

[59] de Baere T, Teriitehau C, Deschamps F, Catherine L, Rao P, Hakime A, Auperin A, Goere D, Elias D, Hechelhammer L. Predictive factors for hypertrophy of the future remnant liver after selective portal vein embolization. Annals of Surgical Oncology. 2010;17:2081–2089.

[60] Giraudo G, Greget M, Oussoultzoglou E, Rosso E, Bachellier P, Jaeck D. Preoperative contralateral portal vein embolization before major hepatic resection is a safe and efficient procedure: a large single institution experience. Surgery. 2008;143:476–482.

[61] Elias D, Ouellet JF, De Baère T, Lasser P, Roche A. Preoperative selective portal vein embolization before hepatectomy for liver metastases: long-term results and impact on survival. Surgery. 2002;131:294–299.

[62] Broering DC, Hillert C, Krupski G, Fischer L, Mueller L, Achilles EG, Schulte am Esch J, Rogiers X. Portal vein embolization vs. portal vein ligation for induction of hypertrophy of the future liver remnant. Journal of Gastrointestinal Surgery. 2002;6:905–913; discussion 913.

[63] Nagino M, Kamiya J, Nishio H, Ebata T, Arai T, Nimura Y. Two hundred forty consecutive portal vein embolizations before extended hepatectomy for biliary cancer: surgical outcome and long-term follow-up. Annals of Surgery. 2006;243:364–372.

[64] Liem MS, Liu CL, Tso WK, Lo CM, Fan ST, Wong J. Portal vein embolisation prior to extended right-sided hepatic resection. Hong Kong Medical Journal. 2005;11:366–372.

[65] Schnitzbauer AA, Lang SA, Goessmann H, Nadalin S, Baumgart J, Farkas SA, Fichtner-Feigl S, Lorf T, Goralcyk A, Hörbelt R, Kroemer A, Loss M, Rümmele P, Scherer MN, Padberg W, Königsrainer A, Lang H, Obed A, Schlitt HJ. Right portal vein ligation combined with in situ splitting induces rapid left lateral liver lobe hypertrophy enabling two-staged extended right hepatic resection in small-for-size settings. Annals of Surgery. 2012;255:405–414.

[66] Alvarez FA, Ardiles V, Sanchez Claria R, Pekolj J, de Santibañes E. Associating liver partition and portal vein ligation for staged hepatectomy (ALPPS): tips and tricks. Journal of Gastrointestinal Surgery. 2013;17:814–821.

[67] Li J, Girotti P, Königsrainer I, Ladurner R, Königsrainer A, Nadalin S. ALPPS in right trisectionectomy: a safe procedure to avoid postoperative liver failure? Journal of Gastrointestinal Surgery. 2013;17:956–961.

[68] Dokmak S, Belghiti J. Which limits to the "ALPPS" approach? Annals of Surgery. 2012;256:e6. (e16–17).

[69] Machado MA, Makdissi FF, Surjan RC. Totally laparoscopic ALPPS is feasible and may be worthwhile. Annals of Surgery. 2012;256:e13. (e16–19) doi:10.1097/SLA.Ob013e318265ff2e

[70] Donati M, Stavrou GA, Basile F, Gruttadauria S, Niehaus KJ, Oldhafer KJ. Combination of in situ split and portal ligation: lights and shadows of a new surgical procedure. Annals of Surgery. 2012;256:e11–12. (e16–9).

[71] Andriani OC. Long-term results with associating liver partition and portal vein ligation for staged hepatectomy (ALPPS). Annals of Surgery. 2012;256:e5 (e16–9).

[72] Govil S. Rapid improvement in liver volume induced by portal vein ligation and staged hepatectomy: the ALPPS procedure. HPB (Oxford). 2012;14:874 Doi:10.1111/j.1477-2574.2012.00573.x.

[73] Oldhafer KJ, Donati M, Maghsoudi T, Ojdanić D, Stavrou GA. Integration of 3D volumetry, portal vein transection and in situ split procedure: a new surgical strategy for inoperable liver metastasis. Journal of Gastrointestinal Surgery. 2012;16:415–416.

[74] Conrad C, Shivathirthan N, Camerlo A, Strauss C, Gayet B. Laparoscopic portal vein ligation with in situ liver split for failed portal vein embolization. Annals of Surgery. 2012;256:e14–5 (e16–7).

[75] Cavaness KM, Doyle MB, Lin Y, Maynard E, Chapman WC. Using ALPPS to induce rapid liver hypertrophy in a patient with hepatic fibrosis and portal vein thrombosis. Journal of Gastrointestinal Surgery. 2013;17:207–212.

[76] Alvarez FA, Ardiles V, de Santibanes E. The ALPPS approach for the management of colorectal carcinoma liver metastases. Current Colorectal Cancer Reports. 2013. Doi:10.1007/s11888-013-0159-4

Chapter 10

Living Donor Liver Transplantation for Hepatocellular Carcinoma

Chih-Che Lin,
Ahmed Mohammed Abdel Aziz Elsarawy and
Chao-Long Chen

Additional information is available at the end of the chapter

http://dx.doi.org/10.5772/65109

Abstract

Hepatocellular carcinoma (HCC) is a major worldwide health problem, which is expected to increase steadily due to different underlying liver diseases. Surgical treatment modalities including liver transplantation (LT) or liver resection (LR) are the mainstay options for early cases of HCC. Liver transplantation for well-selected cases provides excellent survival outcomes comparable to nonmalignant indications of LT. Living donor liver transplantation (LDLT) is an alternative option or even the sole one in the current era of organ shortage problem and in some Asian countries where deceased organ donation is markedly reduced due to various reasons. The adoption of LDLT for HCC treatment elicited many dynamic changes and debates to the dilemma of LT as a whole. In this chapter, we focus on different perspectives of LDLT for HCC, including selection criteria evolution, controversial topics, ethical considerations, operative highlights, and other points.

Keywords: hepatocellular carcinoma, living donor, liver, transplantation, criteria, loco-regional therapy

1. Introduction

Hepatocellular carcinoma (HCC) is the sixth most common cancer and the third leading cause of deaths globally. The selection of treatment modalities for HCC is challenging because it depends not only on the stage of tumor and the patient's performance but also on the underlying liver function. Though the staging systems of HCC are clinically useful for treatment allocation, the decision making should be tailored to each patient, taking into account morphological, pathological, and biological tumor criteria. Liver resection (LR) or liver transplantation (LT) can be adopted as a surgical curative therapy for early disease. Ablative therapies such as radiofrequency ablation (RFA) and percutaneous ethanol injection (PEI) can also cure small tumors. Transarterial chemoembolization (TACE), transarterial radio embolization (TARE), and external beam radiation therapy (EBRT) can control locally advanced disease that is no longer amenable to cure [1].

Liver transplantation has been considered theoretically the best treatment for HCC since it cures the cancer and its underlying pathology. Milan criteria (MC) were the cornerstone for LT because patient selection according to them resulted in survival outcome comparable to LT for nonmalignant cases. More cases of HCC were subjected to LT with the changes made in 2002 in western countries when additional points were added to the model for end-stage liver disease (MELD) scoring system for HCC patients that are within MC. However, the protracted waiting list for deceased donor liver transplantation (DDLT) took many patients beyond MC and hence lost their chance of LT [2].

The incorporation of living donor liver transplantation (LDLT) into the treatment roadmaps of HCC not only gave a new horizon to more patients, but also elicited many dynamic scientific debates and opened different perspectives for the field of LT in general and the treatment of HCC in particular. Thanks to the extensive research and experience of many groups working on LDLT, especially the Asian transplantation groups, most LT centers now are achieving excellent results.

Specifically to the treatment of HCC, LDLT has several major advantages including: avoidance of prolonged waiting times, allowing elective timing of transplantation under best circumstances both for the patient and the tumor burden, not consuming the public donor pool that may reduce the chance of LT for nonmalignant cases awaiting transplant, and providing organ replacement therapy in parts of the world where brain death and deceased donation are less commonly accepted [3].

In addition to the conventional hepatitis virus-related HCC, a steadily increasing burden of HCC will be witnessed with the emergence of alcohol-related cirrhosis and nonalcoholic steatohepatitis (NASH) as potential major causes of HCC, adding more burden to the transplantation demands and worsening the worldwide problem of organ shortage. It has been recognized that fine-tuning and timing of liver transplantation for HCC are only possible with live organ donation. For these reasons, the need for implementation and optimization of LDLT program will continue in the near future [4–6].

In the following sections, we will discuss basic concepts, criteria evolution, ethical considerations, and controversial topics regarding LDLT for HCC treatment, some of them are commonplace among LDLT and DDLT. The technical details of the procedure of LDLT in general are beyond the scope of this chapter. However, surgical details that are related to the oncologic outcome of the patients with HCC are highlighted.

http://dx.doi.org/10.5772/65109

2. Current practice of LDLT for HCC

HCC represents more than 90% of primary liver cancers and It has a well-remarked geographic distribution. Around 85% of cases occur in East Asia, sub-Saharan Africa, and Melanesia. The great burden of HCC is most prevalent among the less developed world. In developed regions, the incidence is low, except for Southern Europe where the incidence is significantly higher [7, 8].

By and large, LDLT has emerged as an alternative to DDLT and it is the only option for patients with HCC in many Asian countries, where the problem of organ shortage is commonly faced. It also provides a suitable option for patients exceeding the MC in western countries such as the United States and Europe, and in the absence of legislative regulations and setup for DDLT in some developing countries especially in the Middle East and North Africa [9–11].

At the beginning of this century, it was estimated that LDLT would represent a significant proportion of the patients transplanted with HCC. Unfortunately, the risks of death and major complications for the healthy donors at the early experience (0.3 and 2%, respectively) reduced its practice on a wide scale. With the cumulative experiences over the past two decades, LDLT is now practiced smoothly in centers of excellence with experience of hepatobiliary surgery and transplantation medicine [7, 12].

2.1. Western experience

Since 2002, HCC patients who are within Milan criteria gain additional points under the MELD organ allocation policy. This resulted in shorter waiting time for HCC patients in many regions of the United States, obviating the need for LDLT. In some regions, however, longer waiting times with higher dropout rates support the use of LDLT for cases of HCC within the Milan criteria and in candidates who do not meet criteria for waiting list priority [13].

The situation of LDLT within the western experience can be configured from the 2012 release of European Association of Study of the Liver (EASL) guidelines, that mentioned "Living donor liver transplantation is an alternative option in patients with a waiting list exceeding 6–7 months, and offers a suitable setting to explore extended indications within research programs" [7].

In the United States, approximately 7000 new patients with HCC are put on the waiting list for LT every year, 10–15% of whom die during the waiting period. In Europe and the United States, the dropout rate at various centers ranges between 15 and 35%. From this perspective, LDLT offer a survival advantage to a significant proportion of HCC patients in the western world [14].

2.2. Eastern experience

The liver transplantation setup in Asia differs from that in the West, in the fact that no priority is given to HCC patients. This setup is formulated to avoid the inevitable shift of most of the deceased grafts to the persistently increasing HCC cases on the expense of nonmalignant cases waiting LT. The resultant wait-list lead Asian centers to practice various approaches to cover the needs, including bridging treatment for HCC, salvage transplantation after prior hepatectomy and LDLT for HCC. Shortage of donors in Asian countries is attributed to many factors including cultural and religious beliefs [10, 15].

3. Basic concepts

3.1. Philosophy

The most prominent advantage of LDLT for HCC treatment is the reduction of waiting time on the list for all cases including other etiologies of liver failure with nearly no effect on public donor pool. Living donor liver grafts are dedicated gifts to the recipients and are generally of good quality taking into account that most of living donors are healthy young individuals [15, 16].

The concept of "gifting" allowed LDLT for HCC patients who are beyond MC or any other proposed criteria and opened the door for liberal expansion. This concept is not accepted in the wait list of DDLT in which the procedure is conditioned to the "within criteria" cases only. The concept of "gifting" must not be taken for granted in the case of LDLT. Since the risk of a living donor is taken, selection criteria must be adopted for HCC patients with optimization of the pretransplantation conditions to ensure a high survival outcome. In other words, the readily available willing donor does not justify the ultramajor procedure of transplantation in the absence of a survival benefit for the recipient. In addition, donor safety remains the other pillar of a sound decision of LDLT [17].

3.2. Indications

LDLT is indicated in HCC patients, who are within accepted universal or regional criteria for transplantation. In view of organ scarcity, the indications can be described currently to be result-oriented in terms of overall and recurrence-free survival. Consequently, there is marked variation between different regions and institutions for applied indications. In essence, cases fitting Milan criteria are indicated for LDLT if waiting list would be >7 months or if there is a willing available donor. Milan criteria form the solid base of morphological indications for HCC. As discussed later, LDLT has allowed transplantation for patients who are outside Milan criteria according to the dynamically changing criteria in different institutions [18, 19].

3.3. Contraindications

Likewise, there is heterogeneity in the contraindications between different regions according to criteria limits for patient selection. However, there is a body of evidence that LDLT is absolutely contraindicated in the following conditions: cases of HCC that show major vascular invasion as evidenced by pretransplant imaging, the presence of extrahepatic metastases including suspicious porta hepatis nodal disease and cases with ruptured HCC. Absolute contraindications of LDLT in nonmalignant cases hold true for HCC and include cases with uncontrolled systemic infection or lethal uncontrolled medical comorbidities [20].

4. Terminology

With the implementation of LDLT programs and better understanding of the clinical course and biological nature of HCC, various clinical settings have emerged. In addition, the current progress of the interventional anticancer therapies enforced the armamentarium of the HCC management for all clinical scenarios. The following are different settings rather than different types of LDLT.

4.1. Primary LDLT

It is the procedure of LDLT performed upfront for the treatment of the cancer and underlying primary liver disease. In this setting, no previous liver resection is performed but initial ablative loco-regional therapies like RFA or PEI may have been performed. It is carried out for nonresectable HCC cases fitting the standard Milan criteria, UCSF criteria or other established and justified criteria for individual institutions. According to Barcelona Clinic Liver Cancer (BCLC) guidelines, primary LDLT is conducted for early cases of HCC with poor liver functions that cannot tolerate initial resection or ablation [7].

4.2. Salvage LDLT

In this setting, LT is performed when there is tumor recurrence or deterioration of liver functions after initial hepatectomy. The integral point in salvage LDLT is that it is performed aiming at a similar outcome to nonrecurrent cases. The pretransplant setting in the case of salvage LT after previous hepatectomy differs from that of primary LT in the availability of tissue pathology, so that almost all factors that determine tumor's behavior (grade, the presence or absence of microvascular invasion, the grade of necrosis in response to loco-regional therapy) are determined beforehand. That is why the predictive power of outcome of salvage LT should be more precise. Very importantly, we should consider that patients who have "within criteria" recurrence after hepatectomy, and hence amenable to salvage LT, are not more than 25% in some series. This means that nearly 70% of cases may miss the chance of a curative LT at all. The transplantability at the time of recurrence has been found to be an important variable determining the final outcome [21]. Noteworthy that when salvage LT is considered due to transplantable recurrence, the recurrence pattern should be evaluated before embarking into LT even if the liver functions and tumor burden are amenable to LT. Intrahepatic recurrent tumors after hepatectomy originates from either primary tumor metastases or de novo tumor foci. The interval and histopathological analysis of hepatectomy specimens give a clue to the pattern of recurrence. Tumors recurring in the first 12 months are most likely tumor metastases within the liver, while those arising after 12 months represent newly developed tumor foci. At histopathological analysis of hepatectomy, the presence of satellite nodules and portal vein invasion herald tumor metastases and early recurrence. The transplantation team should not rush to salvage LDLT except after considering the biological aggressiveness of the recurrent tumor and the likelihood of re-recurrence into the implanted neo-liver [22].

4.3. Sequential LDLT and preemptive LDLT

They are new categories with no consensus, performed in some centers within institutional protocols. In preemptive LDLT, cases that underwent initial hepatectomy and showed adverse histopathological criteria like microvascular invasion or satellite tumor nodules are prepared for LDLT without unnecessary waiting for the inevitable expected recurrence [21, 23, 24].

In sequential LDLT, pretransplant loco-regional therapy (LRT) is administered aiming at complete pathological necrosis of the index tumor before LDLT for cases within accepted criteria. Moreover, LDLT is performed after a scheduled short interval due to donor availability. The exact duration of the interval is not yet determined. Some centers perform LDLT after 3 months from the time of pretransplant therapy. This concept developed from the cumulative experience of histopathological assessment of explanted livers and the impact of pathological necrosis on post LT outcomes. HCC patients who achieve pathological necrosis ≥60% have significantly better overall survival and recurrence-free survival [25].

> *The employment of salvage LDLT is sometimes controversial. Some transplant surgeons, in view of certain radiological, pathological and biological hallmarks, don't prefer to wait for the inevitable recurrence or deterioration of patient or liver conditions to occur (preemptive LDLT). Some argue that the readily available donor associated with vigilant surveillance can always tailor the transplantation in the right time for the best outcome (salvage LDLT).*

5. Evolution of selection criteria

Over the previous two decades, criteria of LT had been expanded and modified from morphological and nonmorphological perspectives. Nevertheless, Milan criteria (MC) keep their place as the gold standard for LT. The long-term outcome and prognostic impact of LT within MC had been reproducibly studied with consistent excellent results [19, 26].

5.1. Why the criteria for LDLT had been expanded?

The MC advocated by Mazzaferro et al. [27] in 1996 are considered the base upon which several centers around the world validated their experiences in liver transplantation. These first clear-cut criteria were published in the *New England journal of medicine* as a practice changing and ground breaking progress in HCC treatment. That is because MC provided posttransplant survival rates of 75–95% at 2 years and 70–80% at 5 years in several studies. Indeed, a meta-analysis of published data has confirmed the survival advantage of MC and its association with a low risk of selecting patients with aggressive tumors [19, 27–29].

However, Milan criteria have been expanded and modified steadily for the following reasons:

http://dx.doi.org/10.5772/65109

1. They were considered too restrictive and many reports showed similar outcomes for cases beyond Milan [13, 30].

2. The growing evidence of the clear contribution of nonmorphological tumor characteristics to the outcome of patients after transplantation. So, the static "morphological" Milan criteria were expanded and modified. The other pathological and biological tumor criteria include: micro-vascular invasion, alpha-feto protein (AFP) level, deoxy-gamma carboxy prothrombin (dGCP) level and tumor avidity on PET scan [31–35].

3. The observation of two incorrectly estimated groups: an underestimated group that had been transplanted within MC but showed worse outcome and an overestimated group that was beyond MC and had comparable outcome after LDLT [35, 36].

5.2. Selection criteria according to different centers of excellence (Table 1) [27, 37–45]

Selection criteria of liver transplantation in different series and centers of excellence			
Criteria	**Parameters**	**Type of parameters**	**Over-all survival**
Milan	Solitary tumor ≤ 5 cm[T1], up to 3 tumors non >3 cm, no macrovascular invasion	Morphological only	85% (4-year)
UCSF	Solitary HCC ≤ 6.5 cm, or ≤ 3 nodules with the largest lesion ≤ 4.5 cm and a total tumor diameter ≤ 8 cm	Morphological only	75% (5-year)
Modified Milan (Up to 7)	Tumor number + size of the largest tumor (cm) ≤ 7	Morphological only	71% (5-year)
Toronto	Any tumor size or number, if pretransplant tumor biopsy showed no poor differentiation, no major vascular invasion, no extrahepatic disease	Morphological-pathological	72% (5-year)
Kyoto University	≤ 10 tumors, all ≤ 5 cm and the serum level of des. Gama carboxy prothrombin (d.GCP) ≤ 400 mIU/ml	Morphological-biological	87% (5-year)
Kyushu University	HCC ≤ 5 cm and a serum d.GCP ≤ 300 mIU/ml. It had been refined by adding neutrophil to lymphocyte ratio (NLR) >4	Morphological-biological	83% (5-year)
Tokyo University	5-5 rule: HCC not larger than 5 cm and no more than 5 nodules	Morphological only	75% (5-year)
Asan Medical Center	HCC not larger than 5 cm, 6 or fewer nodules without gross vascular invasion	Morphological only	82% (5-year)
Hangzhou	HCC ≥ 8 cm if serum alpha-fetoprotein level ≤ 400 ng/ml and only grade I or II	Morphological, biological, and pathological	72.% (5-year)

Table 1. Different selection criteria for liver transplantation adopted in most of transplantation in the world. Note that the main western criteria (Milan, UCSF, UP to 7) depend largely on morphology. Eastern-based criteria (Kyoto-Kyushu-Hangzhou) had modified by incorporating biological behavior of the tumors. The Toronto criteria are unique in its sole dependence on pretransplant biopsy.

Milan criteria were based on preoperative imaging and validated in many institutions all over the world [27]. In 2001, Yao et al. in the University of California San Francisco (UCSF) expanded the morphological criteria based on pathological assessment of explanted livers and then they prospectively validate their criteria based on pretransplant imaging in 2007 [37, 46]. Though this set of criteria is applied successfully in many regions, it has not been applied on a wide scale because they allow transplantation for large HCCs (6.5 cm, representing a tumor volume of 144 cm^3), which had been associated with worse outcomes in some studies. UCSF criteria (like Milan criteria) also exclude all patients with more than three lesions, some of whom may have the same outcome as those within criteria [47]. The 3- and 5-year survival rates after LDLT based on the UCSF criteria range between 78–96% and 66–90%, respectively, in different centers [28]. This wide variation of survival outcomes may also be attributed to variations of the surgical outcome and early mortality.

It should be emphasized that there are no consensus criteria for LDLT allocation. Each individual institution adopts one of the current criteria, tailoring treatment to their unique patient and general circumstances. Most of centers with high experience in LDLT for HCC currently focus on modification rather than numerical expansion of the number and size of tumors. The incorporation of biological factors (tumor markers, inflammatory markers) or available pathological factors from previous hepatectomy help select best candidates and hence predict the outcome and protect against recurrence [29, 35, 48].

6. Preoperative evaluation

Liver transplantation under optimal circumstances is a clear benefit of LDLT. The procedure can be carried out in a timely fashion after exhaustive assessment of tumor burden by different imaging modalities and biological markers. The tumor burden can then be manipulated by pretransplant therapies using the different loco-regional treatment options. Preoperative evaluation of the donor is not much different from the nonmalignant cases of LDLT except for some additional ethical perspectives as discussed previously. For the recipient, the details of preoperative assessment are beyond the scope of this chapter. However, we consider some important points in the pretransplant setting.

6.1. Imaging

Preoperative imaging of the recipient aims at assessment of tumor burden and suitable metastatic workup, for occult HCC or other cancer types. Dynamic CT or MRI with arterial enhancement is the standard of care according to high level of evidence. Extrahepatic staging should include CT chest and CT or MRI of abdomen and pelvis [12, 23].

The discrepancy between preoperative imaging and real tumor burden in explanted livers had been investigated in many centers. The state-of-the-art imaging modalities are not 100% accurate. CTA and MRI were both accurate to determine whether patients fit within the Milan or UCSF criteria, but CTA was slightly better than MRI to evaluate tumor number and size [49]. In the current era of pretransplant invasive therapies, the liver background became more confusing due to the presence of regenerative nodules, necrotized tumors, and other small tumors [35].

The incidental finding of pulmonary nodule(s) on pretransplant CT warrants appropriate evaluation. Many studies had determined a cutoff point to the size of pulmonary lesion at 5 mm. A lesion < 5 mm is less likely to be malignant and if remained stable or showed regression over a period of 3–6 months, liver transplantation is performed. For a lesion > 5 mm, a biopsy is needed to rule out malignant nature that contraindicates transplantation. If this lesion was the same in repeated images over previous 2 years, the possibility of infection is most likely and management is done accordingly. Video-assisted thoracic surgery (VATS) is perfectly employed for an excision biopsy of these small pulmonary nodules [50].

6.2. Alpha-feto protein (AFP)

This biological tumor marker plays important role in the assessment of tumor burden and aggressiveness although many other markers have been used in clinical practice over the past two decades. The AFP value has its clinical significance either in the preoperative or the posttransplant settings. In addition, the dynamic changes to its value in relation to downstaging therapy had been explored. An important question in the preoperative setting is its role as an exclusion tool, either alone or in combination of other radiological, biological, or pathological markers.

Some studies check the cutoff level above which patients should not undergo LT. At an AFP level >1000 ng/ml, approximately 5% of patients would be excluded from LT with 20% reduction in the rate of HCC recurrence. If a lower cut-off level is applied, this would result in a greater reduction in the recurrence rate but at the expense of excluding many more patients from LT who might not have tumor recurrence and would have benefited from LT. Also, patients who had decline of an initial AFP level >1000 ng/ml after loco-regional therapy had a more favorable prognosis after LT. Alpha feto-protein level <1000 has thus been combined to the UCSF criteria for patient selection in some centers [51].

More recently, a prospective multicenter study has explored the use of a combination of total tumor volume (TTV) ≤ 115 cm^3 and AFP ≤ 400 ng/ml as an exclusion tool from LT in centers with a median waiting time of 8 months. This study took an advantage from a previous observation of the inferior survival outcome of patients who are within MC but have the AFP level ≥400 ng/ml. In this study, patients who were beyond MC but within TTV/AFP had survival outcome similar to cases within MC [29].

Many other biomarkers can be evaluated in the pretransplant setting to predict the posttransplant outcome. A recent study in our center showed that repeated measurement of serum levels of novel biomarkers including fibroblast growth factor-2 (FGF-2), survivin, Ki67, endostatin, and vascular endothelial growth factor (VEGF), before and after LDLT for HCC, could predict HCC recurrence [52].

6.3. Fludro-deoxy glucose-positron emission tomography (FDG-PET) scan

Pretransplant 18F-FDG uptake on PET scan in liver transplant candidates with HCC is a useful additional parameter for the evaluation of tumor biology. Positive preoperative PET scans are significantly associated with an increased risk of posttransplant HCC recurrence and inferior outcome, an observation that relates a positive PET status with the presence of microvascular invasion in explant tumor pathology [31]. In a recent Korean study, the combination of the positive FDG-PET study and AFP level >200 ng/ml could predict tumor recurrence more precisely after LDLT than Milan criteria [35]. More recently, a retrospective study at our center has showed that the combination of UCSF criteria with the FDG-PET status can predict tumor recurrence after LDLT and that tumor recurrence is earlier in cases with positive FDG-PET results. On the basis of the maximal standardized uptake value (SUVmax), high-risk group cases (positive study with $SUV_{max} \geq 5$) had worse recurrence-free survival compared with low-risk cases (positive study with $SUV_{max} < 5$) [53].

6.4. Donor characteristics

In addition to the previously discussed controversy of impact of donor type (living or deceased) on HCC recurrence, other donor factors have been studied. A recent review of the American Scientific Registry of Transplant Recipients (SRTR) that involved 9724 patients revealed that the following donor factors were independently associated with high risk of HCC recurrence after transplantation: high BMI, history of DM, and severe graft steatosis. All the previous factors are evident at the time of organ allocation and must be considered before transplantation [54].

7. Loco-regional therapy (LRT)

The pretransplant therapies are implemented heavily for HCC, being an essential component of HCC treatment algorithms in most of treatment guidelines. Earlier in the treatment of HCC roadmaps, they were considered "bridging" tools to keep the patient chances of LT during the waiting time. Currently, a realized value of LRT is their ability to probe the tumor's internal milieu, acting as a selecting tool based on the degree of tumor's response as an indicator of its aggressiveness. So, adopting such therapies gives the time to observe the tumor's behavior before the ultramajor costly step of liver transplantation [55]. Bypassing such an observation period in the setting of multifocal or locally advanced tumor risks transplanting patients with systemic disease.

7.1. HCC downstaging before liver transplantation

The difference between downstaging and neoadjuvant therapies is that in the former the tumor status is beyond the proposed criteria for transplantation and LRT is administered to reduce the tumor burden and to render the case fit for transplantation. In neoadjuvant therapy, the patient is already within criteria but treatment is given to prevent tumor progression to the

http://dx.doi.org/10.5772/65109

"beyond criteria" state while waiting for the donor and to induce tumor necrosis aiming at better long-term outcome [56].

In different series from Asian centers, more than 30% of patients who were beyond Milan/UCSF criteria were effectively downstaged to the "within criteria" state with a 5-year survival rate similar to the initially fit cases [57, 58]. A meta-analysis explored the effect of downstaging to Milan criteria, and the success rate exceeded 40%. However, the recurrence rate was as high as 16% [59].

TACE and RFA are the main tools of downstaging. TACE mediates its effect by inducing complete pathological necrosis with response rates ranging between 27 and 57%. RFA is used For accessible lesions to induce coagulative necrosis, either alone or in combination with liver resection [60]. In LDLT, timing of transplantation after a period of waiting from the time of LDLT is possible. Most centers wait for a period of 3–6 months to evaluate tumor progression as an indicator of aggressiveness before embarking into LDLT.

Though widely applicable in most HCC guidelines, there are no unified criteria either for selecting cases for downstaging or for determining them as good responders and hence listing them for LT. This fact highlights the wide variation of transplantation criteria among different regions and centers. As a rule of thumb, the criteria to enter a downstaging program should include patients who have well-defined and acceptable chances of good outcomes after transplantation if the downstaging goal is achieved [56]. In our center, not only we apply downstaging for cases beyond UCSF criteria, but also we consider cases with high AFP or high FDG uptake on PET scan for downstaging. In our early experience, patients were downstaged to fit Milan criteria. Our initial results of 35 patients were encouraging with a 5-year survival rate of 90% and those patients are still disease-free up to date, after follow-up of 10 years. Since July 2006, our criteria were extended to UCSF criteria. In our experience of 161 HCC patients, 51 (31.6%) were successfully downstaged to fit the UCSF criteria. The overall 1- and 5-year survival rates for downstaged cases were 94.1 and 92.7%, respectively. The recurrence rate was 9.2%. The survival rates were similar for different pretransplantation downstaging procedures [57].

8. Operative/surgical highlights

The first successful case of liver transplantation in Asia was performed by Chen in 1984 in Chang Gung Memorial Hospital, Taiwan. From the cumulative experience at our center, we would like to emphasize that a sound surgical procedure is mandatory for the best outcome. It has been postulated that the experience of the transplant team is an important factor that independently affects the outcome though the learning curve of liver transplant can be steep and painful in some centers launching an LDLT program. In essence, we prefer not to correct recipient coagulopathy before surgery, because many studies showed no value of preoperative correction. Donor hepatectomy should be accomplished with minimal blood loss, obviating the need for blood transfusion. The routine use of microsurgical procedure is performed in our center for arterial anastomosis as well as biliary reconstruction. Surgical outcome largely affects survival and hence final outcome. Early postoperative vascular complications are the main reasons of graft loss and in-hospital mortality and must be managed vigorously [49, 61–64].

8.1. Timing of donor and recipient surgeries

In nonmalignant cases of LDLT, the recipient surgery is usually begun after the donor surgery commenced till confirmation of feasible biliary anatomy by cholangiography. In the early experience of LDLT for HCC, some surgeons preferred to confirm resectability of the liver containing cancer and the absence of lymph node metastases through a smaller incision before proceeding with graft harvesting from the donor [65, 66]. However, the current imaging modalities surpass this step and allow precise decision in advance. Most experienced centers largely depend on high quality CT or MRI images and the timing is adopted like nonmalignant cases of end-stage liver failure.

8.2. Safety margin

A proper safety margin is an integral part of the sound oncological surgical procedure. Some peripheral lesions may be found in very close proximity to or even adherent to parietal peritoneum, diaphragm, omentum, or less commonly small or large bowl loops. A previous hepatectomy increases the adhesions with the aforementioned structures. It is thus convenient to take a proper safety margin through excision of parts of peritoneum and diaphragmatic muscle. Very infrequently, small or large bowl resection and anastomosis may be required. Re-exploration for additional safety margin after final pathological assessment is a very hazardous procedure for such a frail patient, but may be warranted in some conditions according to institutional experience.

8.3. Management of nodal disease

In a recent review from the International Registry of Hepatic Tumors in Liver Transplantation, the incidence of lymph node metastases in cirrhotic patients with HCC undergoing LT was 6.5%. Hilar lymph node (LN) involvement in cases of HCC constitutes a contraindication for liver transplantation because of dismal prognosis. Recent imaging techniques are able to identify enlarged suspicious lymph nodes in the pretransplant setting. However, the frequent presence of LN enlargement due to chronic inflammation in cases of hepatitis C-induced cirrhosis may make the diagnosis less clear. It is convenient to perform frozen section evaluation for suspicious nodes unexpectedly encountered during recipient operation. The decision to proceed or abort the procedure in the case of inconclusive frozen section analysis or the unavailability of frozen section depends largely on the experience of the transplant team. According to a meta-analysis study, systematic hilar lymphadenectomy during LT for HCC should routinely be undertaken, especially in the context of coexisting hepatitis C or secondary biliary cirrhosis. Some centers recommend harvesting of at least four lymph nodes at the time of liver transplantation but the debate remains open with no available consensus on the extent of such lymphadenectomy [67, 68].

http://dx.doi.org/10.5772/65109

8.4. The middle hepatic vein (MHV)

The MHV is a controversial topic within the LDLT procedure in general. In the case of LDLT for HCC, this issue should be taken more seriously. It has been postulated that the resultant venous congestion from improper management of tributaries of MHV is a possible factor favoring tumor recurrence. Congestion of the graft leads to impediment of portal inflow with subsequent ischemia in the congested region and compensatory accelerated regeneration of the well-drained areas of the graft. Consequently, the cellular changes in response to both processes may enhance tumor recurrence [69].

8.5. IVC management (see Figure 1)

The observation of HCC recurrence after LDLT in the hepatic vena-caval wall has shed light on the possibility of microvascular infiltration with consequent local and distant recurrence. This finding triggered the concept of aggressive en-bloc caval resection and reconstruction during LDLT. This step is also justified by another two facts: first, it prevents a positive margin of latent cancer in caval branches; second, the least amount of manipulation of the native liver with HCC should be employed to avoid and control distant metastasis after LDLT [70].

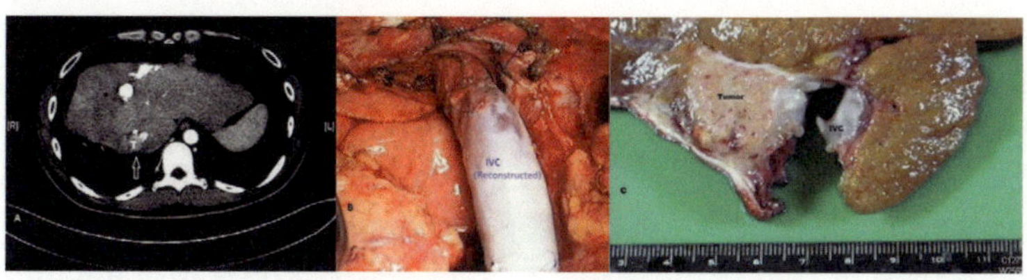

Figure 1. A case of HCC subjected to LDLT. The tumor (T) was intimately adherent to the IVC wall without apparent invasion in pretransplant CT angiography (A; arrow). During the recipient operation, the liver was explanted en-bloc with the IVC segment adjacent to the tumor. Reconstruction of the IVC was carried out using cryo-preserved iliac v. graft (B). Final gross pathology shows no intraluminal transgression by the tumor (C).

8.6. Complications of LDLT of the manipulated liver, i.e., after loco-regional therapy

Extensive adhesions are commonly encountered following previous liver resection in case of salvage liver transplantation. Tough vascular adhesions usually form between a large hepatectomy site and small intestine and omentum. Sharp dissection and meticulous hemostatic control would reduce the difficulty of subsequent transplantation and decrease the incidence of postoperative complications [71]. Laparoscopic liver resection is now performed on a wide scale in many centers. One of the most prominent advantages of laparoscopic initial hepatectomy is the marked reduction of adhesions as evidenced in subsequent liver transplantation in many series thus facilitating the procedure [72].

Intimal dissection (ID) of the recipient hepatic artery has emerged as a grave complication that may occur after TAE or TACE. Intimal dissection if not discovered and managed properly may end up in graft loss. Gentle handling of HA is mandatory during LT to prevent aggravation or precipitation of dissection in the fragile HA. Once this complication is suspected intraoperatively, microscopic assessment is needed for proper decision. Either trimming and discarding the dissected segment or discarding the whole native HA and reconstruction may be considered, hence the importance of microvascular expertise in the LDLT team [73].

9. Ethical considerations

Two main ethical pillars of the decision of LDLT for management of HCC must be considered. First, donor safety and optimizing his or her care is no different in LDLT for HCC compared to that for nonmalignant cases of liver failure. Second, the procedure must provide an acceptable outcome to the recipient compared to DDLT. From the ethical point of view, LDLT is justified, as long as the proposed regional criteria are strictly followed, being MC or any scientifically justified institutional expanded or modified criteria. Noteworthy that there is no consensus about what risk to the living donor might be considered acceptable for a given risk of recurrence [13, 74].

With increased awareness and patient education facilities, the ethical responsibilities regarding patient counseling became more complex. It is not all about the perioperative complications. Recently, ethical considerations took a very different perspective, that is offering LDLT to high-risk patients and excluding others who are low-risk patients based on imaging criteria only. As mentioned earlier, two wrongly estimated groups are revealed: cases within criteria that have aggressive biological behavior and cases beyond criteria with indolent tumors. Two ethical situations subsequently ensued; the first is the risk of recurrence of biologically aggressive tumors even when strict criteria are adhered to, i.e., the underestimated group. The second is about the loss of chance of LT in the other group. The transplantation team should never rush to transplantation in response to family pressure and readily available donor without proper discussion of all that issues [35].

When the partial graft fails for any reason, a special—but very uncommon—ethical situation is encountered because normally it requires an urgent deceased donor retransplantation. It has been established that if LDLT was used in a situation where a deceased donor is contraindicated, such as exceeding the accepted criteria for deceased donation, the patient should not be retransplanted because he/she would not be transplanted initially if on wait-list for DDLT [12, 66]. Finding another living donor must be balanced against the expected outcome of the procedure. There are no clear-cut decisions to such situations and the institutional experience would tailor the right decision.

When talking about salvage LDLT, the patient may be reluctant to undergo the procedure even with the availability of a donor. Some patients may argue that they want to be alive more but do not want to harm anyone. In these circumstances, the transplant team should alert the patient about how long can he/she delay the procedure without a considerable risk of tumor progression or being transferred into the nontransplantable state. A study from Japan revealed that patients who receive downstaging therapy can wait no more than 12 months. However, the exact duration is not determined and the management plan should be tailored to each case [75].

http://dx.doi.org/10.5772/65109

10. Controversial topics

The increasing number of HCC cases, the parallel progress in expertise of LDLT, and the dynamic changes in the selection criteria all enriched the liver transplantation community with many important topics and debates. A lot of studies were carried out to find answers or to reach a consensus in many of these topics. However, the retrospective nature of most studies, the different reporting methodologies and small sample sizes are all flaws that hampered the appearance of high level of evidence to address all topics.

10.1. What is the best treatment option of early HCC? Resection or liver transplantation? Primary or salvage approach?

- The surgical decision can be either LR or LT in 20–25% of cases of HCC amenable for surgery. Liver transplantation is hypothetically superior to resection because it removes the cancer and its underlying pathology. For many patients it is not possible to perform resection because of the tumor size, anatomical location of the tumor, or poor liver function, and liver transplantation is the only surgical option [76]. However, even in many Asian centers which perform LDLT on regular basis, up to 50% of early HCC cases may not have suitable donors or be concerned about the risk to donor. So, many Asian centers adopt the policy of offering LR to patients with resectable tumors with compensated cirrhosis and deferring LT to the salvage setting [13, 23, 77, 78].
- The controversy regarding LR or LT in HCC patients is largely confined to early cases with a well-preserved liver function. There are no randomized controlled trials that addressed this issue through a head-to-head comparison. Given that organ shortage for LT is a persistent challenge worldwide and also the presence of underserved areas with deficient LT programs, the identification of cases that would obtain similar survival outcomes when either submitted to LR or to LT is of paramount importance [79, 80].
- The strategy of offering LR for simultaneously resectable and transplantable cases was based on the observation from many studies that 20–30% of HCC cases that had LR may not witness recurrence for >5 years. In addition, with vigilant surveillance programs, most of recurrent cases would fit into the MC and can be transplanted under optimal conditions due to the availability of the living donor, with no negative impact on the outcome. This obviates many patients the downside of early immunosuppression [5]. In addition, the mortality rate of LR at an experienced center is less than 2–5%, and overall survival rates were comparable to primary LT [4, 24].
- **The Barcelona Clinic Liver Cancer approach**: Resection is the treatment of choice in patients with very early stage HCC and normal bilirubin levels as well as the absence of portal hypertension. If the liver functions are impaired, LT is recommended as a primary treatment approach. In the early stage of HCC, it has been found that the 10-year outcome after LT is superior to LR in view of the latter's well-known higher recurrence risk. So, the choice of primary LT is recommended. The same approach is adopted by the American Association of Study of Liver Disease (AASLD) guidelines that prefer liver resection for very early cases with the optimal liver profile [7, 78, 81, 82].

- A meta-analysis of studies that involved patients within MC revealed a survival advantage for LT over LR [83]. In a more recent meta-analysis that involved 1572 patients in whom both LR and LT are feasible, the authors did not find any survival advantage of LT compared with LR. They concluded—based on low quality evidence—that LR is preferable to LT in patients who are feasible for both options [84].

- Conclusion: the overall survival advantage of LT is unclear, though recurrence-free survival is definitely better with LT. The main drawback for LT—especially LDLT—is the relatively increased mortality in the early postoperative period. In high volume centers where LDLT is performed at high rates, perioperative mortality is reduced significantly. So, a clear overall survival advantage for LT may be evident [85]. For a definite evidence-based conclusion, a randomized controlled trial comparing LT and LR is needed, a condition that is very difficult due to practical and ethical restrictions. Proper patient selection and optimization of criteria according to the pretransplant setting (primary or secondary) would help make a treatment roadmap.

10.2. Living donor or deceased donor for HCC?

One of the most critical controversies in the transplantation field is the possibility of an increased rate of recurrence of HCC after LDLT compared to DDLT.

Several hypotheses have been postulated to figure out this possibility:

- The fast tract effect: due to the shortened waiting time for LDLT, progression of HCC with aggressive tumor biology might not be recognized during such a short-waiting time. This is in contrary to the situation in DDLT, where the long-waiting time can naturally select cases with indolent behavior.

- The growth factors and cytokines released during rapid regeneration of the partial grafts might contribute to tumor progression and recurrence.

- The extensive dissection and mobilization of the liver might increase the feasibility of tumor dissemination through the hepatic vein and increased potential for leaving residual tumor cells.

- The exaggerated vascular inflow associated with small size grafts elicits vast angiogenesis with subsequent carcinogenic effect.

- The less radical hepatectomy in LDLT with the native IVC left in place may constitute a suboptimal oncologic procedure [15, 55, 86–88].

A multi-center study was carried out on the database of China Liver Transplant Registry (CLTR) to highlight this issue. They explored the data of 6860 patients (6471 (DDLT) and 389 LDLT and concluded that both overall survival and recurrence-free survival were comparable between both approaches [89]. In an international consensus conference of liver transplantation (Zurich 2012), it had been stated that no convincing difference in outcome could be identified according to the type of graft, although a higher risk of recurrence was noted in fast-tracked patients. The experts advised an interval of observation for the biological behavior of the tumor to manifest. A period of 3 months had been suggested [12]. Many other groups reported similar recurrence rates after LDLT and DDLT and also similar long-term outcomes [14, 87].

However, others have found significantly higher rates of tumor recurrence after LDLT compared with DDLT for HCC. The Adult to Adult Living Donor Liver transplantation (A2ALL) study reported a significantly higher 3-year tumor recurrence rate after LDLT [15, 88, 90, 91]. One should consider that many studies that reported better outcome of DDLT than LDLT are conducted in the west and some of them were flawed by small sample sizes and the possibility of selection bias since DDLT was applied mostly on cases within Milan criteria only and those beyond Milan criteria are relegated to LDLT [92].

A systematic review and meta-analysis addressed this question (Is the regenerating liver of LDLT a fertile environment for HCC recurrence?). Though no randomized controlled trials were included, they came to a similar conclusion; disease-free survival (DFS) is worse after LDLT compared with DDLT but there was no difference observed in overall survival (OS). In the same meta-analysis, there was a concern that the follow-up periods in the included studies are probably too brief to detect a major impact on survival resulting from differences in disease recurrence. The same study revealed that the overall survival after LDLT vs. DDLT was better —though not statistically significant—in studies from eastern centers compared with studies from western centers. This may reflect differences between these regions in patient selection or case-volumes effects on surgical outcomes [6]. In conclusion, to date there is no definite evidence supporting higher recurrence after LDLT than DDLT [55, 92].

10.3. Pre-LDLT liver biopsy, can the trend be changed?

Because the risk of tumor seeding may be 2–4% along the needle biopsy tract and thus increasing the risk of metastases, liver biopsy should be considered only when there is uncertainty as to the diagnosis. This might occur, for example, in the presence of an HCC arising in the noncirrhotic liver or contradictory clinical, laboratory, and radiological findings [81]. However, a biopsy has the potential problems of sampling error. For example, different nodules may have different grades within the index tumor. It has also been demonstrated that even in a single-needle biopsy, adjacent tumor cells can be of different degrees of differentiation. Nevertheless, if transplantation is planned for HCC beyond the standard criteria, tumor biopsy appears to be a logical approach if there is suspicion of diagnosis [28].

Dubay et al. [44] have provided their experience in the University of Toronto based solely on a liver biopsy before LT. They have no size or number restriction for LT. They concluded that a protocol using a biopsy to exclude poorly differentiated tumors achieved excellent survival rates (70% at 5 years) [44].

10.4. Can we exclude morphological selection criteria in the coming era?

Morphological criteria of HCC describe the appearance, while biological criteria describe the concealed behavior. Ultimately, the behavior of HCC is the final-deciding factor on patient outcome. As shown earlier, modification of morphological criteria is pursued in many studies with the incorporation of biological factors [13]. In a study from Korea, the recipient selection based on pure biological factors was proposed. The group showed that FDG PET positivity with a cutoff point of maximum systemic uptake value (SUV_{max}) of 1.1 combined with the AFP serum level at 400 ng/ml is able—alone—to predict patient outcome more precise than morphological criteria [35]. More studies are needed to explore nonmorphological selection processes.

11. Conclusions

LDLT is a robust treatment pathway for HCC. Indeed, it may be the only pathway in this era of organ shortage especially in some Asian countries. The employment and dynamic application of selection criteria of LDLT for HCC are the cornerstone to acquire the best outcome. The number and size of the tumor(s) are not the only factors to consider for patient selection but some other factors are also present. Most of transplantation centers are combining biological (AFP-tumor avidity in PET scan) and pathological (pretransplant biopsy) factors of the tumors to the morphological factors aiming at refined patient selection for the optimal outcome. In the current era of personalized medicine, treatment of HCC should be tailored according to each individual patient and tumor criteria. A sound oncological surgical procedure is the core of successful LDLT and has its direct impact on the final outcome.

Author details

Chih-Che Lin[1*], Ahmed Mohammed Abdel Aziz Elsarawy[2] and Chao-Long Chen[1]

*Address all correspondence to: immunologylin@gmail.com

1 Department of general surgery and liver transplant center, Chang Gung Memorial Hospital, Kaohsiung, Taiwan

2 Liver transplant center, Chang Gung Memorial Hospital, Kaohsiung, Taiwan

References

[1] Knox JJ, Cleary SP, Dawson LA. Localized and systemic approaches to treating hepatocellular carcinoma. J Clin Oncol. 2015;33(16):1835–44. Available from: http://jco.ascopubs.org/content/33/16/1835.long

[2] Bruix J, Gores GJ, Mazzaferro V. Hepatocellular carcinoma: clinical frontiers and perspectives. Gut. 2014;844–55.

[3] Sonnenday CJ. Recurrent hepatocellular carcinoma after living donor liver transplantation: a preventable problem or an acceptable risk? Ann Surg Oncol. United States; 2010;17:2262–3.

[4] de Villa VH, Lo C-M, Chen C-L. Ethics and rationale of living-donor liver transplantation in Asia. Transplant. 2003;75(3 Suppl):S2–5. Available from: http://www.ncbi.nlm.nih.gov/pubmed/12589129

[5] Chen C-L, Concejero AM. Liver transplantation for hepatocellular carcinoma in the world: the Taiwan experience. J Hepatobil Pancreat Sci. Japan. 2010;17(5):555–8.

[6] Grant RC, Sandhu L, Dixon PR, Greig PD, Grant DR, McGilvray ID. Living vs. deceased donor liver transplantation for hepatocellular carcinoma: a systematic review and meta-analysis. Clin Transplant. Denmark; 2013;27(1):140–7.

[7] Dufour JF, Greten TF, Raymond E, Roskams T, De T, Ducreux M, et al. EASL–EORTC clinical practice guidelines: management of hepatocellular carcinoma. J Hepatol. 2012;56(4):908–43. Available from: http://linkinghub.elsevier.com/retrieve/pii/S0168827811008737

[8] Torre LA, Bray F, Siegel RL, Ferlay J. Global cancer statistics. CA Cancer J Clin. 2015;65(2):87–108.

[9] Shirabe K, Taketomi A, Morita K, Soejima Y, Uchiyama H, Kayashima H, et al. Comparative evaluation of expanded criteria for patients with hepatocellular carcinoma beyond the Milan criteria undergoing living-related donor liver transplantation. Clin Transplant. Denmark; 2011;25(5):E491–8.

[10] Chen C-L, Kabiling CS, Concejero AM. Why does living donor liver transplantation flourish in Asia? Nat Rev Gastroenterol Hepatol. 2013;10(12):746–51. Available from: http://www.ncbi.nlm.nih.gov/pubmed/24100300

[11] Khalaf H, Marwan I, Al-Sebayel M, El-Meteini M, Hosny A, Abdel-Wahab M, et al. Status of liver transplantation in the Arab world. Transplantation. 2014;97(7):722–4. Available from: http://www.ncbi.nlm.nih.gov/pubmed/24603475

[12] Clavien P-A, Lesurtel M, Bossuyt PMM, Gores GJ, Langer B, Perrier A. Recommendations for liver transplantation for hepatocellular carcinoma: an international consensus conference report. Lancet Oncol. England; 2012;13(1):e11–22.

[13] Mazzaferro V, Chun YS, Poon RTP, Schwartz ME, Yao FY, Marsh JW, et al. Liver transplantation for hepatocellular carcinoma. Ann Surg Oncol. United States; 2008;15(4):1001–7.

[14] Bhangui P, Vibert E, Majno P, Salloum C, Andreani P, Zocrato J, et al. Intention-to-treat analysis of liver transplantation for hepatocellular carcinoma: living versus deceased donor transplantation. Hepatology. United States; 2011;53(5):1570–9.

[15] Ng KK, Lo CM. Liver transplantation in Asia: past, present and future. Ann Acad Med Singapore. Singapore; 2009;38(4):310–22.

[16] Chen C, Cheng Y, Yu C, Ou H, Tsang LL, Huang T, et al. Living donor liver transplantation: the Asian perspective. Transplantat. 2014;97 Suppl 8: S3.

[17] Barr ML, Belghiti J, Villamil FG, Pomfret EA, Sutherland DS, Gruessner RW, et al. A report of the vancouver forum on the care of the live organ donor: lung, liver, pancreas, and intestine data and medical guidelines. Transplantat. 2006;81(10):1373–85. Available from: http://content.wkhealth.com/linkback/openurl?sid=WKPTLP:landingpage&an=00007890-200605270-00004

[18] Nadalin S, Bockhorn M, Malagó M, Valentin-Gamazo C, Frilling A, Broelsch CE. Living donor liver transplantation. HPB (Oxford). 2006;8(1):10–21. Available from: http://www.pubmedcentral.nih.gov/articlerender.fcgi?artid=2131378&tool=pmcentrez&rendertype=abstract

[19] Mazzaferro V, Bhoori S, Sposito C, Bongini M, Langer M, Miceli R, et al. Milan criteria in liver transplantation for hepatocellular carcinoma: an evidence-based analysis of 15 years of experience. Liver Transpl. United States; 2011;17 Suppl 2:S44–57.

[20] Farkas S, Hackl C, Schlitt HJ. Overview of the indications and contraindications for liver transplantation. Cold Spring Harb Perspect Med. United States; 2014;4(5).

[21] Majno PE, Sarasin FP, Mentha G, Hadengue A. Primary liver resection and salvage transplantation or primary liver transplantation in patients with single, small hepatocellular carcinoma and preserved liver function: an outcome-oriented decision analysis. Hepatology. United States; 2000;31(4):899–906.

[22] Lee HS, Choi GH, Joo DJ, Kim MS, Choi JS. The clinical behavior of transplantable recurrent hepatocellular carcinoma after curative resection: implications for salvage liver. Transplantation. 2014;2717–24.

[23] Concejero A, Chen C-L, Wang C-C, Wang S-H, Lin C-C, Liu Y-W, et al. Living donor liver transplantation for hepatocellular carcinoma: a single-center experience in Taiwan. Transplantation. United States; 2008;85(3):398–406.

[24] Cherqui D, Laurent A, Alain. Liver resection for transplantable hepatocellular carcinoma. Ann Surg. 2009;250(5). 738–46.

[25] Chan K-M, Yu M-C, Chou H-S, Wu T-J, Lee C-F, Lee W-C. Significance of tumor necrosis for outcome of patients with hepatocellular carcinoma receiving locoregional therapy prior to liver transplantation. Ann Surg Oncol. United States; 2011;18(9):2638–46.

[26] Yoshizumi T, Harimoto N, Itoh S, Okabe H, Kimura K, Uchiyama H, et al. Living donor liver transplantation for hepatocellular carcinoma within milan criteria in the present era. Anticancer Res. Greece; 2016;36(1):439–45.

[27] Mazzaferro V, Regalia E, Doci R, Andreola S, Pulvirenti A, Bozzetti F, et al. Liver transplantation for the treatment of small hepatocellular carcinomas in patients with cirrhosis. N Engl J Med. United States; 1996;334(11):693–9.

[28] Chan SC, Fan ST. Selection of patients of hepatocellular carcinoma beyond the Milan criteria for liver transplantation. Hepatobiliary Surg Nutr. China (Republic: 1949); 2013;2(2):84–8.

[29] Toso C, Meeberg G, Hernandez-Alejandro R, Dufour J-F, Marotta P, Majno P, et al. Total tumor volume and alpha-fetoprotein for selection of transplant candidates with hepatocellular carcinoma: a prospective validation. Hepatology. United States; 2015;62(1):158–65.

[30] Majno P, Mazzaferro V. Living donor liver transplantation for hepatocellular carcinoma exceeding conventional criteria: questions, answers and demands for a common language. Vol. 12, Liver transplantation: official publication of the American Association for the Study of Liver Diseases and the International Liver Transplantation Society. United States; 2006. p. 896–8.

[31] Kornberg A, Freesmeyer M, Barthel E, Jandt K, Katenkamp K, Steenbeck J, et al. 18F-FDG-uptake of hepatocellular carcinoma on PET predicts microvascular tumor invasion in liver transplant patients. Am J Transplant. Denmark; 2009;9(3):592–600.

[32] Hirakawa M, Yoshimitsu K, Irie H, Tajima T, Nishie A, Asayama Y, et al. Performance of radiological methods in diagnosing hepatocellular carcinoma preoperatively in a recipient of living related liver transplantation: comparison with step section histopathology. Jpn J Radiol. Japan; 2011;29(2):129–37.

[33] Piardi T, Gheza F, Ellero B, Woehl-Jaegle ML, Ntourakis D, Cantu M, et al. Number and Tumor Size Are Not Sufficient Criteria to Select Patients for Liver Transplantation for Hepatocellular Carcinoma. Ann Surg Oncol. 2012;19(6):2020–6.

[34] Na GH, Kim DG, Han JH, Kim EY, Lee SH, Hong TH, et al. Inflammatory markers as selection criteria of hepatocellular carcinoma in living-donor liver transplantation. World J Gastroenterol. United States; 2014;20(21):6594–601.

[35] Hong G, Suh K-S, Suh S-W, Yoo T, Kim H, Park M-S, et al. Alpha-fetoprotein and (18)F-FDG positron emission tomography predict tumor recurrence better than Milan criteria in living donor liver transplantation. J Hepatol. Netherlands; 2016;64(4):852–9.

[36] Ito T, Takada Y, Ueda M, Haga H, Maetani Y, Oike F, et al. Expansion of selection criteria for patients with hepatocellular carcinoma in living donor liver transplantation. Liver Transpl. United States; 2007;13(12):1637–44.

[37] Yao FY, Ferrell L, Bass NM, Watson JJ, Bacchetti P, Venook A, et al. Liver transplantation for hepatocellular carcinoma: expansion of the tumor size limits does not adversely impact survival. Hepatology. United States; 2001;33(6):1394–403.

[38] Lee S-G, Hwang S, Moon D-B, Ahn C-S, Kim K-H, Sung K-B, et al. Expanded indication criteria of living donor liver transplantation for hepatocellular carcinoma at one large-volume center. Liver Transpl. United States; 2008;14(7):935–45.

[39] Zheng S-S, Xu X, Wu J, Chen J, Wang W-L, Zhang M, et al. Liver transplantation for hepatocellular carcinoma: Hangzhou experiences. Transplantation. United States; 2008;85(12):1726–32.

[40] Sugawara Y, Tamura S, Makuuchi M. Living donor liver transplantation for hepatocellular carcinoma: Tokyo University series. Dig Dis. Switzerland; 2007;25(4):310–2.

[41] Mazzaferro V, Llovet JM, Miceli R, Bhoori S, Schiavo M, Mariani L, et al. Predicting survival after liver transplantation in patients with hepatocellular carcinoma beyond the Milan criteria: a retrospective, exploratory analysis. Lancet Oncol. 2009;10(1):35–43. Available from: http://dx.doi.org/10.1016/S1470-2045(08)70284-5

[42] Taketomi A, Sanefuji K, Soejima Y, Yoshizumi T, Uhciyama H, Ikegami T, et al. Impact of des-gamma-carboxy prothrombin and tumor size on the recurrence of hepatocellular carcinoma after living donor liver transplantation. Transplantation. United States; 2009;87(4):531–7.

[43] Takada Y, Uemoto S. Liver transplantation for hepatocellular carcinoma: the Kyoto experience. J Hepatobiliary Pancreat Sci. Japan; 2010;17(5):527–32.

[44] DuBay D, Sandroussi C, Sandhu L, Cleary S, Guba M, Cattral MS, et al. Liver transplantation for advanced hepatocellular carcinoma using poor tumor differentiation on biopsy as an exclusion criterion. Ann Surg. United States; 2011;253(1):166–72.

[45] Yoshizumi T, Ikegami T, Toshima T, Harimoto N, Uchiyama H, Soejima Y, et al. Two-step selection criteria for living donor liver transplantation in patients with hepatocellular carcinoma. Transplant Proc. United States; 2013;45(9):3310–3.

[46] Yao FY, Xiao L, Bass NM, Kerlan R, Ascher NL, Roberts JP. Liver transplantation for hepatocellular carcinoma: validation of the UCSF-expanded criteria based on preoperative imaging. Am J Transplant. 2007;7(11):2587–96.

[47] Toso C, Asthana S, Bigam DL, Shapiro AMJ, Kneteman NM. Reassessing selection criteria prior to liver transplantation for hepatocellular carcinoma utilizing the scientific registry of transplant recipients database. Hepatology. 2009;49(3):832–8.

[48] Yang SH, Suh KS, Lee HW, Cho EH, Cho JY, Cho YB, et al. A revised scoring system utilizing serum alphafetoprotein levels to expand candidates for living donor transplantation in hepatocellular carcinoma. Surgery. 2007;141(5):598–609.

[49] Lu C-H, Chen C-L, Cheng Y-F, Huang T-L, Tsang LL-C, Ou H-Y, et al. Correlation between imaging and pathologic findings in explanted livers of hepatocellular carcinoma cases. Transplant Proc. United States; 2010;42(3):830–3.

[50] Wu Y-J, Lin C-C, Lin Y-H, Wang S-H, Lin T-L, Chen C-L, et al. Incidentally small pulmonary nodule in candidates for living donor liver transplantation. Ann Transplant. Poland; 2015;20:734–40.

[51] Hameed B, Mehta N, Sapisochin G, Roberts JP, Yao FY. Alpha-fetoprotein level> 1000 ng/mL as an exclusion criterion for liver transplantation in patients with hepatocellular carcinoma meeting the milan criteria. Liver Transpl. 2014;20(8):945–51.

[52] Chiu KW, Nakano T, Chen KD, Hsu LW, Lai CY, Huang CY, et al. Repeated-measures implication of hepatocellular carcinoma biomarkers in living donor liver transplantation. PLoS One. 2015;10(5):1–12. Available from: <Go to ISI>://WOS:000354916100020

[53] Hsu C-C, Chen C-L, Wang C-C, Lin C-C, Yong C-C, Wang S-H, et al. Combination of FDG-PET and UCSF criteria for predicting HCC recurrence after living donor liver transplantation. Transplantat. 2016 Sep;100(9):1925–32.

[54] Orci LA, Berney T, Majno PE, Lacotte S, Oldani G, Morel P, et al. Donor characteristics and risk of hepatocellular carcinoma recurrence after liver transplantation. Br J Surg. England; 2015;102(10):1250–7.

[55] Park G-C, Song G-W, Moon D-B, Lee S-G. A review of current status of living donor liver transplantation. Hepatobiliary Surg Nutr. China (Republic: 1949); 2016;5(2):107–17.

[56] Toso C, Mentha G, Kneteman NM, Majno P. The place of downstaging for hepatocellular carcinoma. J Hepatol. 2010;52(6):930–6. Available from: http://dx.doi.org/10.1016/j.jhep.2009.12.032

[57] Yu CY, Ou HY, Huang TL, Chen TY, Tsang LLC, Chen CL, et al. Hepatocellular carcinoma downstaging in liver transplantation. Transplant Proc. 2012;44(2):412–4.

[58] Na GH, Kim EY, Hong TH, You YK, Kim DG. Effects of loco regional treatments before living donor liver transplantation on overall survival and recurrence-free survival in South Korean patients with hepatocellular carcinoma. HPB (Oxford). England; 2016;18(1):98–106.

[59] Parikh ND, Waljee AK, Singal AG. Downstaging hepatocellular carcinoma: a systematic review and pooled analysis. Liver Transplant. 2015;21(9):1142–52. Available from: http://www.ncbi.nlm.nih.gov/pubmed/25981135 [cited 2015 Nov 17].

[60] Xu D-W, Wan P, Xia Q. Liver transplantation for hepatocellular carcinoma beyond the Milan criteria: a review. World J Gastroenterol. United States; 2016;22(12):3325–34.

[61] Majeed TA, Wai CT, Rajekar H, Lee KH, Wong SY, Leong SO, et al. Experience of the transplant team is an important factor for posttransplant survival in patients with hepatocellular carcinoma undergoing living-donor liver transplantation. Transplant Proc. United States; 2008;40(8):2507–9.

[62] Chen C-L, Concejero AM. Early post-operative complications in living donor liver transplantation: prevention, detection and management. HBPD INT. China; 2007;6(4): 345–7.

[63] Chen C-L, Concejero AM, Cheng Y-F. More than a quarter of a century of liver transplantation in Kaohsiung Chang Gung Memorial Hospital. Clin Transpl. United States; 2011;213–21.

[64] Jawan B, Wang C-H, Chen C-L, Huang C-J, Cheng K-W, Wu S-C, et al. Review of anesthesia in liver transplantation. Acta Anaesthesiol Taiwanica. Taiwan LLC; 2014;52(4):185–96. Available from: http://linkinghub.elsevier.com/retrieve/pii/S1875459714001088

[65] Nadalin, S., Bockhorn, M., Malagó, M., Valentin-Gamazo, C., Frilling, A., & Broelsch, C. E. (2006). Living donor liver transplantation. *HPB* :8(1), 10–21. http://doi.org/10.1080/13651820500465626.

[66] Abdeldayem HM, editor. Living Donor Liver Transplantation, Liver Transplantation - Technical Issues and Complications. InTech. 2012. Available from: http://www.intechopen.com/books/liver-transplantation-technical-issues-and-complications/living-donor-livertransplantation

[67] Ercolani G, Grazi GL, Ravaioli M, Grigioni WF, Cescon M, Gardini A, et al. The role of lymphadenectomy for liver tumors. Ann Surg. 2004;239(2):202–9.

[68] Sotiropoulos GC, Malago M, Molmenti EP, Losch C, Lang H, Frilling A, et al. Hilar lymph nodes sampling at the time of liver transplantation for hepatocellular carcinoma: to do or not to do? Meta-analysis to determine the impact of hilar lymph nodes metastases on tumor recurrence and survival in patients with hepatocellular carcin. Transpl Int. 2007;20(2):141–6. Available from: http://www.ncbi.nlm.nih.gov/pubmed/17239022\nhttp://onlinelibrary.wiley.com/doi/10.1111/j.1432-2277.2006.00412.x/abstract?systemMessage=Wiley+Online+Library+will+be+disrupted+on+7+July+from+10:00-12:00+BST+(05:00-07:00+EDT)+for+essential+maintenance

[69] Suh S-W, Lee J-M, You T, Choi YR, Yi N-J, Lee K-W, et al. Hepatic venous congestion in living donor grafts in liver transplantation: is there an effect on hepatocellular carcinoma recurrence? Liver Transplant Off Publ Am Assoc Study Liver Dis Int Liver Transplant Soc. United States; 2014;20(7):784–90.

[70] Matsuda H, Sadamori H, Shinoura S, Umeda Y, Yoshida R, Satoh D, et al. Aggressive combined resection of hepatic inferior vena cava, with replacement by a ringed expanded polytetrafluoroethylene graft, in living-donor liver transplantation for hepatocellular carcinoma beyond the Milan criteria. J Hepatobiliary Pancreat Sci. Japan; 2010;17(5):719–24.

[71] Pahari H, Li W-F, Lin T-S, Wang C-C, Yong C-C, Lin T-L, et al. Extensive adhesions in living donor liver transplantation: a retrospective analysis. World J Surg. 2015;40(2): 427–32. Available from: http://link.springer.com/10.1007/s00268-015-3219-x

[72] Memeo R, De'Angelis N, de Blasi V, Cherkaoui Z, Brunetti O, Longo V, et al. Innovative surgical approaches for hepatocellular carcinoma. World J Hepatol. United States; 2016;8(13):591–6.

[73] Lin T-S, Chiang Y-C, Chen C-L, Concejero AM, Cheng Y-F, Wang C-C, et al. Intimal dissection of the hepatic artery following transarterial embolization for hepatocellular carcinoma: an intraoperative problem in adult living donor liver transplantation. Liver Transplant Off Publ Am Assoc Study Liver Dis Int Liver Transplant Soc. United States; 2009;15(11):1553–6.

[74] Pomfret EA, Lodge JPA, Villamil FG, Siegler M. Should we use living donor grafts for patients with hepatocellular carcinoma? Ethical considerations. Liver Transplant Off Publ Am Assoc Study Liver Dis Int Liver Transplant Soc. United States; 2011;17 Suppl 2:S128–32.

[75] Mizuno S, Yokoi H, Shiraki K, Usui M, Sakurai H, Tabata M, et al. Prospective study on the outcome of patients with hepatocellular carcinoma registered for living donor liver transplantation: how long can they wait? Transplantat. United States; 2010;89(6): 650–4.

[76] Taefi a, Abrishami a, Eghtesad B, Sherman M. Surgical resection versus liver transplant for patients with hepatocellular carcinoma (Review). Cochrane Database Syst Rev. 2013;(6).

[77] Ho C, Lee P, Chen C, Ho M. Long-Term outcomes after resection versus transplantation for hepatocellular carcinoma within UCSF criteria. Ann Surg Oncol. 2012;19(3):826–33.

[78] Dai WC, Chan SC, Chok KSH, Cheung TT, Sharr WW, Chan ACY, et al. Good longterm survival after primary living donor liver transplantation for solitary hepatocellular carcinomas up to 8 cm in diameter. HPB (Oxford). England; 2014;16(8):749–57.

[79] Blumgart LH, Jarnagin WR, Belghiti J, Buchler MW, Chapman WC, M.I. D, et al., editors. Liver Transplantation: Indications and General Considerations. In: Blumgart's Surgery of the Liver, Biliary Tract, and Pancreas. 5th ed. Philadelphia: Elsevier; 2012.

[80] Silva MF, Sapisochin G, Strasser SI, Hewa-geeganage S, Chen J, Wigg AJ. Liver resection and transplantation offer similar 5-year survival for Child-Pugh-Turcotte A HCC-patients with a single nodule up to 5 cm: a multicenter, exploratory analysis. Eur J Surg Oncol. 2013;39(4):386–95. Available from: http://dx.doi.org/10.1016/j.ejso.2012.12.011

[81] Bruix J, Sherman M. Management of hepatocellular carcinoma: an update. Hepatol. United States; 2011;53(3):1020–2.

[82] Sapisochin G, Castells L, Dopazo C. Single HCC in cirrhotic patients: liver resection or liver transplantation?? Long-term outcome according to an intention-to-treat basis. Ann Surg Oncol. 2013;20(4):1194–202.

[83] Dhir M, Lyden ER, Smith LM, Are C. Comparison of outcomes of transplantation and resection in patients with early hepatocellular carcinoma: a meta-analysis. Hpb. 2012;14(9):635–45.

[84] Proneth A, Zeman F, Schlitt HJ, Schnitzbauer A. Is resection or transplantation the ideal treatment in patients with hepatocellular carcinoma in cirrhosis if both are possible? A systematic review and metaanalysis. Ann Surg Oncol. 2014;21(9):3096–107. Available from: http://www.ncbi.nlm.nih.gov/pubmed/24866437

[85] Kaido T, Morita S, Tanaka S, Ogawa K, Mori A, Hatano E, et al. Long-term outcomes of hepatic resection versus living donor liver transplantation for hepatocellular carcinoma: a propensity score-matching study. Dis Markers. United States; 2015;2015:425926.

[86] Dionigi R. One Liver for Two: Split and Living Donor Liver Transplantation for Adult and Pediatric Patients. In: Recent Advances in Liver Surgery. Austin, TX: Landes Bioscience; 2009.

[87] Di Sandro S, Slim AO, Giacomoni A, Lauterio A, Mangoni I, Aseni P, et al. Living donor liver transplantation for hepatocellular carcinoma: long-term results compared with deceased donor liver transplantation. Transplant Proc. United States; 2009;41(4):1283–5.

[88] Lee S-G, Moon D-B, Shin H, Kim K-H, Ahn C-S, Ha T-Y, et al. Living donor liver transplantation for hepatocellular carcinoma: current status in Korea. Transplant Proc. United States; 2012;44(2):520–2.

[89] Hu Z, Qian Z, Wu J, Zhou J, Zhang M, Zhou L, et al. Clinical outcomes and risk factors of hepatocellular carcinoma treated by liver transplantation: a multi-centre comparison of living donor and deceased donor transplantation. Clin Res Hepatol Gastroenterol. 2015; 2016 Jun;40(3):315–26

[90] Fisher RA, Kulik LM, Freise CE, Lok ASF, Shearon TH, Brown RSJ, et al. Hepatocellular carcinoma recurrence and death following living and deceased donor liver transplantation. Am J Transplant. Denmark; 2007;7(6):1601–8.

[91] Park M-S, Lee K-W, Suh S-W, You T, Choi Y, Kim H, et al. Living-donor liver transplantation associated with higher incidence of hepatocellular carcinoma recurrence than deceased-donor liver transplantation. Transplant J. 2014;97(1):71–7. Available from: http://content.wkhealth.com/linkback/openurl?sid=WKPTLP:landingpage&an=00007890-201401150-00012

[92] Ninomiya M, Shirabe K, Facciuto ME, Schwartz ME, Florman SS, Yoshizumi T, et al. Comparative study of living and deceased donor liver transplantation as a treatment for hepatocellular carcinoma. J Am Coll Surg. United States; 2015;220(3):297–304.e3.